WH120

Prognostic Markers
in Hematologic Oncology

Dedication

To my wife, Elżbieta, and my daughters, Marta, Ewa and Małgorzata

Contents

© 2006 Taylor & Francis, an imprint of the Taylor & Francis Group

First published in the United Kingdom in 2006
by Taylor & Francis,
an imprint of the Taylor & Francis Group,
2 Park Square, Milton Park
Abingdon, Oxon OX14 4RN, UK

Tel.:   +44 (0) 20 7017 6000
Fax.:   +44 (0) 20 7017 6699
Email: info.medicine@tandf.co.uk
Website: http://www.tandf.co.uk/medicine

British Library Cataloguing in Publication Data

Data available on application

Library of Congress Cataloging-in-Publication Data

Data available on application

ISBN10 1-84184-554-X
ISBN13 9-78-1-84184-554-8

Distributed in North and South America by

Taylor & Francis
2000 NW Corporate Blvd
Boca Raton, FL 33431, USA

Within Continental USA
Tel.: 800 272 7737; Fax.: 800 374 3401
Outside Continental USA
Tel.: 561 994 0555; Fax.: 561 361 6018
E-mail: orders@crcpress.com

Distributed in the rest of the world by
Thomson Publishing Services
Cheriton House
North Way
Andover, Hampshire SP10 5BE, UK
Tel.: +44 (0) 1264 332424
E-mail: salesorder.tandf@thomsonpublishingservices.co.uk

Composition by C&M Digitals (P) Ltd., Chennai, India
Printed and bound by T.G. Hostench, S.A., Spain

Prognostic Markers
in Hematologic Oncology

Wojciech Gorczyca MD PhD
Genzyme Genetics, New York, NY, USA

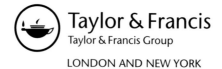

Taylor & Francis
Taylor & Francis Group

LONDON AND NEW YORK

Acknowledgments

The author would like to thank Robert Peden (commissioning editor at Taylor and Francis, London, UK) for help and support for this book, Michael Lorenzo (Genzyme Genetics, New York) for cytogenetic and FISH images, Bobi-Jo Rainey (Genzyme Genetics, New York) for molecular (PCR) images and Moya Costello (Genzyme Genetics, Los Angeles) for the cover design.

Preface

The tumors of the hematopoietic system, which include such diverse entities as chronic lymphocytic leukemia (B-CLL), diffuse large B-cell lymphoma, chronic myeloid leukemia, myelodysplastic syndrome and acute leukemia, belong to the most common human malignancies. Based on the morphology, immunophenotype and chromosomal/genetic markers, the hematologic cancers are divided into general categories of lymphoid, myeloid, histiocytic/dendritic and mast cell tumors. Their classification and diagnosis, from both a clinical and a pathologic point of view, are complicated and require a multimethodology approach. Clinical behavior, response to treatment and prognosis vary greatly, not only between separate entities, but also within individual disorders (e.g. ALK$^+$ vs. ALK$^-$ T-cell lymphoma). Establishing the proper diagnosis is just a first step in patients' management. The type of treatment, which can range from observation (no treatment) to aggressive chemotherapy followed by stem cell transplantation, is often dictated by additional parameters (e.g. presence of IgV_H mutations in B-CLL). In an organized way, this book presents numerous predictive and prognostic parameters valid in today's practice of hematologic oncology. Part I discusses the most relevant clinical, morphologic, chromosomal, genetic and immunophenotypic markers. Part II discusses the prognostic parameters in major hematologic malignancies. There is no need to emphasize the fact that prognostication is a complex matter. Results on prognostic markers from retrospective studies may be blurred, owing to differences in treatment regimens. Many previously well-established biomarkers require reanalysis coincident with the improvement in therapy. Some of the prognostic markers lose their predictive power with new treatment regimens (e.g. new data suggest that treatment with imatinib (Gleevec) overcomes the adverse prognostic significance of der(9) deletions in patients with CML). Expression of favorable and unfavorable markers in the same patient requires careful correlation in order to draw a prognostic conclusion. Patients with t(15;17)$^+$ AML respond to ATRA regardless of secondary molecular changes. On the other hand, some ALL patients with favorable genetic abnormalities (e.g. *TEL-RUNX1*) are not cured, whereas those with an unfavorable profile (e.g. certain *MLL* rearrangements) are cured. Recent improvements in technologies, including molecular tests for minimal residual disease (MRD) and DNA microarray, change our understanding of the biology of specific tumors, enable quantitative monitoring of responses to treatment at molecular levels and allow a targeted and customized approach to the management of hematologic cancers.

PART I

Overview of prognostic markers in hematologic oncology

CHAPTER 1

Clinical and laboratory parameters

PROGNOSTIC INDICES

The International Prognostic Index for malignant lymphoma

The International Prognostic Index (IPI) was developed using data from similarly treated patients with diffuse large B-cell lymphoma to correlate clinical parameters with prognosis[1]. Based on age, performance status, stage, number of extranodal sites of involvement, and serum level of lactate dehydrogenase (LDH), patients were separated into four prognostically distinct groups: low risk (0–1 adverse factor), low-intermediate risk (2 factors), high-intermediate risk (3 factors) and poor risk (4–5 adverse factors). The IPI is strongly predictive of outcome in diffuse large B-cell lymphoma (DLBCL)[2] with 5-year survival rates of 83%, 69%, 46% and 32% for low, low-intermediate, high-intermediate and poor risk groups, respectively[1]. The risk stratification of DLBCL patients with a favorable IPI score can be further improved by the additional use of age (>50 years) and stage (II) as adverse factors. Patients without these adverse factors had an excellent prognosis, with a survival rate of 90% and 80% at 5 and 15 years, respectively. In contrast, patients with both adverse factors had poor outcome, with survival at 5 and 15 years of 70% and 29%, respectively[3]. IPI appears to be more useful in predicting survival than the Ann Arbor staging classification and is currently the most widely accepted prognostic factor system

for patients with aggressive non-Hodgkin's lymphoma (NHL). The basic prognostic markers included to construct the IPI are thought to be surrogates for biological factors that ultimately determine outcome. New diagnostic procedures, better supportive care and new treatment protocols are changing the significance of some of the parameters (e.g. age). The addition of rituximab to the chemotherapy including cyclophosphamide, adriamycin, vincristine and prednisone (CHOP) regimen increases the complete-response rate and prolongs event-free and overall survival in elderly patients with diffuse large B-cell lymphoma[4,5].

Although IPI was designed for aggressive NHL, it can also be used in indolent lymphomas[6–11]. When the IPI was included in a multivariate analysis, along with the main initial variables, IPI and sex (male, worse) were the main parameters related to survival in low-grade lymphomas[8], and IPI and achievement of complete remission were the most important factors predicting response to therapy[8]. In multivariate analysis, the IPI score was the main significant predictor of overall survival in B-small lymphocytic lymphoma[12]. Anemia and B-symptoms were predictive of poor overall survival in patients with low IPI scores. A variant of the IPI score for follicular lymphoma (FL), referred to as the Follicular Lymphoma IPI (FLIPI)[13], discriminates the patients within stage III/IV, patients under and over the age of 60 years, and within IPI subgroups, and therefore

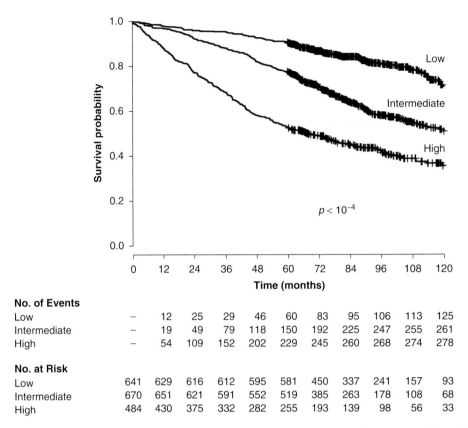

No. of Events										
Low	–	12	25	29	46	60	83	95	106	113	125
Intermediate	–	19	49	79	118	150	192	225	247	255	261
High	–	54	109	152	202	229	245	260	268	274	278

No. at Risk										
Low	641	629	616	612	595	581	450	337	241	157	93
Intermediate	670	651	621	591	552	519	385	263	178	108	68
High	484	430	375	332	282	255	193	139	98	56	33

Figure 1.1 Survival of the 1795 patients according to risk group as defined by the Follicular Lymphoma International Prognostic Index

From: Solal-Celigny P, et al. Follicular lymphoma international Prognostic Index. Blood 2004;104:1258–65. © 2004 by The American Society of Hematology, used with permission

more closely reflects the heterogeneity of FL and can provide the basis for risk-adapted stratification of FL management. FLIPI, along with the presence of bulky disease and B-symptoms, predict survival in patients with relapse/progression[14]. Figure 1.1 presents survival of the patients with FL according to risk group as defined by the FLIPI. The value of IPI in mantle cell lymphoma is not well established, partly because most of the patients are within high-risk categories[15]. Stratification of patients with lymphoplasmacytic lymphoma/Waldenström's macroglobulinemia according to the IPI has limited value[16].

The IPI has been applied to peripheral T-cell lymphoma and it appears to predict outcome,

independent of T-cell phenotype[17]. The IPI proved to be a significant prognostic factor for both progression-free and overall survival in peripheral T-cell lymphomas[18,19]. Although liver and/or bone marrow involvement are significant (poor) prognostic factors in the univariate analysis, only the IPI remained significant in the multivariate analysis of patients with peripheral T-cell lymphoma[19]. In peripheral T-cell lymphoma (unspecified) and anaplastic large cell lymphoma (ALCL) clinical separation of patients into good-risk (IPI 0–1) and poor-risk (IPI ≥ 2) subsets can be demonstrated[20]. Generally, patients with T-cell lymphoma have inferior survival in all IPI risk groups when compared with diffuse

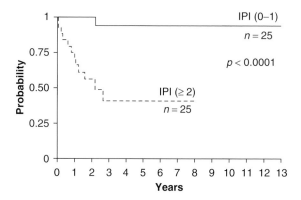

Figure 1.2 Overall survival of anaplastic lymphoma kinase-positive (ALK+) lymphoma according to age-adjusted International Prognostic Index (0 to 1, low/low intermediate-risk group; 2, high/high intermediate-risk group)

From: Falini B, *et al.* ALK+ lymphoma: clinico-pathological findings and outcome. Blood 1999;93:2697–706. © 1999 by The American Society of Hematology, used with permission

large B-cell lymphoma[21]. In the category of anaplastic lymphoma kinase (ALK)+ ALCL, 5-year survival in patients in the low/intermediate-risk group (IPI < 2) was 94%, and in patients in the high/intermediate-risk group (IPI ≥ 2) it was 41%[22]. Figure 1.2 presents the overall survival of ALK+ lymphoma according to the age-adjusted IPI.

International Prognostic Scoring System for myelodysplastic syndromes

In patients with myelodysplastic syndromes (MDS), several different multiparameter scoring systems (the Mufti, Aul, Sanz, Morel and Toyama scores, and the International Prognostic Scoring System (IPSS)) are highly predictive for survival and transformation to acute myeloid leukemia (AML). The IPSS is based on the percentage of blasts in the bone marrow, cytogenetic abnormalities and the degree and number of cytopenias[23]. The IPSS divides MDS into four risk

groups (Table 1.1): low, 0; intermediate-1 (INT-1), 0.5–1.0; INT-2, 1.5–2.0; and high, ≥ 2.5. The IPSS separates patients according to the risk of transformation into acute leukemia and distinctive groups for median survival (low, 5.7 years; INT-1, 3.5 years; INT-2, 1.2 years; and high, 0.4 year)[23]. Stratification for age, the presence of abnormal localization of immature precursors (ALIP) and CD34-positivity further improves the prognostic value of the IPSS, with respect to overall, as well as leukemia-free survival, in particular within the lower-risk categories[24]. In multivariate analysis of patients with MDS, the percentage of bone marrow blasts, hemoglobin level, platelet count, neutrophil count, LDH and karyotype are found to be independent single variables for survival, and bone marrow blasts, neutrophil count, platelet count and karyotype for AML evolution[25]. The highest predictive values were found for the Aul, Sanz and Toyama scores for overall survival, and the IPSS, Toyama and Morel scores for AML-free survival. Karyotype-based multiparameter systems appear to be particularly effective in defining MDS patients who are at high risk of transforming to acute leukemia.

Prognostic systems for B-chronic lymphocytic leukemia

Two staging system, Rai and Binet, are being used in B-chronic lymphocytic leukemia (B-CLL) patients (Table 1.2). Both systems are useful for prognosis in B-CLL. The median survival for patients in stage 0 (low risk; Rai) or A (Binet) is more than 10 years, whereas it drops to 5 years in stage IV (high risk; Rai) or C (Binet). Both staging systems have contributed significantly to the identification of major prognostic groups in B-CLL, although they fail to predict disease progression accurately at the individual level. Biologic factors, such as the mutational status of the immunoglobulin heavy-chain variable genes (IgV_H), cytogenetics, CD38 expression and some serum markers have recently improved prognostic assessment in B-CLL. There are significant survival

Table 1.1   The International Prognostic Scoring System (IPSS) for myelodysplastic syndromes (MDS)

	Score value				
Prognostic variable	0	0.5	1	1.5	2
Bone marrow blasts	<5	5–10	—	11–20	21–30
Karyotype*	Good	Intermediate	Poor		
Cytopenias	0/1	2/3			

Low risk, 0; INT-1, 0.5–1; INT-2, 1.5–2; high, ≥2.5
*Good, normal, −Y, del(5q), del(20q); poor, complex (≥3 abnormalities) or chromosome 7 abnormalities; intermediate, other abnormalities

Table 1.2   Staging systems for B-chronic lymphocytic leukemia

Staging system	Risk	Stage	Clinical features
Rai	Low	0	Lymphocytosis
	Intermediate	I	Lymphocytosis; lymphadenopathy
		II	Lymphocytosis; splenomegaly and/or hepatomegaly
	High	III	Lymphocytosis; hemoglobin <11 g/dl
		IV	Lymphocytosis; platelets <100×10^9/l
Binet	Low	A	No cytopenia; <3 lymph node areas enlarged
	Intermediate	B	No cytopenia; ≥3 lymph node areas enlarged
	High	C	Hemoglobin; <10 g/dl platelets <100×10^9/l

differences observed between the IgV_H mutational status among stage A and stage B and C patients, indicating that Binet classification and status of IgV_H genes are independent prognostic variables and are most likely to be complementary[26].

Other staging and prognostic systems

The Ann Arbor staging classification divides lymphomas into four groups (Table 1.3 presents a current update of the Ann Arbor – the Cotswold Staging System). This system is used predominantly for staging of Hodgkin's lymphoma (HL), since NHL are infrequently localized at the time of diagnosis and more often than HL involve extranodal sites. The Ann Arbor classification does not correlate well with prognosis. Hasenclever and Diehl identified seven adverse prognostic factors in HL: a serum albumin level of <4 g/dl, hemoglobin <10.5 g/dl, male sex, age ≥45 years, stage IV (Ann Arbor), leukocytosis >15×10^9/l and lymphocytopenia <0.6×10^9/l[27]. These factors

failed to identify a distinct group of patients at very high risk. Disease stage remains the major prognostic factor in HL.

Sokal and Hasford's prognostic scoring system for chronic myeloid leukemia (CML) is presented in Chapter 10 (Table 10.1).

MINIMAL RESIDUAL DISEASE

Minimal residual disease (MRD) is defined as a submicroscopic disease detectable in bone marrow and/or blood in patients in complete clinical remission (CR). Detection of MRD has prognostic value in acute lymphoblastic leukemia (ALL) and AML. Cytogenetic/fluorescent *in situ* hybridization (FISH), molecular and immunological techniques that are more sensitive than morphology are increasingly being used to assess and quantify MRD[28–35]. Immunological marker analysis allows the detection of aberrant or unusual immunophenotypes (e.g. CD45$^-$, CD33$^+$ B cells), while real-time quantitative polymerase

Table 1.3 The Cotswold Staging Classification for Hodgkin's lymphoma

Stage I	Involvement of a single lymph node region or lymphoid structure (e.g. spleen, thymus, Waldeyer ring)
Stage II	Involvement of ≥ 2 lymph node regions on the same side of the diaphragm
Stage III	Involvement of lymph node regions on both sides of the diaphragm
III$_1$	With or without splenic, hilar, celiac or portal nodes
III$_2$	With para-aortic, iliac or mesenteric nodes
Stage IV	Involvement of extranodal site(s) (not due to direct extension from a nodal site)
A	No symptoms
B	Fever, sweats, weight loss
X	Bulky disease (>10 cm lymph node; > 1/3 widening of the mediastinum)
E	Involvement of a single extranodal site, contiguous or proximal to a known nodal site

chain reaction (PCR) techniques (RQ-PCR) target fusion regions of chromosome aberrations (e.g. *BCR–ABL, IGL–MYC, TEL– AML1(RUNX1), NPM–ALK*), chimerism (e.g. short tandem repeats) and clone-specific immunoglobulin and T-cell receptor gene rearrangements[32,36–39]. Analysis of the patient-specific fusion sequences may be more useful for MRD monitoring in certain acute leukemias associated with numerous chromosomal translocations of one gene (e.g. *MLL*)[40]. Immunophenotyping by multiparameter four- or six-color flow cytometry or allele-specific PCR for the immunoglobulin gene rearrangement, allow detection of one leukemic cell in 10^5 normal cells[41,42]. Immunophenotypes that allow detection of one leukemic cell in 10^4 normal cells can be identified in at least 90% of patients with acute lymphoblastic leukemia; immunophenotypes that allow detection of one leukemic cell in 10^3–10^4 normal cells can be identified in at least 85% of patients with acute myeloid leukemia[43]. The combination of cell sorting based on leukemia-specific immunophenotype and PCR analysis of short tandem repeats (STR) has also been successfully used for MRD detection[36]. The rationale underlying MRD studies is to improve measurement of treatment response (especially early after induction therapy), to provide independent prognostic information and to optimize therapeutic strategies adapted to the molecular response by identification of low-risk and high-risk patients, who may benefit from treatment reduction or treatment intensification, respectively. Persistence of MRD during treatment reflects drug resistance and signals clinical recurrence.

Minimal residual disease in lymphoma/ chronic lymphocytic leukemia

Although current treatment protocols, especially stem cell transplantation, lead to a complete remission (CR) in most patients with NHL and some patients with B-CLL, many of the patients relapse. This implies that CR is compatible with the presence of residual malignant cells. In patients with B-CLL and NHL, the prognostic significance of MRD is still a matter of debate, as the majority of patients remain MRD$^+$ after conventional treatment[44]. This is changing, however, with the implementation of new treatment modalities, such as application of monoclonal antibodies (e.g. rituximab (Rituxan) and alemtuzumab (Campath)), where a significant proportion of patients convert to MRD negativity and experience prolonged remission.

In B-CLL patients, flow cytometry immunophenotyping (e.g. based on CD19/CD5/CD20/CD79b expression, CD5$^+$/CD20$^+$ co-expression, abnormal Igκ/Igλ ratio) reveals residual leukemic cells in the majority of patients after standard chemotherapy[35,45,46]. Both flow cytometry and PCR yield clinically relevant information in monitoring B-CLL patients, with clonotypic PCR detecting MRD more often than flow cytometry[34,47,48]. MRD detection by flow and RQ-PCR were equally suitable to monitor MRD kinetics after allogeneic stem cell transplantation, but the PCR method detected impending relapses after autologous stem cell transplantation earlier[47]. The long-term prognostic impact of phenotypic remission in B-CLL patients in CR is not yet fully established. The normalized phenotype after conventional chemotherapy is associated with significantly longer relapse-free survival, but does not translate into prolonged overall survival[49]. The presence of MRD in patients with B-CLL in CR after treatment with alemtuzumab or autologous stem cell transplantation correlates with a shorter survival compared with that of patients achieving MRD$^-$ complete remission[35,50]. Patients with $>0.01\times10^9/l$ circulating leukemic cells have significant ($>5\%$) marrow disease. In patients achieving CR by National Cancer Institute criteria[51], the detection of residual bone marrow disease (at more than 0.05% of leukocytes) predicts significantly poorer event-free and overall survival[35]. Brugiatelli et al. reported that phenotypic identification of leukemic cells preceded overt clinical relapse by 3–14 months[49]. The persistence of PCR$^+$/MRD after stem cell transplantation is associated with increased probability of relapse[52]. Esteve et al. reported that the persistence of MRD in B-CLL appeared to have different implications depending on the type of marrow transplantation – autologous or allogeneic[33]. Persistence of MRD after autologous transplantation is highly predictive of clinical progression, but the detection of MRD after allogeneic transplantation does not necessarily predict clinical relapse[33]. It appears that MRD status at the end of therapy is more predictive of duration of remission than conventional response criteria and identifies the patients at risk of early disease progression[50]. MRD$^-$ remission in CLL is achievable with alemtuzumab, leading to an improved overall and treatment-free survival[53]. In the series reported by Moreton et al., complete remission, partial remission and no response to alemtuzumab were observed in 36%, 19% and 46% of CLL patients, respectively[53]. Among purine analog-refractory patients, 50% responded to alemtuzumab[53].

Follicular lymphoma (FL) is associated with a frequent bone marrow involvement at diagnosis, typically with a paratrabecular pattern. Most patients with FL achieve a CR after treatment, but eventually most of them, particularly those with stage IV, relapse because of MRD. The impact of measuring MRD in the bone marrow or blood by RQ-PCR of t(14;18) (BCL2-IGH RQ-PCR) on survival is not clear; i.e. some patients have molecular remission without complete clinical remission (most probably due to preferential elimination of tumor cells from blood or bone marrow over nodal sites with new therapy). Molecular negativity in peripheral blood is not associated with a better survival[54]. Lambrechts et al. reported that the presence or absence of t(14;18)$^+$ cells in the circulation in stage III and IV FL treated with conventional remission induction therapy showed no obvious correlation with the clinical remission status and the remission duration[55]. Also, Mandigers et al. did not show any correlation between clinical response and quantitation of circulating t(14;18)$^+$ cells in patients with stage II–IV FL treated with standard chemotherapy and interferon-α. However, the progression-free survival was significantly prolonged in patients with >1 log decrease in circulating t(14;18)$^+$ cells[54]. Patients who achieve a molecular remission after autologous transplant and/or chemotherapy do not necessarily have a better disease-free survival[56,57]. By multivariate analysis, β_2-microglobulin level and molecular response are important variables associated with clinical outcome in patients with FL. Serial PCR analysis to determine the molecular response in FL correlates well with outcome, especially when combined with pretreatment β_2-microglobulin level[56]. Figure 1.3 presents blood involvement by FL.

Mantle cell lymphoma (MCL) appears to be largely resistant to complete eradication by conventional chemotherapy[58]. The majority of patients have positive MRD (BCL1-IGH-PCR) in bone marrow irrespective of histological involvement[59]. A new treatment regimen with rituximab and combination chemotherapy may transiently clear blood or bone marrow of detectable tumor cells, but molecular remission does not translate into prolonged progression-free survival (16.5 months in MRD$^+$ vs. 18.8 months in MRD$^-$)[60]. Brugger et al. showed that a single course

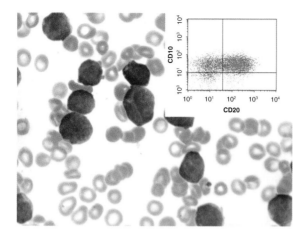

Figure 1.3   Follicular lymphoma in 'leukemic phase' (blood)

of rituximab consolidation given after autologous stem cell transplantation may help to eliminate MRD and may translate into improved event-free survival in both FL and MCL patients[61].

Minimal residual disease in multiple myeloma

Flow cytometry (DNA ploidy and cytoplasmic Ig, light scatter distribution and reactivity patterns to CD138, CD38 and CD45) and patient-specific reverse transcriptase (RT-PCR) can be applied to monitor MRD in multiple myeloma (MM) patients. Flow cytometry immunophenotyping of plasma cells might be useful for detecting MRD in cases with aberrant antigen expression and for selection of therapeutic agents that have specific membrane targets[62]. Patients with MM in CR after chemotherapy or autologous stem cell transplantation frequently have positive MRD results[63,64], and only 5–15% of patients attain durable PCR-negativity[64–66]. The time-to-progression of patients with pre-transplantation IgH/2b-actin ratio of >0.03% in bone marrow was significantly shorter than that of patients with lower MRD levels[67]. The subset of MM patients in long-term CR after high-dose chemotherapy and allogeneic stem cell transplantation who are PCR/MRD⁻ is higher and approaches 70%[65,68,69].

The cumulative risk of relapse at 5 years was 0% for PCR/MRD⁻ patients, 33% for PCR/mixed patients and 100% for PCR/MRD⁺ patients[68]. MRD/PCR-negativity is associated with a very low rate of clinical relapse[69,70]. Allogeneic stem cell transplantation offers the potential ability to induce sustained serological and molecular CR in selected patients with MM. Patient-specific real-time IgH-PCR detects molecular disease prior to the clinical diagnosis of progression or relapse and provides the opportunity for earlier treatment intervention[71].

Minimal residual disease in acute myeloid leukemia

In multivariate analysis, MRD level is the most powerful independent prognostic factor in AML patients, followed by cytogenetics and number of cycles to achieve CR[72]. MRD in the first bone marrow in morphologic CR obtained after induction therapy provides important information for risk assessment in patients with AML[72]. Based on the level of MRD (number of residual tumor cells per normal cell determined by flow cytometry), San Miguel suggested four risk categories for disease-free and overall survival in AML: very low risk ($<10^{-4}$), low risk (10^{-3}–10^{-4}), intermediate risk (10^{-2}–10^{-3}) and high risk ($>10^{-2}$)[72]. The relapse-free survival rates at 3 years for these risk groups were 100%, 85%, 55% and 25%, respectively. In the series by Venditti et al., MRD level of $\geq 3.5 \times 10^{-4}$ cells at the end of consolidation therapy strongly predicted relapse and was significantly associated with an *MDR1* phenotype and intermediate or unfavorable cytogenetic findings[73]. The pre-autologous stem cell transplantation MRD status predicts successful outcome in patients receiving transplantation. In a series reported by Venditti et al., a high-dose chemotherapy conditioning regimen followed by autologous stem cell transplantation had no impact on the unfavorable prognostic value of high pre-transplant MRD level[74].

The association of long-term clinical remission and molecular disease eradication is well established in AML patients with t(15;17) and inv(16)[75–79].

The MRD-positivity by qualitative RT-PCR after consolidation therapy in patients with acute promyelocytic leukemia (APL) or reappearance of *PML–RARα* transcripts after negative results is highly predictive of relapse. In patients with t(8;21)$^+$ AML molecular remission was a prerequisite but not a guarantee for long-term disease-free survival. The long-term complete remission in those patients was associated with persistent molecular disease eradication[80]. Owing to the slow kinetics of *AML1(RUNX1)–ETO* after consolidation chemotherapy, the value of qualitative RT-PCR (nested RT-PCR) to predict early relapse is limited. Additionally, in patient with t(8;21) AML, the *AML1(RUNX1)–ETO* fusion may be present in non-leukemic stem cells, monocytes and lymphocytes[81]. In this situation RQ-PCR might help to define individual relapse risk and to improve as well as facilitate clinical decision-making[80]. The large majority of patients with AML associated with t(16;16)/inv(16) in long-term complete remission were found to be MRD$^-$ by RT-PCR. However, similarly to AML with t(8;21), some long-term survivors remained PCR/MRD$^+$.

Minimal residual disease in acute lymphoblastic leukemia

MRD plays a significant role in the measurement of response to treatment in childhood B- and T-cell acute lymphoblastic leukemia (ALL) and in adult B-ALL (the ability to predict relapse based on MRD is weaker in adult T-ALL)[82–85]. Although MRD levels measured by flow cytometry and PCR correlate well[84], these techniques differ in their applicability and sensitivity and MRD results obtained by one method cannot yet easily be compared with MRD results obtained by another method[39,86]. The discordant results between flow cytometry and RQ-PCR are due to the limited sensitivity of flow cytometry analysis within the range of 0.01–0.001% and less often due to the unstable or subclonal Ig/TCR gene rearrangements or a limited quantitative range of the applied RQ-PCR targets[86]. In T-ALL, bone marrow sampling might be replaced by blood sampling,

because the dissemination of T-ALL cells to bone marrow and blood appears to be comparable[87]. The complete disappearance of leukemic cells (or their reduction to <1/100 000 cells) may be necessary to achieve a cure of ALL[88]. Low levels or negative MRD after completion of induction therapy predicts good outcome in ALL, and the risk of relapse is associated with MRD level[89–93]. Combined information on MRD from the first 3 months of treatment (especially at the end of induction treatment and before consolidation treatment) distinguishes patients with good prognoses from those with poor prognoses[90]. The quantification of residual leukemic cells in serial marrow aspirates during therapy may allow the early detection of relapse. Negative MRD at the end of induction therapy and before consolidation is associated with a 2% relapse rate at 5 years (low risk), whereas patients with an intermediate (10^{-3}) or high ($\geq 10^{-2}$) level of positive MRD at both measurements have a 5-year relapse rate of 80% (high risk)[90]. MRD is highly predictive of the relapse in B-ALL patients undergoing stem cell transplantation[94]. Using multiparameter flow cytometry to quantify MRD before transplant, estimated disease-free survival for the MRD$^+$ and MRD$^-$ patients was 33.3% and 73.5%, respectively[95]. Also, in patients after bone marrow transplant MRD is predictive of the relapse. Patients who subsequently relapsed were MRD$^+$ in 88%, and those in long-term complete remission were MRD$^+$ in only 22% in post-transplant analysis[96]. MRD in childhood ALL appears to be an independent prognostic factor, allowing a precise risk group classification[44]. The finding of terminal deoxynucleotidyl transferase (TdT)$^+$ cells or cells with aberrant phenotype in an erythrocyte-free cerebrospinal fluid (CSF) sample with a negative cytomorphology is highly predictive for impending central nervous system (CNS) relapse[97,98]. Despite clinical and morphological remission being achieved by over 80% of adult patients with ALL, 5-year survival is limited to 40% of patients, clearly indicating that morphology is insufficient in predicting the outcome. Analysis of disease-free survival rates for MRD$^+$ and MRD$^-$ patients shows that MRD positivity is associated with increased relapses (being most significant at 3–5 months post-induction and beyond). The association of MRD test results and disease-free survival better predicts the outcome than other standard parameters and is therefore important in determining managements of individual patients[89,99].

Minimal residual disease in chronic myeloid leukemia

MRD status by molecular cytogenetics (FISH) or PCR is included in treatment strategies in patients with CML. FISH, whose results are more sensitive than standard cytogenetics and correlate well with those by PCR[100], allows identification of the BCR–ABL fusion gene (both p210 and p190) and monitoring of response to treatment[101]. Patients with positive results after standard treatment and/or allogeneic transplantation may benefit from new treatment strategies. El-Rifai et al. suggested that consecutive findings of equal amounts of residual leukemic cells did not necessarily predict a relapse; however, careful follow-up at shorter intervals was suggested[102]. An increasing number of leukemic cells predicted an ensuing relapse[102]. RT-PCR is very sensitive (10^{-5}–10^{-6}) and therefore allows for MRD evaluation in patients in CR after chemotherapy as well as those undergoing allogeneic or autologous stem cell transplantation[103]. The significance of PCR-MRD-positivity after stem cell transplantation is uncertain, since most of the patients are PCR$^+$ within 6 months after treatment, and detection of BCR–ABL$^+$ cells even several years after transplantation does not translate to disease progression. These limitations of the applicability of RT-PCR for predicting relapse in CML patients can be overcome by either competitive RT-PCR or RQ-PCR (Figure 1.4). Olavarria et al. showed that RQ-PCR performed early after stem cell transplantation was useful for predicting outcome, and that the risk of relapse correlated with the number of BCR–ABL transcripts[104]. They classified the results as (1) negative (no BCR–ABL transcripts), (2) positive at low level (<100/μg RNA and/or the BCR–ABL/ABL ratio of <0.02%) or (3) positive at high level (transcript levels

exceeded the thresholds defined above)[104]. Three years after stem cell transplantation, the cumulative incidence of relapse was 16.7%, 42.9% and 86.4%, for negative, positive at low level and positive at high level PCR results, respectively. Using RQ-PCR, Radich et al. showed that the median BCR–ABL level of patients who relapsed was significantly greater (40 443 copies/μg RNA) than those who remained in remission (24 copies/μg RNA)[105].

AGE

Age is strongly associated with prognosis in hematopoietic malignancies. Presentation and prognosis in HL, NHL and MM varies based on staging and age at the time of diagnosis. In NHL older age is usually associated with a poorer outcome. In DLBCL relapse-free survival is influenced by age, being worse in older patients[106,107]. In Burkitt's lymphoma, age >10 years is a poor prognostic factor[108,109]. Adult patients with Burkitt's lymphoma with bone marrow and/or CNS involvement have 5-year survival rates below 30%[110,111]. The median overall survival among patients with multiple myeloma aged ≤65 years is 42 months, and >65 years is 18 months[112]. In MM, deletions of chromosome 13 (Delta 13) and t(14;16) are associated with shorter survival in patients ≤70 years old but no effect of survival is seen for those over 70 years. In younger patients t(4;14) and p53 deletions are also significant poor prognostic markers.

The incidence of myeloid disorders, including both AML and chronic myeloproliferative disorders, increases dramatically with age. Generally, an age of ≥ 60 years is an unfavorable prognostic factor for overall survival in patients with AML. Older patients with AML have a high frequency of leukemic cells with multidrug resistance as determined by the expression of MDR1[113,114] as well as an increased frequency of unfavorable karyotypes[115–119] when compared with younger patients. For the patients of <60 years, multivariate analysis showed that the FLT3 gene mutation was the strongest prognostic factor for overall survival[120,121], whereas in patients aged >60 years, the mutational status of FLT3 did not influence overall survival[122].

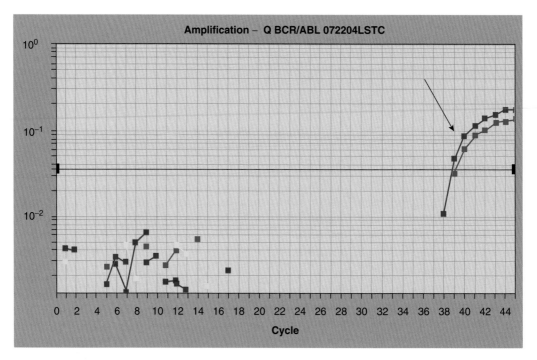

Figure 1.4 Chronic myeloid leukemia, minimal residual disease by *BCR–ABL* RNA detection (real-time quantitative polymerase chain reaction). Note low level of *BCR–ABL* (arrow)

In MDS, patients of <60 years have improved survival in the individual risk categories (IPSS, *see above*) compared with patients of >60 years.

In adult ALL the two most important clinical prognostic factors are patient age and total white cell or blast count. Patients aged over 50–60 years are regarded as a prognostically unfavorable group. The 5-year survival for patients 15–45 years old is 37%, and for those 75 years or older is 3%[123]. Among patients with ALL, not only is the frequency of MRD in adults higher than in pediatric patients, but the levels of MRD are significantly higher than in comparably treated children. As age increases, the percentage of patients having the t(9;22) rises. Philadelphia (Ph) chromosome-positive ALL is associated with a poor prognosis. Young adult patients (16–21 years old) have a lower incidence of favorable cytogenetic hyperdiploidy and an increased incidence of the T-cell phenotype when compared with patients 1–9 years old. Prognosis is much worse for ALL patients <1 years old and >10 years old.

LABORATORY PARAMETERS

β₂-microglobulin

The β_2-microglobulin, a low-molecular-weight polypeptide, is derived from turnover by tumor cells. High serum levels are found in highly proliferative lymphomas. The β_2-microglobulin, similarly to LDH, has been identified as a prognostic marker in malignant lymphoma. The β_2-microglobulin serum level predicts relapse and survival in large cell lymphomas[124] and is a good predictor of complete response and time to treatment failure in low-grade B-cell lymphomas[125] and in cutaneous lymphoma/Sézary's syndrome[126].

In MM patients, the serum β_2-microglobulin measurement is a prognostic predictor for complete response to treatment and overall survival[127–129]. The median survival is 36 months for patients with pretreatment serum β_2-microglobulin values of less than 6 mg/l, as compared with a median survival of 23 months for patients with a β_2-microglobulin level of ≥6 mg/l. Serum β_2-microglobulin correlates with stage: median values ranged from 3.7 mg/l for stage IA, to 10.1 for stage IIIB. Serum β_2-microglobulin level appears to be a powerful prognostic factor for MM[129]. Low β_2-microglobulin level (≤ 2.7 mg/l) is associated with a significantly better complete response rate compared with high levels (54 vs. 19%). Similarly, the complete response rate is 39% when the bone marrow plasma cell percentage is low (<40%) and 21% with greater involvement. Complete response rate is 50% when β_2-microglobulin and bone marrow plasma cell percentages are low, 36% if either is high, and 12% when both are high[127,128]. The β_2-microglobulin level, in combination with hemoglobin level, plays a pivotal role in predicting the need to start therapy in asymptomatic patients with Waldenström's macroglobulinemia and in predicting the overall survival[130–132].

Elevated serum β_2-microglobulin level (1.25 times the upper limit of normal) is an independent adverse prognostic factor for an overall survival in classical HL[133].

Cancer antigen 125

Cancer antigen 125 (CA125) is a glycoprotein expressed in normal tissues derived from celomic epithelium and is commonly used as a tumor marker. Serum CA125 levels are elevated in malignant tumors, including lymphoma. Elevated levels of CA125 in NHL are associated with advanced disease stage, bulky tumors, poor response to treatment, bone marrow involvement, extranodal disease, serosal involvement, high levels of serum LDH and β_2-microglobulin, elevated IPI and poor survival rates[134,135]. CA125 level in conjunction with serum LDH and β_2-microglobulin serve as surrogate markers of the tumor load, proliferative activity and invasive potential. High serum CA125 level at diagnosis in lymphoma patients is associated with decreased event-free and overall survival[134,135]. CA125 is significantly high in patients with serous membrane involvement[136].

Cytokines

Cytokines are short-acting mediators by which cellular immune responses are regulated. They can act in an endocrine manner by stimulating cells at a distance or in a paracrine manner, in which they act on cells in their immediate vicinity. Interaction of cytokines with their receptors results in the activation of intracellular tyrosine kinase activity. Apart from the cytokine receptor superfamily, there are also the receptor tyrosine kinases (RTKs), which have intrinsic tyrosine kinase activity. Hematopoietic cytokines include colony stimulating factors (CSFs), erythropoietin (EPO), thrombopoietin (TPO), stem cell factor (SCF), Flt3 ligand and certain interleukins (IL). The specific actions of cytokines include hematopoiesis (through CSF), natural immune responses (through IL-1, tumor necrosis factor (TNF)-α, interferons and IL-8), stimulation of lymphocyte growth and activation (through IL-2, and others) and activation of non-specific inflammatory cells. The cytokine IL-6 has been identified as a major growth factor responsible for MM cells' growth and survival. IL-6 stimulates the proliferation of plasma cells (S-phase fraction), prevents apoptosis (blocks caspase-9 activation) and confers resistance to chemotherapeutic agents. The IL-6 activity is in part mediated through the activation of nuclear factor kappa B (NF-κB). IL-18 plays a role in the host's response to tumors and angiogenesis. Mutations in genes encoding cytokine receptors and RTKs are associated with several hematopoietic disorders. The best known are c-*Kit* mutations in AML and mastocytosis (but also in solid tumors, such as gastrointestinal stromal tumor) and *FLT3* mutations in AML (*see below*).

Cytokines in NHL can reflect production by the tumor cell, the host immune response or both. In lymphoma patients, there is a correlation between high risk according to the IPI criteria and high levels of serum cytokines (IL-2, IL-6, IL-10); high-risk patients have higher serum levels of cytokines when compared with the low-risk group[137]. IL-6 plays a role in B-cell growth and differentiation. Prognostic value has been shown for IL-6, IL-10 and TNF-α. Increasing levels of IL-6 in B-CLL significantly correlate with patient age, severity of anemia, Rai stage, white blood cell count and β_2-microglobulin level[138]. Using an IL-6 level of 3 pg/ml as a cut-off, patients with low IL-6 levels had a significantly longer overall survival than those with high IL-6 levels[138]. TNF-α is

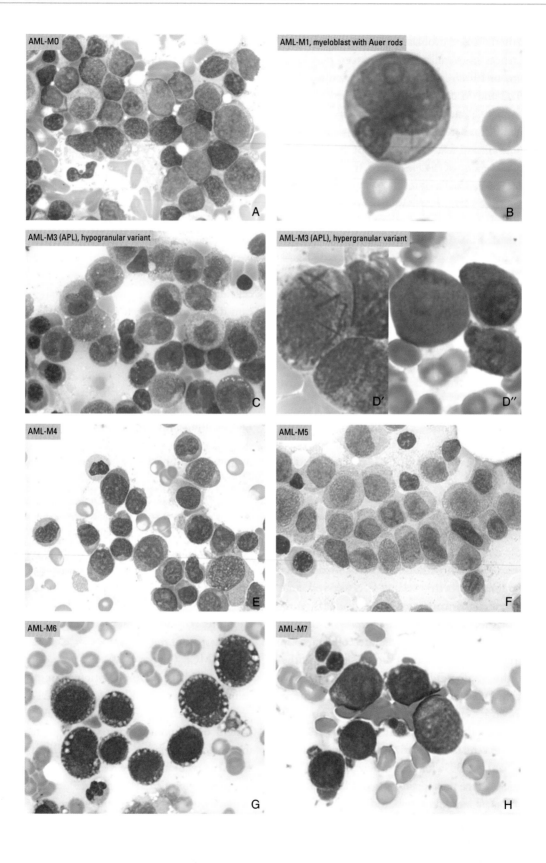

AML-M0

AML-M1, myeloblast with Auer rods

AML-M3 (APL), hypogranular variant

AML-M3 (APL), hypergranular variant

AML-M4

AML-M5

AML-M6

AML-M7

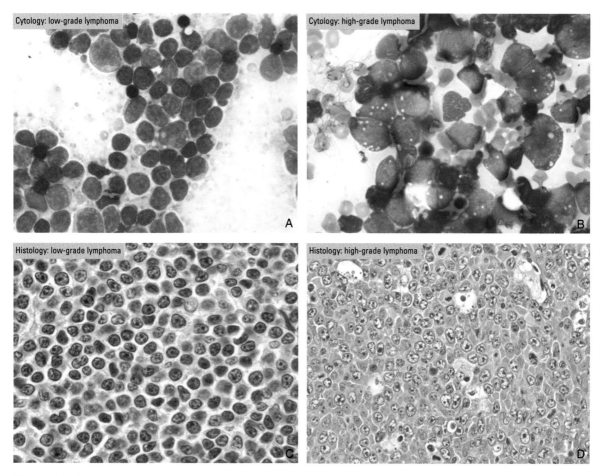

Figure 1.6   Low- vs. high-grade lymphoma. A–B, cytology; C–D, histology. Low-grade lymphomas are composed of small to medium-sized lymphocytes with dense chromatin and inconspicuous nucleoli (A, follicular lymphoma; C, B-small lymphocytic lymphoma). High-grade lymphomas are composed of medium to large lymphocytes with hyperchromatic nuclei, prominent nucleoli and vacuolated cytoplasm (B and D, diffuse large B-cell lymphoma)

On the molecular level, the transformation is associated with accumulations of genetic alterations most often involving tumor suppressor genes such as $p16^{INK4a}$, $p53$ and $p27^{KIP1}$. Levels of retinoblastoma protein (pRb) are low in low-grade lymphoma and are higher in most high-grade lymphomas[206,207]. The

higher frequency of $p53$ mutations in high-grade lymphomas when compared with low-grade tumors suggests that $p53$ inactivation is one of the events leading to lymphoma progression. Mutations of $p53$ are associated with large cell transformation of mucosa-associated lymphoid tissue (MALT)

Figure 1.5   Acute myeloid leukemia (AML), FAB categories. A, AML, minimally differentiated (M0); B, AML without maturations (M1); C, hypogranular variant of acute promyelocytic leukemia (AML-M3); D, acute promyelocytic leukemia (APL), hypergranular variant (D′, numerous Auer rods in faggot cell; D″ hypergranular promyelocytes); E, acute myelomonocytic leukemia (AML-M4); F, acute monoblastic leukemia (AML-M5); G, acute erythroid leukemia (AML-M6); H, acute megakaryoblastic leukemia (AML-M7)

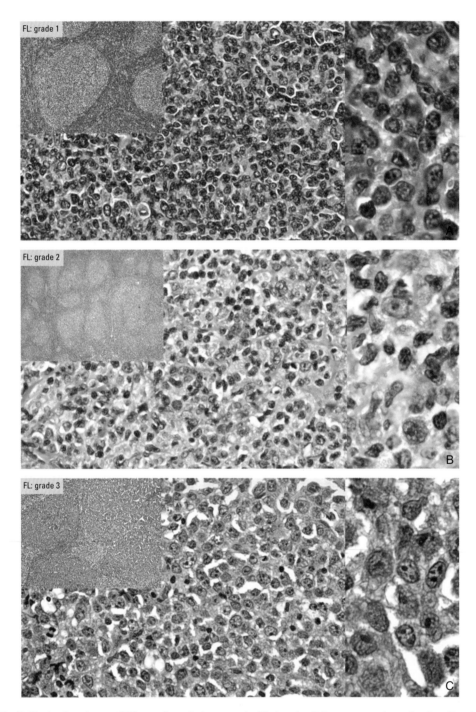

Figure 1.7   Follicular lymphoma (FL), grading. A, Low-grade FL (grade 1) is composed predominantly of small cells with irregular nuclei. B, Intermediate-grade FL (grade 2) has a mixture of small (centrocytes) and larger (centroblasts) lymphocytes. C, High-grade FL (grade 3) has predominantly large lymphocytes. Depending on the presence of a few scattered small lymphocytes, grade 3 FL can be subdivided into 3a (small cells present) and 3b (small cells absent)

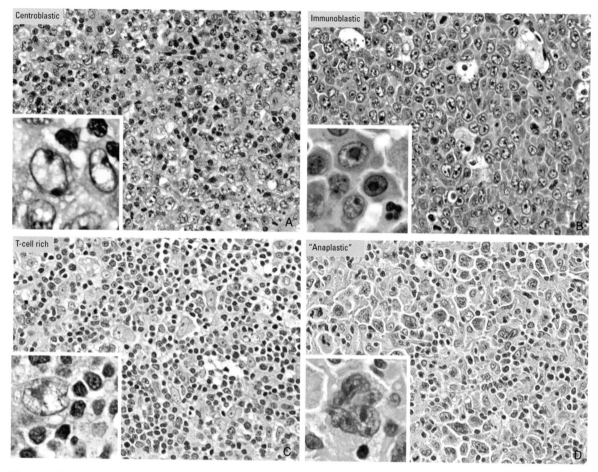

Figure 1.8 Diffuse large B-cell lymphoma, cytologic variants. A, centroblastic; B, immunoblastic, C, T-cell rich; D, 'anaplastic'

lymphoma[208], FL[209,210] and blastoid variants of mantle MCL[211].

In B-SLL/CLL transformation to high-grade lymphoma (Richter's syndrome; Figure 1.17) occurs in approximately 3–5% of cases[212]; these are mostly DLBCL, but Hodgkin-like transformation also occurs. Transformation of splenic marginal zone B-cell lymphoma (SMZL) to large cell lymphoma is comparable to other low-grade lymphomas[213], and is slightly lower than in FL or MCL, but higher than in B-SLL/CLL. In SMZL most disease-related deaths are associated with transformation to DLBCL[214]. The transformation of FL to high-grade tumors is often associated with deletion of 9p21,

which results in reduction or loss of $p16^{INK4a}$ expression[215]. The high frequency and exclusive occurrence of deletions involving $p16$ in the DLBCL evolved form of FL suggests that genetic loss at 9p21 is an important secondary genetic event in the histologic progression of FL[215]. FL may undergo transformation into a blastic variant with expression of TdT (Figure 1.18). Blastic variants of MCL shows higher numbers of pRb-positive cells than the typical cases[206].

The majority of T-large granular lymphocyte (T-LGL) leukemias have an indolent, non-progressive course, but occasional cases progress to aggressive T-LGL leukemia or systemic T-cell lymphoma of large

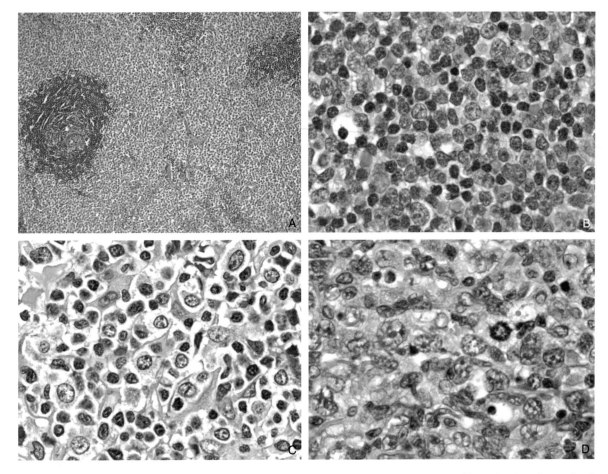

Figure 1.9   Cytologic variants of peripheral T-cell lymphoma, unspecified. A, T-zone pattern; B, predominantly small cell type; C, mixed small and large cell type; D, predominantly large cell type

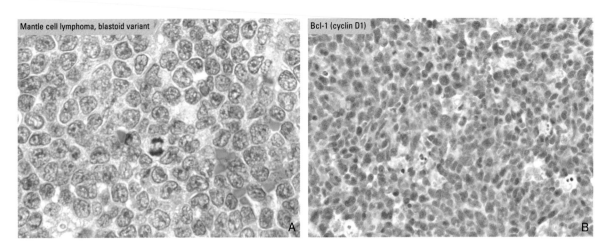

Figure 1.10   Mantle cell lymphoma, blastoid variant. A, histology; B, Bcl-1 (cyclin D1) immunostaining

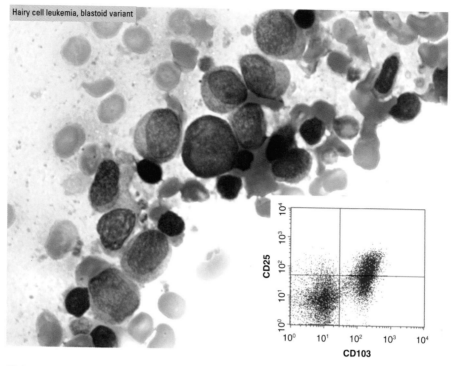

Figure 1.11　Hairy cell leukemia, blastoid variant

cells. Only very rare cases of indolent NK-cell lymphoproliferative disorder progress to aggressive NK-cell leukemia. Smoldering and chronic variants of adult T-cell leukemia/lymphoma (ATCL) may progress to highly aggressive lymphomatous or acute variants of ATCL. Angioimmunoblastic T-cell lymphoma may display morphologic progression to Epstein–Barr virus (EBV)-associated DLBCL. Mycosis fungoides may transform into a large cell T-cell lymphoma with aggressive behavior. Lymphomatoid papulosis occasionally is associated with development of HL, cutaneous anaplastic large cell lymphoma or mycosis fungoides[216–220].

HL, both classical and nodular lymphocyte predominant HL (NLPHL) may progress into DLBCL[221,222]. NLPHL shows a tendency for progression to an increasingly more diffuse pattern over time (increased number of lymphocyte and histiocyte (L&H) cells in internodular areas > T-cell-rich large

B-cell lymphoma- like pattern > overt DLBCL)[223]. Progression of NLPHL to large B-cell lymphoma has been reported in 3–5% of cases[222,224].

Unifocal Langerhans cell histiocytosis (solitary eosinophilic granuloma) may progress to multifocal/multisystem disease (Letterer–Siwe disease) in about 10% of cases. Similarly, mast cell disease may progress from indolent localized disease to highly aggressive systemic mastocytosis. The clinical course of CML typically displays progression from chronic phase to accelerated phase and finally to blast crisis/acute leukemia (*for details, see Chapter 10*). Transformation of non-CML chronic myeloproliferative disorders into acute leukemia is much less common than in CML and is often therapy-related. Progression of chronic myelomonocytic leukemia (CMML) into AML is reported in 15–30% of cases[225]. Among MDS, progression into acute leukemia occurs in about 1–14% of refractory anemia with ringed sideroblasts (RARS),

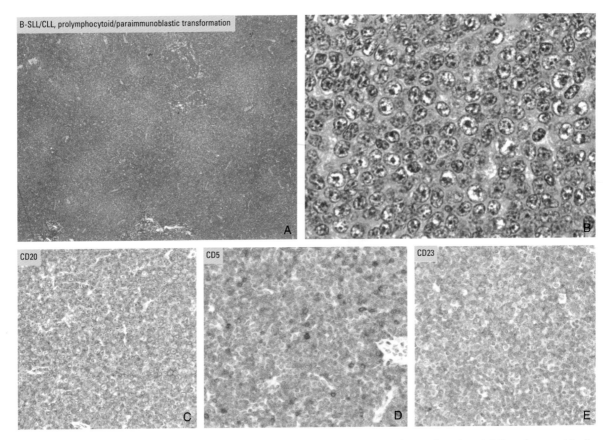

Figure 1.12 B-small lymphocytic lymphoma/chronic lymphocytic leukemia, prolymphocytoid/paraimmunoblastic transformation. A, low magnification; B, high magnification; C–E, immunohistochemistry (C, CD20; D, CD5; E, CD23)

in 6–26% of refractory anemia (RA), in 11% of refractory cytopenia with multilineage dysplasia (RCMD) and in 25–38% of refractory anemia with excess blasts (RAEB)[226,227]. Among patients with primary MDS under the age of 50 years, 47% progressed to AML, with an overall median time to progression of 2 months[228]. The risk of death due to leukemic evolution is decreased in IPSS low-risk MDS as compared with that for the more advanced IPSS groups (19% vs. 30–45%)[23]. Transformation of MDS to ALL is extremely rare[229].

Table 1.4 presents the spectrum of morphologic progression/transformation in different types of hematopoietic tumors.

Angiogenesis

Angiogenesis plays an important role in tumor progression and dissemination. Increased microvessel density has also been reported in hematopoietic tumors[230]. In MM, there is a correlation between increased angiogenesis (microvessel density) and survival[127,231–233]. Increased bone marrow microvessel density correlates with proliferation fraction (Ki-67) and with deletion of 13q14, but not with other cytogenetic, clinical and laboratory parameters of MM[232,234]. Overall survival is reported to be significantly different among MM patients with high-, intermediate- and low-grade angiogenesis, with

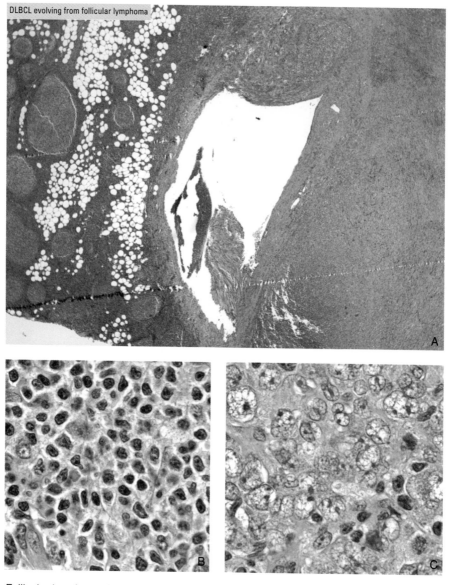

Figure 1.13 Follicular lymphoma (FL) transforming into diffuse large B-cell lymphoma (DLBCL). A, Low magnification shows both components: FL on the left and DLBCL on the right. B–C, high magnification shows different cytomorphologic features of two components: FL is composed of small lymphocytes (B) and DLBCL is composed of large cells with nucleoli (C)

median survival times of 2, 4 and 4.4 years, respectively[235]. Increased angiogenesis has been found in AML, ALL, MDS, CML, B-CLL and NHL. Molica *et al.* showed a significant increase of bone marrow angiogenesis in patients with Binet stage

A B-CLL[236]. Kini *et al.* reported that microvessel number, bone marrow cellularity and Binet stages were interrelated[237]. In a Molica series, a cut-off value of $0.90 \, \text{mm}^3 \times 10^{-2}$ or greater of the microvessel area identified patients with earlier upstaging and shorter

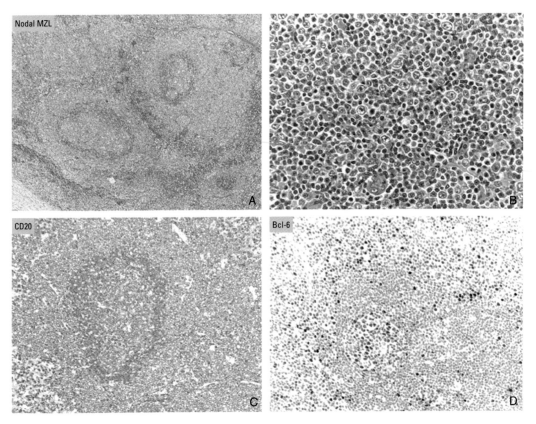

Figure 1.14 Nodal marginal zone B-cell lymphoma with transformation into diffuse large B-cell lymphoma. A, low magnification shows expanded marginal zone around residual follicles. B, high magnification shows increased number of large cells. C–D, immunohistochemistry reveals expression of CD20 (C) and focally Bcl-6 (D) by transformed cells

progression-free survival[236]. Simultaneous elevation of serum vascular endothelial growth factor (S-VEGF) and basic fibroblast growth factor (S-bFGF) is associated with poor survival in various types of lymphomas, including DLBCL[238]. S-VEGF and S-bFGF have independent influences on survival in multivariate models when tested together with the components of the IPI[238].

CELL PROLIFERATION

In the hematopoietic system, the correct proportion of immature and mature cells, and the numbers of cells of each lineage, depend on cell division (Figure 1.19), apoptosis (programmed cell death), replicative senescence and differentiation. Disruption of the physiologic

balance between cell division and apoptosis is characteristic for all cancers. Cell proliferation is controlled at the entry to the cell cycle, in proliferating cells, and at the exit from the cell cycle by a family of serine/threonine kinases called the cyclin-dependent kinases (cdks)[239]. At least 15 cyclins, proteins synthesized and degraded in a cyclical fashion during the cell cycle, have been identified. The mitotic cyclins (cyclins A, B1, B2 and B3) accumulate during S and G_2 phases and are destroyed in mitosis. The G_1 cyclins (cyclins C, D1, D2, D3 and E), as the name implies, accumulate during entry into G_1. All types of cyclin D initiate activation of cdks required for progression through G_1 and S phases. On the other hand, cdks or a cdk–cyclin complex can associate with specific cdk inhibitors, leading to cell cycle arrest. The cyclin kinase

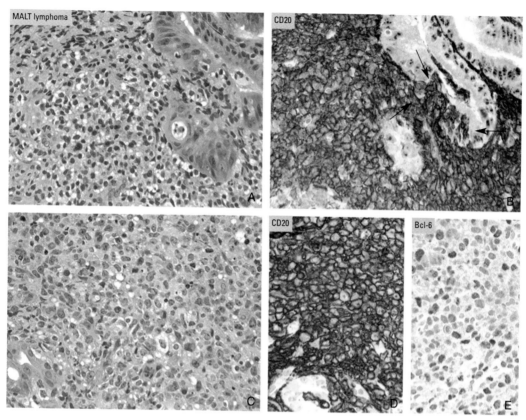

Figure 1.15 Gastric marginal zone B-cell lymphoma (MALT) with transformation into diffuse large B-cell lymphoma. A, low-grade component with lymphoepithelial lesions. B, CD20 expression by lymphomatous cells (*note infiltration of benign epithelium by B cells; arrows*). C, high-grade component. D–E, transformed cells express CD20 (D) and Bcl-6 (E)

inhibitors (CKI) include $p16^{INK4A}$, $p15^{INK4B}$, $p18^{INK4C}$, $p21^{Cip1}$, $p27^{Kip1}$ and $p57^{Kip2}$ [239]. The substrates for the cdks include pRb (encoded by the *RB1* gene), p107 and p130. The phosphorylation status of those substrates determines their activity and cell cycle regulation. Apart from its role in proliferation, pRb is also involved in differentiation, apoptosis and replicative senescence.

The cell proliferative fraction, as determined by mitotic count (Figure 1.20), S-phase, thymidine labeling, or immunohistochemistry (Ki-67/MIB1), predicts the outcome in malignant lymphomas[240–245]. Additionally, the proliferative status appears to be an important factor in predicting the efficacy of treatment. Ki-67 expression was shown to be a predictor of efficacy of rituximab plus chemotherapy[246].

Based on the proliferation index, lymphomas are divided into low grade (low-growth fraction) and high grade (high-growth fraction). It appears that the accumulation of tumor cells in low-grade lymphomas is due to alteration of apoptosis regulation rather than disruption of the cell cycle with subsequent increase in proliferation. The opposite is associated with high-grade lymphomas characterized by high proliferation and often also increased number of apoptotic cells. Overall, survival is significantly reduced in lymphoma patients with a high Ki-67 proliferative index compared with those with a low proliferative index. One-year survival estimates are 82% for lymphomas with low-growth fraction versus 18% for those with a high proliferative index[241]. In DLBCL, a high proliferative fraction as defined by

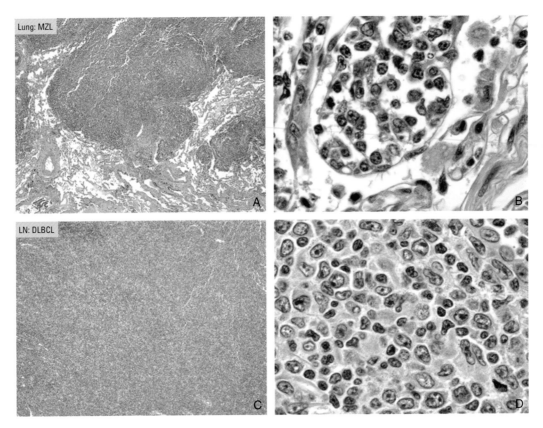

Figure 1.16 Marginal zone B-cell lymphoma of lung (BALT/MALT lymphoma; A–B) with transformation into diffuse large B-cell lymphoma (C–D) after 1 year. A, C, low magnification; B, D, high magnification. Molecular studies revealed clonal peak (polymerase chain reaction for immunoglobulin rearrangements) at exactly the same location in both lymphomas

the expression of Ki-67 (>60% of malignant cells) is associated with increased risk of relapse and shorter survival[241]. In FL, p53 and Ki-67 expressions do not provide sufficient information to predict the risk of transformation to a higher grade[247]. However, high Ki-67 expression in FL correlates with an inferior response to treatment with rituximab (Rituxan)[246]. In gastric MALT lymphomas, the Ki-67/MIB1 index has limited independent value for predicting outcome[248]. Patients with MCL with a high Ki-67 index and increased number of mitoses have less favorable prognoses than patients with low proliferation[15,249]. Increased expression of Ki-67 in MCL is associated with deregulation of several cell cycle regulatory components[250]. Patients with MCL with

Ki-67 expression in ≥26% of the lymphoma cells had median survival of only 13 months as compared with 45 months in the rest of the patients (<26% Ki-67+ cells)[15]. A significantly higher mitotic index and Ki-67 index were found in blastoid MCL as compared with typical MCL[251]. A multivariate regression analysis incorporating commonly used clinical prognostic features confirmed the independent effect of cell proliferation on survival in lymphoma patients. Figure 1.21 presents Ki-67/MIB1 expression in malignant lymphomas.

Determination of the Ki-67 fraction is useful in predicting prognosis in patients with plasma cell neoplasms[252]. There is a marked difference in survival between patients with MM with Ki-67 >8% as

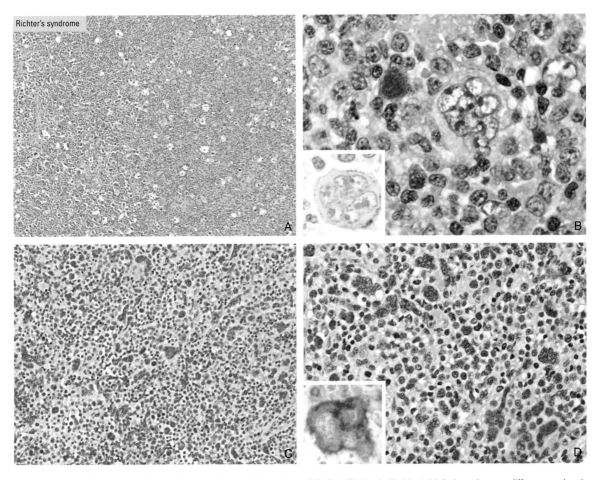

Figure 1.17   Richter's syndrome (large cell transformation of B-CLL/SLL). A–B, Hodgkin's lymphoma: diffuse predominantly small cell infiltrate (A) with scattered large cells. High magnification reveals typical multinucleated Reed–Sternberg cells with nucleoli (B; *inset: Epstein–Barr virus (EBV) expression by R–S cell*). C–D, diffuse large B-cell lymphoma with anaplastic features (low magnification, C; high magnification, D; *inset: CD22 expression by large atypical cell*)

compared to patients with Ki-67 <8%[253]. MM patients with a high S-phase fraction (>3%) show a significantly increased incidence of anemia and hypercalcemia; higher values of β_2-microglobulin and creatinine are found, as well as a poor prognosis as assessed both by response duration and overall survival[166]. In MM, apart from being a marker of proliferative activity, Ki-67 is also associated with bone marrow angiogenesis and tumor burden[232,253]. Figure 1.22 presents dual immunostaining of MM for Ki-67 (proliferation marker) and CD138 (plasma cell marker).

In classical HL, a high proliferation index (Ki-67/MIB1) and loss of pRb expression are found to be adverse prognostic factors influencing respectively lower overall survival and failure to achieve complete remission[254,255].

APOPTOSIS

Growth of malignancies depends on an imbalance between the rate of cell production and the rate of cell death. Cell death occurs by two main methods: necrosis and apoptosis. Apoptosis is a genetically

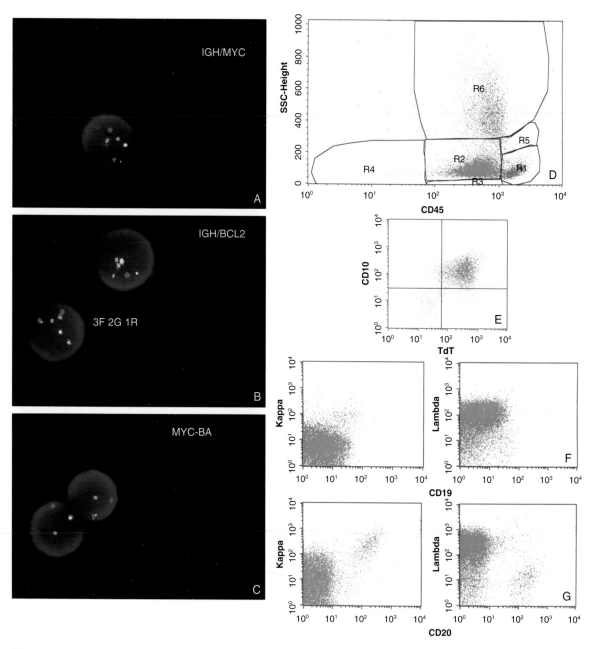

Figure 1.18   Blastic transformation of follicular lymphoma. A–C, fluorescence *in situ* hybridization (FISH) analysis showing c-*MYC* translocation (A), *BCL2* translocation (B) and break-apart dual color with split signals (C; red and green split signals; yellow/orange, normal signal). D–G, flow cytometry analysis shows leukemic cells in blastic region (D) co-expressing CD10 and TdT (E) with clonal lambda expression (F–G), dim CD19 (F), and negative CD20 (G)

Table 1.4 Types of morphologic progression/transformation in hematopoietic tumors

Neoplasm	Morphological progression
B-CLL/SLL	Prolymphocytic/paraimmunoblastic transformation Classical Hodgkin's lymphoma Diffuse large B-cell lymphoma
Follicular lymphoma	Diffuse large B-cell lymphoma Precursor B-lymphoblastic leukemia (B-ALL)
Marginal zone B-cell lymphoma, MALT type	Diffuse large B-cell lymphoma
Splenic marginal zone B-cell lymphoma	Diffuse large B-cell lymphoma
Mantle cell lymphoma	Blastoid variant of mantle cell lymphoma
Hairy cell leukemia	Blastic variant of hairy cell leukemia
Mycosis fungoides	T-cell lymphoma, large cell type
Adult T-cell leukemia (ATCL), smoldering and chronic types	ATCL, acute and lymphomatous types
Lymphomatoid papulosis	Mycosis fungoides Cutaneous anaplastic large cell lymphoma Systemic T-cell lymphoma Hodgkin's lymphoma
T-large granular lymphocyte leukemia (T-LGL)	Aggressive T-LGL T-cell lymphoma, large cell type
Multiple myeloma	Plasma cell leukemia Anaplastic multiple myeloma
Classical Hodgkin's lymphoma	Diffuse large B-cell lymphoma
Nodular lymphocyte predominant Hodgkin's lymphoma	Diffuse large B-cell lymphoma
Myelodysplastic syndrome, low grade	Refractory anemia with excess blasts Acute myeloid leukemia
Myelodysplastic syndrome, high grade	Acute myeloid leukemia
Chronic myeloid leukemia (CML)	Accelerated phase of CML Blast crisis of CML (AML or ALL)
Chronic myeloproliferative disorders (polycythemia vera, essential thrombocythemia, chronic idiopathic myelofibrosis)	Acute myeloid leukemia
Langerhans cell histiocytosis, unifocal	Multifocal, multisystem Langerhans cell histiocytosis (Letterer–Siwe disease)
Chronic myelomonocytic leukemia (CMML)	Acute myeloid leukemia

programmed cell death characterized by distinct, recognizable morphologic features (Figure 1.23), namely shrinking of the cell, membrane blebbing and DNA fragmentation with engulfment of the remnants by macrophages and dendritic cells with no or minimal inflammatory reaction. Programmed cell death is a fundamental requirement for embryogenesis, organ metamorphosis and tissue homeostasis. Apoptosis can be triggered by a variety of physiologic stimuli, growth factor withdrawal, death receptor ligands and toxic insult (e.g. irradiation, ultraviolet (UV) light and cytostatic drugs). Apoptosis must be considered a rescue mechanism that controls the integrity of the cell, erasing aberrant clones. It is likely that failure of apoptosis constitutes a key factor responsible for tumor formation, progression and resistance to drugs. Antitumor drugs, including new molecular targeting therapy (e.g. imatinib in CML, rituximab in $CD20^+$ tumors, alemtuzumab in $CD52^+$ T-/B-lymphomas, gemtuzumab

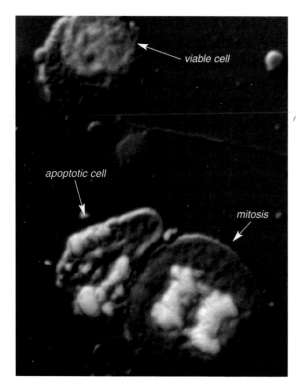

Figure 1.19   Mitosis (cell in metaphase)

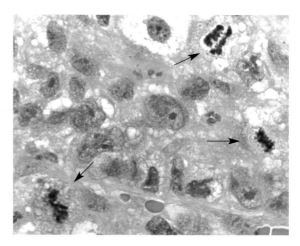

Figure 1.20   High mitotic activity (arrowed) in high-grade malignant lymphoma (anaplastic large cell lymphoma)

in CD33[+] tumors, arsenic trioxide/all-*trans*-retinoic acid (ATRA) in APL and *FLT3* inhibitors in AML) eliminate tumor cells by inducing apoptosis. Several genes (e.g. those encoding survivin, the *BCL2* family, and *p53* (*TP53*)), are involved in apoptotic regulation and execution. *p53* is activated in response to DNA damage, and loss of its function (mutation, chromosome deletion) increases the threshold of DNA damage at which the cell will commit to apoptosis[256]. *p53* mutations are frequently observed in hematologic cancer during disease progression and are associated with high resistance to treatment[256]. The *BCL2* proto-oncogene encodes a mitochondrial protein that blocks apoptosis. High expression of *BCL2* is associated with drug resistance and poor prognosis in NHL and AML[257,258]. Dysfunction of the p53/BAX/caspase 3 apoptosis signaling pathway has been shown to play a role in carcinogenesis, tumor progression and the development of acquired drug resistance.

Upon activation of apoptosis, series of caspases (cysteine-containing aspartic acid-specific proteases) are activated through cleavage of the proenzymes[259]. Inhibitors of apoptosis proteins (IAPs) are a family of related proteins that suppress apoptosis by inhibiting caspases. Survivin, a unique member of the IAP family, links cell death and proliferation. Survivin is not expressed in terminal differentiated tissues, but is expressed in many malignancies. Disruption of survivin expression causes cell death and cell division defects. The elevated survivin expression is associated with poor prognosis and increased tumor recurrence in many cancers[260,261]. Another widely expressed IAP is XIAP, which is one of the most potent inhibitors of caspases.

The apoptotic signal can be amplified through the mitochondria and inhibited through the action of competing molecules such as the inhibitor c-FLIP, which binds to the receptor complex in place of caspase 8. Two major apoptotic pathways are recognized. The (stress-induced) 'intrinsic' or mitochondrial pathway is thought to be triggered by the translocation into mitochondria of Bcl-2 family members, leading to alterations in mitochondrial permeability and cytochrome c release, with subsequent activation of caspase 9. Release of mitochondrial cytochrome c leads to the cytosolic

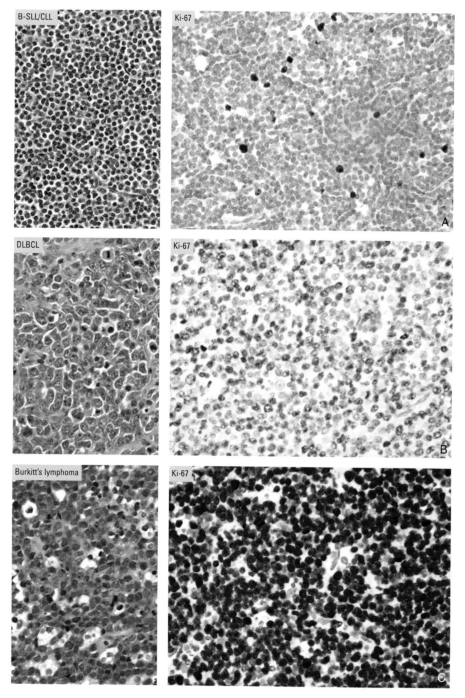

Figure 1.21   Ki-67 (MIB1) staining in malignant lymphoma. Low (A), intermediate (B) and high (C) proliferation (Ki-67 index)

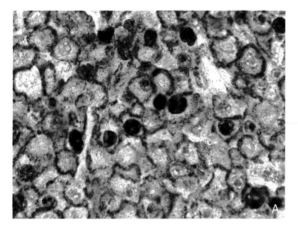

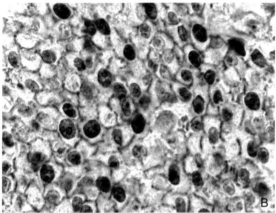

Figure 1.22 Plasma cell myeloma. Dual staining for CD138 (plasma cell marker; red cytoplasmic membrane staining) and Ki-67 (proliferation marker; brown nuclear staining) in two cases of multiple myeloma. A, rare plasma cells co-express Ki-67 (low proliferation fraction). B, numerous plasma cells express Ki-67 (high proliferation fraction)

assembly of the apoptosome – a caspase activation complex involving Apaf1 and caspase 9 that induces hallmarks of apoptosis. The Bcl-2 family of proteins are the most prominent targets for cancer therapy (Bcl-2, Bcl-X$_L$, Bcl-W, Mcl-1, Bfl-1 and Bcl-B). These proteins are often overexpressed in hematologic malignancies including Bcl-2 overexpression in the majority of follicular lymphomas and in about one-third of DLBCL. The second (cell surface death receptor signaling) 'extrinsic' pathway involves death receptors, such as tumor necrosis factor (TNF)

receptors or Fas (CD95), whose binding to their ligands leads to activation of caspase 8[262–265]. Binding of TNF to its cellular receptor, TNFR1, triggers two signaling pathways, one resulting in activation of the caspase family of proteases, triggering apoptosis, while the other triggers activation of NF-κB which interferes with the caspase pathway and induces an inflammatory reaction. The TNF family of cytokines, Fas ligand (FasL) and TRAIL (Apo2 ligand) trigger activation of the caspase pathways without concomitant involvement of NF-κB. c-FLIP (FLICE-inhibitory protein) plays an essential role in regulation of death receptor-induced apoptosis; it inhibits Fas-mediated apoptosis. The overexpression of c-FLIP is tumor-specific, which may be one of the *in vivo* mechanisms by which tumor cells escape from apoptotic death during malignant transformation. A favorable response to chemotherapy depends on an intact apoptosis cascade, and poor response to therapy in lymphomas or leukemias may be caused by inhibition of the apoptosis cascade, including caspase 3. The inhibition of the caspase 9-mediated pathway, but not the caspase 8-mediated pathway, plays a significant role in therapy resistance in patients with nodal DLBCL[266].

Apoptosis in lymphoproliferative disorders

The apoptotic index in lymphomas increases with malignancy grade and proliferative activity, but is not related to location, cell of origin, clinical stage, bone marrow involvement or *p53* expression[267]. Increased resistance to apoptosis promotes lymphomagenesis, with aberrant expression of cell survival proteins such as Bcl-2 and c-Myc occurring in distinct lymphoma subtypes. A subset of B-cell neoplasms, including DLBCL, primary effusion lymphoma (PEL) and MM, express galectin 3, another antiapoptotic protein[268]. NF-κB, which is a transcription factor belonging to the *REL* family, induces the expression of antiapoptotic factors such as the *IAP*, c-*FLIP* and *TRAF1–2*, as well as members of the *BCL2* family such as *BCL-X$_L$*[269]. Bai *et al.* identified distinct clusters of DLBCL with respect to the combined expression

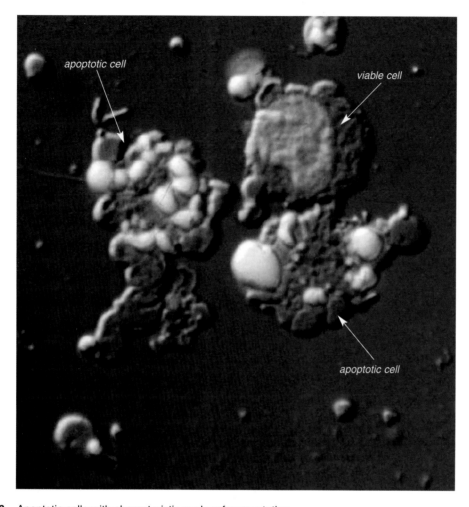

Figure 1.23   Apoptotic cells with characteristic nuclear fragmentation

levels of the apoptosis-associated Bcl-2 family of proteins[270]. The high expression pro-apoptotic proteins (BAX, Bak and Bid) and low expression of anti-apoptotic proteins was significantly associated with the germinal center B-like phenotype[270,271]. In a study reported by Gascoyne *et al.*, *BCL2* gene rearrangement status could not be shown to have an impact on outcome, but expression of anti-apoptotic Bcl-2 protein was a strong significant predictor of overall survival, disease-free survival and relapse-free survival in DLBCL[272]. The c-*REL* proto-oncogene in amplified in a subset of DLBCL[273,274] of germinal center cell origin, especially in extranodal tumors and in primary mediastinal lymphoma[275]. The *IAP* family (*XIAP*, c-*IAP1*, c-*IAP2*) encodes a group of proteins involved

in the suppression of apoptosis by blocking caspase activity. *BCL6* suppresses the expression of the *p53* (*TP53*) tumor suppressor gene and modulates DNA damage-induced apoptotic responses in germinal center B-cells. Muris *et al.* reported that caspase 9 inhibition was strongly associated with a poor response to chemotherapy and usually with a fatal outcome, whereas caspase 8 inhibition was associated with an excellent clinical outcome in patients with DLBCL[266].

Low-grade B-cell malignancies, particularly FL and B-CLL represent neoplasms characterized primarily by a problem with cell death rather than the cell cycle[276]. Dipeptidyl peptidase 2 (DPP2), a serine protease that plays a key role in keeping cells in the quiescent state, is involved in cell-cycle control in B-CLL. Inhibition of DPP2 results in apoptosis of normal lymphocytes. Based on the susceptibility of leukemic cells to apoptosis after exposure to DPP2, two distinct subsets of B-CLL can be identified: those susceptible and those resistant to DPP2 inhibition-induced apoptosis[277]. If resistant to apoptosis (42.1%), the CLL cells have higher expression of ZAP-70 and exhibit a worse prognosis, such as a shorter treatment-free time period[277]. Thus, resistance versus susceptibility to DPP2 inhibition-induced apoptosis is suggested as a novel prognostic factor in B-CLL.

Bcl-2 and other antiapoptotic proteins (Bcl-X, Bcl-X$_L$) are frequently expressed in FL[278,279]. Zhao *et al.* reported that a high *BCL-X$_L$* level was significantly associated with multiple sites of extranodal involvement, elevated LDH level and high IPI, and *BCL-X$_L$* gene overexpression was linked to short overall survival in FL[278].

The chromosomal translocation t(11;18)(q21;q21), which has been identified as a recurring cytogenetic abnormality in gastric MALT lymphoma, leads to fusion of the *API2* gene at 11q21 and the *MALT2* gene at 18q21[280–282]. *API2* (c-*IAP2*) is a member of the *IAP* gene family with a caspase-inhibitory function and is essential for the suppression of apoptosis and giving tumor cells survival advantages[283,284]. *API2–MALT1* fusion transcripts lead to an increased inhibition of apoptosis, thereby helping lymphoma cells to survive[285]. It is also suggested that *Helicobacter pylori* eradication therapy itself induces apoptosis in leukocytes in the gastric mucosa[286].

In T-cell lymphomas, similarly to B-cell lymphoproliferations, identification of relevant protooncogenes and tumor suppressor genes involved in cell-cycle progression and apoptosis (e.g. *Nucleophosmin–ALK* fusion, *p53* and *RB1*) represent potential candidates for molecular based therapy. In ALCL, a high number of caspase 3-positive tumor cells predicted a highly favorable clinical outcome[287]. Poor prognosis was strongly related to a high number of Bcl-2$^+$ neoplastic cells. ALK$^+$ ALCL had significantly higher levels of active caspase 3, while high expression of the antiapoptotic proteins Bcl-2 and

protease inhibitor 9 (PI9) was almost completely restricted to ALK$^-$ tumors[287].

Antilymphoma activity of rituximab (an anti-CD20 antibody) and alemtuzumab (an anti-CD52 antibody) is mediated by antibody-dependent cytotoxicity (ADCC), by complement-mediated cytotoxicity (CDC) and by activating apoptotic cell death. The latter effect can be enhanced by conjugating anti-CD20 antibody with cytotoxic agents. Deregulation of the ubiquitin–proteasome pathway by proteasome inhibitor bortezomib (PS-341) induces apoptosis through the upregulation of specific proapoptotic proteins and has been associated with significant clinical responses in a variety of hematologic malignancies, including multiple myeloma and NHL[288].

Apoptosis in multiple myeloma

Resistance to apoptosis plays an important role in both pathogenesis and resistance to treatment of MM[289]. Distinct gene expression patterns have been found to be associated with different lesions: the overexpression of *CCND2* and genes involved in cell adhesion pathways was observed in cases with deregulated *MAF* and *MAFB*, whereas genes upregulated in cases with the t(4;14) showed apoptosis-related functions[290]. The apoptotic index is very low in MM[291]. Most malignant plasma cells overexpress Bcl-2, which contributes to resistance against apoptosis induced by dexamethasone and other anticancer agents. New chemotherapeutic and biologic agents currently available for MM (e.g. proteasome inhibitors) may inhibit proliferation and induce apoptosis in MM cells characterized by overexpression of Bcl-2[292]. Patients with refractory MM showed response rates of 50%, including complete remissions after treatment with bortezomib (a selective inhibitor of the 26S proteasome)[293]. Oblimersen sodium (Genasense), an antisense oligonucleotide that specifically binds to Bcl-2 messenger RNA, decreases production of Bcl-2 protein in MM cells and enhances the cytotoxicity of dexamethasone and doxorubicin. Combining oblimersen with other anticancer agents represents a therapy-enhancing strategy to reverse the multidrug resistance seen in MM[294]. The induction of apoptosis or G_1 arrest of the cell cycle (apart from antiangiogenic effects) is listed as a potential mechanism of action of thalidomide – a drug considered a standard approach for the treatment of relapsed and refractory MM[295].

Apoptosis in Hodgkin's lymphoma

Neoplastic cells in HL (Hodgkin cells and Reed–Sternberg cells) shows high expression of cyclins and cdks involved in G_1/S and G_2/M transition and have defective regulation of apoptosis due to overexpression of Bcl-2 (23%), Bcl-X_L (19%) and survivin (89%), loss of BAX expression (3%) and increased nuclear expression of p65/RelA[255]. Bcl-2, Bcl-X_L and NF-κB activation are involved in the resistance to apoptosis by Hodgkin and Reed–Sternberg cells. The presence of NF-κB and its activation is related to changes in the expression of a set of proteins that play a role in the control of cell cycle progression, apoptosis and gene transcription, such as p21, p16, p27, pRb, cyclins E and D3, cdk1, cdk2 and survivin[255]. Shorter survival of patients with HL is related with overexpression of Bcl-2, p53, Bcl-X_L, BAX and high proliferative (Ki-67/MIB1) and apoptotic indexes[255]. Hodgkin/Reed–Sternberg cells resist CD95-induced apoptosis by expression of c-FLIP[296]. c-FLIP, a key regulator of death receptor resistance, is constitutively expressed in HL and may therefore be a major mechanism responsible for Fas-resistance in HL[297].

Apoptosis in acute leukemia

Apoptosis-related proteins are important molecules for predicting chemotherapy response and prognosis in adult AML. Decreased apoptosis and increased angiogenesis can contribute to leukemogenesis and poor prognosis in AML. The inability to undergo apoptosis is a crucial mechanism of multidrug resistance in AML. Caspase activation is an essential step in apoptosis, and cytotoxic drug-induced apoptosis is mediated by caspase 2 and caspase 3. Overexpression of the inactive forms of caspases (caspases 2 and 3) is

frequently observed in the blasts of patients with AML and ALL. Many other genes and enzymes involved in the control and/or execution of apoptosis are expressed at high levels in patients with acute leukemia. The Wilms' tumor gene *WT1* is upregulated in AML. The *BCL2* gene, which encodes a mitochondrial protein that inhibits the onset of apoptosis induced by growth factor withdrawal or cytotoxic agents, is highly expressed on blasts. Suárez *et al.* found high levels of the Bcl-2 antiapoptotic protein and low amounts of the APO2.7 proapoptotic protein on bone marrow CD34+ blasts from AML and high-risk MDS patients[298]. There appears to be a negative correlation between Bcl-2 expression and the number of apoptotic cells, and Bcl-2 expression is increased in chemotherapy-resistant patients when compared with responsive patients[299]. High Bcl-2 expression is related to a poor prognosis in AML[299]. Patients with a higher BAX/Bcl-2 ratio have a significantly higher complete remission rate and a longer overall survival and disease-free survival when compared with patients with low BAX and high Bcl-2 expression (low BAX/Bcl-2 ratio)[300]. At diagnosis, high expression of Bad and BAX predicts adverse outcome, regardless of the response to therapy, particularly in patients who do not enter complete remission, and may serve as prognostic markers in AML[301]. Inhibition of apoptosis in AML is associated with pan-resistance to antileukemic chemotherapy[302]. In childhood *de novo* AML, apoptosis-related molecules (e.g. survivin; *see below*) are associated with maturation stage, cytogenetic risk groups and therapy outcome[303]. Tamm *et al.* reported an inverse correlation of survivin and XIAP expression with survival of patients with AML[303,304]. Adida *et al.* confirmed the association of survivin expression and poor prognosis only after survivin expression was adjusted with the Cox model for established prognostic factors in AML[305]. There was no significant difference in complete remission rate or overall survival between survivin- positive and survivin-negative AML patients[305]. Carter *et al.* suggested that lack of a prognostic impact of XIAP and survivin may be associated with caspase-independent mechanisms of cell death in AML[306].

Gene expression profiling of B-ALL identified sets of differentially expressed genes depending on the resistance or chemosensitivity of leukemic cells to certain drugs[307]. In prednisone-resistant B-ALL there was overexpression of the antiapoptosis gene *MCL1* and underexpression of several transcription-associated genes (e.g. *SMARCB1*, *PRPF18* and *CTCF*)[307]. In ALL both BAX protein expression levels and the BAX/Bcl-2 ratio are significantly lower in samples at relapse as compared with samples at initial diagnosis. Analysis of the downstream effector caspase 3 showed loss of spontaneous caspase 3 processing at relapse, suggesting that severe disturbance of apoptotic pathways occurring both at the level of BAX expression and caspase 3 activation play a role in ALL relapse[308].

Apoptosis in myelodysplastic syndrome

Apoptosis is upregulated in early MDS and involves mainly mature cells in the marrow, leading to ineffective hematopoiesis and contributing to peripheral cytopenias. The CD34[+] blasts are more resistant to apoptosis in high-grade MDS than in low-grade MDS[309–311]. Bcl-2 and c-Myc oncoprotein levels were maturation stage-dependent, with high levels expressed within CD34[+] marrow cells, decreasing markedly with myeloid maturation. The expression of the proapoptotic protein APO2.7 and antiapoptotic Bcl-2 on CD34[+] cells from low-grade MDS are similar to normal marrow[298]. The ratio of expression of c-Myc to Bcl-2 oncoproteins among CD34[+] cells was significantly increased for MDS patients compared with that among cells from normal marrow and patients with AML[310]. Tsoplou *et al.* showed that marrow apoptosis could be detected in both CD34[+] and CD34[−] cells in early MDS and seemed to be restricted to CD34[+] cells in advanced MDS cases[312]. It is postulated that MDS progression is related to accumulation of immature myeloid cells with increased Bcl-2 expression and decreased apoptosis[309]. The association between lower susceptibility to apoptosis and MDS progression (increasing number of CD34[+] cells) was also confirmed by flow cytometry analysis of CD95 and CD95L expression[313]. Analysis of the *IAP* gene family by Yamamoto *et al.* showed significant overexpression of mRNA for survivin, cIAP1, NAIP and XIAP in MDS bone marrow cells compared with control samples[314]. However, the expression of mRNA for survivin, cIAP1 and cIAP2 exhibited a remarkable decrease after the transformation to AML[314].

Apoptosis in chronic myeloid leukemia

In CML, *BCR–ABL* expression inappropriately prolongs the growth factor-independent survival of myeloid progenitors and granulocytes by inhibiting apoptosis, and the decreased rate of programmed cell death appears to be the primary mechanism by which *BCR-ABL* effects expansion of the leukemic clone in CML[315,316]. The transition between the chronic phase of CML and blast crisis is associated with increased resistance to apoptosis correlating with poor prognosis[317]. Patients with the myeloid blast crisis of CML show a progressive expansion of the clone with *p53* loss (associated with a significant reduction in apoptosis), indicating that *p53* loss and point mutations are associated with suppression of apoptosis and progression of CML into myeloid blastic crisis[318].

CHAPTER 2

Chromosomal/genetic aberrations

Cytogenetic aberrations, both structural (translocations and inversions) and numerical (deletion or gain of whole or a portion of a chromosome) occur in the majority of hematopoietic neoplasms. The methods used to detect the genetic changes in cancer include: (1) conventional cytogenetics (karyotyping on cells derived from direct preparations or short-term cultures using banding analysis); (2) molecular cytogenetics, e.g. fluorescence *in situ* hybridization (FISH), multicolor FISH and spectral karyotyping (SKY); and (3) molecular techniques to analyze DNA, RNA or proteins directly, e.g. polymerase chain reaction (PCR), reverse transcriptase PCR (RT-PCR), quantitative real-time PCR (RQ-PCR), Southern blotting and microarray analysis. Many chromosomal and molecular changes define specific hematologic entities and syndromes and have important therapeutic and prognostic impact, e.g. t(15;17)/*PML–RARα* in acute promyelocytic leukemia, t(2;5)/*NPM–ALK* in anaplastic large cell lymphoma, or t(9;22)/*BCR–ABL* in chronic myeloid leukemia (CML), acute myeloid leukemia (AML) and precursor B-lymphoblastic leukemia (B-ALL).

A significant subset of hematopoietic malignancies show lack of chromosomal rearrangements in routine cytogenetics studies and only molecular tests can visualize an underlying genetic defect. *FLT3* length mutation is the most frequent mutation in AML (23.5%) and the majority of patients (70.5%) have a normal karyotype[319]. Similarly, *MLL* mutations occur mainly in cytogenetically normal AML. *MLL*

mutations, similarly to *MLL* translocations, confer a poor prognosis.

GENE EXPRESSION PROFILING (DNA MICROARRAY)

DNA microarray analysis is a highly promising new technique with broad applications, including the prediction of cancer outcomes by simultaneous analysis of the expression of thousands of genes[320,321]. It involves the extraction of RNA from a sample, its conversion to cDNA by labeled probes, hybridization of this labeled cDNA and laser scanning of the hybridized array. A reference RNA is labeled with a different fluorochrome. Spots appear either yellow (if the subject and reference cDNA hybridize equally) or red or green, if either sample cDNA or control probe predominate (Figure 2.1). Microarray technology will most likely lead to identification of new tumors and change the criteria by which current hematopoietic cancers are subclassified. In addition, it will provide new targets for treatment, and identify new prognostic and predictive parameters and markers for monitoring MRD. Microarray analysis has been used to screen for chromosomal aberrations (genomic imbalances, mutations and structural changes) and large-scale gene expression analysis. The prognostic value of published microarray data should be considered with caution, awaiting confirmation by validation studies with repeated random sampling[322].

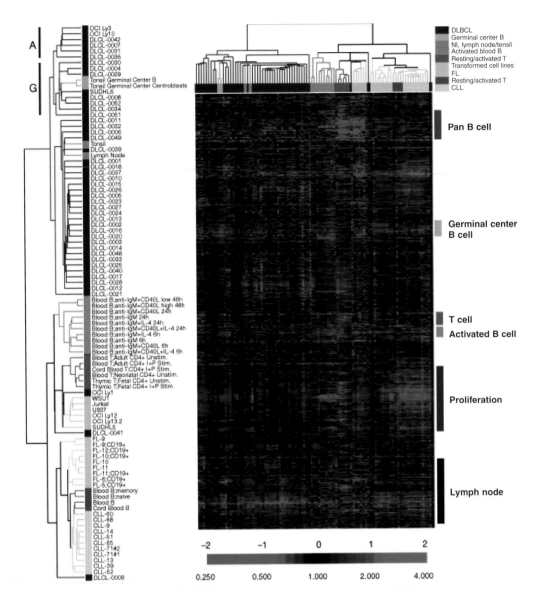

Figure 2.1 DNA microarray (hierarchical clustering of gene expression data). Depicted are the 1.8 million measurements of gene expression from 128 microarray analyses of 96 samples of normal and malignant lymphocytes. The dendrogram at the left lists the samples studied and provides a measure of the relatedness of gene expression in each sample. The dendrogram is color-coded according to the category of mRNA sample studied (see upper right key). Each row represents a separate cDNA clone on the microarray and each column a separate mRNA sample. The results presented represent the ratio of hybridization of fluorescent cDNA probes prepared from each experimental mRNA sample to a reference mRNA sample. These ratios are a measure of relative gene expression in each experimental sample and were depicted according to the color scale shown at the bottom. As indicated, the scale extends from fluorescence ratios of 0.25 to 4 (−2 to +2 in log base 2 units). Gray indicates missing or excluded data

From: Alizadeh AA, *et al.* Distinct types of diffuse large B-cell lymphoma identified by gene expression profiling. Nature 2000;403:503–11. © Nature, used with permission

Diffuse large B-cell lymphoma

Based on microarray-generated gene expression profiles, outcome predictors can be constructed for diffuse large B-cell lymphoma (DLBCL), follicular lymphoma (FL) and mantle cell lymphoma (MCL). Specific expression pattern of a limited number of genes at the time of diagnosis is linked to overall survival in DLBCL and MCL. Such predictors of prognosis may eventually lead to risk-adjusted treatment of lymphomas[323]. In DLBCL (Figures 2.1 and 2.2), gene expression analysis identified three distinct biologic entities (gene-expression subgroups): germinal-center B-cell-like (GCB), activated B-cell-like (ABC) and type 3 DLBCL[199,324–326]. DLBCLs with GCB profile express genes restricted to the germinal center such as *BCL6* and *CD10*, whereas DLBCLs with ABC profile express plasma cell genes such as *XBP1*, *IL4*, *IRF* and *caspase 8*[326]. GCB-type lymphomas are positive for CD10 and/or Bcl-6, and are negative for post-germinal center cell markers typical for plasma cells, such as MUM1 or CD138. ABC-type lymphomas are positive for MUM1 and often CD138. Different subgroups differ also in oncogenic mechanisms: in GCB-type lymphoma, *BCL2* rearrangement by t(14;18) or amplification of the *c-rel* locus are important, whereas in ABC-type lymphoma constitutive NF-κB activation is present[327]. The 5-year survival for GCB-type lymphoma is 60% and for ABC-type lymphoma is 35%. DNA microa ray analysis identified also a preferential survivin–cyclin B relationship in DLBCL, suggesting that cyclin B over-expression, when linked to survivin overexpression in aggressive forms of DLBCL, might demonstrate a specific G_2/M transition promotion[328]. Tissue micro-array (TMA) immunohistochemical analysis can be used to determine the type of DLBCL[329]; the 5-year overall survival for the germinal center B-cell-like group (DLBCL positive for CD10 and/or Bcl-6) was 76% compared with only 34% for the non-germinal center group (positive for MUM1)[329], which is similar to that reported using the cDNA microarray.

Two types of primary cutaneous large B-cell lymphomas recognized recently, primary cutaneous follicle center cell lymphoma and primary cutaneous DLBCL of the leg, differ in gene expression profiling.

Primary cutaneous follicle center cell lymphoma has an expression profile similar to that of GCB whereas DLBCL, leg-type, displays an ABC profile. The prognosis of DLBCL of the leg is worse (5-year survival 52%), when compared with follicle center cell lymphoma (5-year survival > 95%).

Other B-cell lymphoproliferations

FL is a disease characterized by a long clinical course marked by frequent relapses that vary in clinical aggressiveness over time. The selection for more aggressive treatment is currently based on histologic grading and clinical criteria. The results of grading are generally controversial, mainly because of the considerable intra- and interobserver variability[327]. International Prognostic Index (IPI) and Follicular Lymphoma IPI (FLIPI) are currently used for their predictive value at diagnosis. Gene expression profiling may eventually replace histomorphology as a guideline for treatment and prognosis in FL. The major differences in gene expression between indolent and aggressive disease were found in four categories: proliferation markers, metabolism-related genes, signal transduction markers and T-cell and accessory cell-related markers[330]. Glas *et al.* developed an FL stratification gene expression profile to assess the actual clinical behavior in FL to replace current morphologic and clinical systems[196]. This stratification profile contains genes significantly upregulated in the aggressive phase of the disease that are involved in cell cycle control (e.g. *CCNE2*, *CCNA2*, *CDK2*, *CHEK1*, *MCM7*), DNA synthesis (e.g. *TOP2A*, *POLD3A*, *HMGA1*, *POLE2*, *GMPS*, *CTPS*) and genes reflecting increased metabolism (*FRSB*, *RARS*, *HK2*, *LDHA*). The profile based on 81 genes accurately classified 93% of the FL samples (low vs. high grade) in an independent validation set and, in a series of FL cases where histologic grading was ambiguous, precluding meaningful morphologic guidance, the 81-gene profile shows a classification accuracy of 94%[196]. Preliminary data suggest that there may be a molecular profile that can predict early transformation at baseline. Using cDNA microarray analysis, Elenitoba-Johnson *et al.* identified 113 transformation-associated genes whose expression

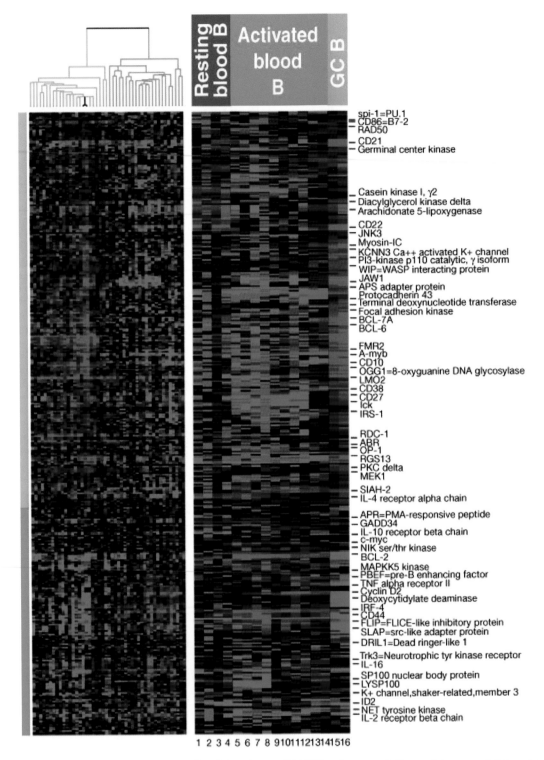

Figure 2.2   Relationship of diffuse large B-cell lymphoma (DLBCL) subgroups (left panel) to normal B-lymphocyte differentiation and activation (right panel). The left panel depicts hierarchical clustering of the genes selectively expressed in germinal center (GC) B-like DLBCL and activated B-like DLBCL. The right panel depicts gene expression

differed between clonally related samples of FL and DLBCL occurring in the same patient[331]. Based on gene-expression profiling, Dave *et al.* found that the length of survival among patients with FL correlated with the molecular features of non-malignant immune cells present in the tumor at diagnosis[332].

DNA microarray of B-cell chronic lymphocytic leukemia (B-CLL) (Figure 2.3) showed significant expression differences in 78 genes compared with the reference tonsillar B lymphocytes. A cluster of genes (*LCP1, PARP, BLR1, DEK, NPM, MCL1, SLP76, STAM, HIVEP1, EVI2B, CD25, HTLF, HIVEP2, BCL2, MNDA, PBX3, EB12, TCF1, CGRP, CD14, ILB, GZMK, GPR17* and *CD79B*) was associated with the unfavorable 11q deletion and also with the unfavorable Binet stages B and C[333]. Using genomic-scale gene expression profiling, Rosenwald *et al.* showed that B-CLL is characterized by a common gene expression profile irrespective of *Ig* mutational status confirming that B-CLL is a single disease with a common mechanism of transformation and/or cell of origin but with two distinct variants (mutated and unmutated)[334]. The expression of hundreds of other genes (Figure 2.3) correlated with the *Ig* mutational status, including many genes that are modulated in expression during mitogenic B-cell receptor signaling[334]. Analysis of 5600 genes in CD38$^+$ vs. CD38$^-$ B-CLL showed a common gene expression profile that is largely independent of CD38 expression, and only the expression of 14 genes (including genes that are involved in the regulation of cell survival) differed significantly between the two groups[335] (CD38 expression in B-CLL is associated with poor response to

therapy and shorter survival). The *ATM* (ataxia telangiectasia mutant)/*p53* (*TP53*)-dependent DNA damage response pathway plays an important role in the progression of lymphoid tumors, including B-CLL. Using microarray analysis of *ATM*-mutant, *p53*-mutant and *ATM/p53* wild-type B-CLLs, Stankovic *et al.* showed that, after exposure to DNA damage, transcriptional responses are entirely dependent on *ATM* function[336]. The *p53* proapoptotic responses comprise only a part of *ATM*-regulated transcription; additionally, ATM regulates prosurvival responses independently of *p53*. Consequently, the greater severity of the *p53*-mutant B-CLLs compared with *ATM*-mutant B-CLLs is consistent with the additive effect of defective apoptotic and elevated survival responses after DNA damage in these tumors[336].

A distinct genetic signature, consisting of 32 genes, was found when comparing MCL with low and high proliferation fractions (Ki-67 index). The signature consisted of genes involved in cellular processes, such as mitotic spindle formation, gene transcription and cell cycle regulation (components of the p53 and retinoblastoma protein (pRb) pathways)[250]. In splenic MZL, cDNA microarray analysis revealed shorter survival to be associated with CD38 expression, naïve *Ig*V$_H$ genes, and the expression of a set of NF-κB pathway genes, including *TRAF5, REL* and *PKCA*.

Multiple myeloma

Multiple myeloma (MM) is characterized by numerous chromosomal abnormalities. Analysis of gene expression identified several distinct subgroups of MM (designated MM1 to MM4), with expression pattern

Figure 2.2 (Continued)

data from the following normal B-cell samples: (1) total CD19$^+$ blood B cells; (2) naive CD27$^-$ blood B cells; (3) memory CD27$^+$ blood B cells; (4) cord blood CD19$^+$ B cells; (5) blood B cells; anti-IgM 6 h; (6) blood B cells; anti-IgM+ IL-4 6 h; (7) blood B cells; anti-IgM+ CD40 ligand 6 h; (8) blood B cells; anti-IgM+ CD40 ligand + IL-4 6 h; (9) blood B cells; anti-IgM 24 h; (10) blood B cells; anti-IgM+ IL-4 24 h; (11) blood B cells; anti-IgM+ CD40 ligand 24 h; (12) blood B cells; anti-IgM+ CD40 ligand + IL-4 24 h; (13) blood B cells; anti-IgM+ CD40 ligand (low concentration) 48 h; (14) blood B cells; anti-IgM+ CD40 ligand (high concentration) 48 h; (15) tonsil germinal center B cells; (16) tonsil germinal center centroblasts

From: Alizadeh AA, *et al.* Distinct types of diffuse large B-cell lymphoma identified by gene expression profiling. Nature 2000;403:503–11. © Nature, used with permission

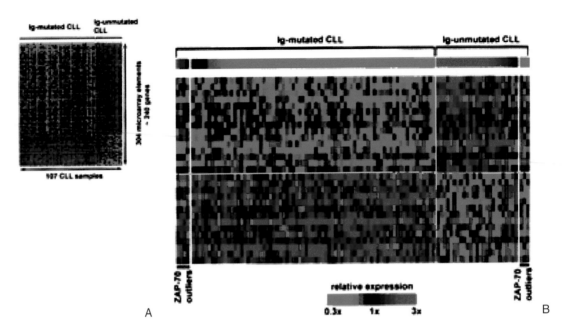

Figure 2.3 DNA microarray analysis identifies genes that are differentially expressed between Ig-mutated and Ig-unmutated chronic lymphocytic leukemia (CLL). The relative level of gene expression is depicted according to the color gradient at the bottom. For each array element, the scale is centered at the best distinction cut-off between the CLL subtypes. Red indicates higher expression, and green indicates lower expression of a given gene in the respective subgroup. (A) Expression profile of CLL subtype distinction genes. Relative expression levels of 304 Lymphochip array elements representing approximately 240 genes that were differentially expressed between Ig-mutated and Ig-unmutated CLL at a significance of $p<0.001$ are shown. Columns represent individual patients ($n=107$), and rows represent individual array elements. (B) ZAP-70 is the best CLL subtype distinction gene. The 30 most differentially expressed ($p<0.00001$) genes between Ig-mutated and Ig-unmutated CLL are shown. Patients are grouped by their IgV_H mutation status and, within subtypes, are arranged by the relative expression level of ZAP-70. Patients discordant for IgV_H mutation status and ZAP-70 expression (ZAP-70 outliers) appear at the left (Ig-mutated CLL, ZAP-70 expression above cut-off) and right (Ig-unmutated CLL, ZAP-70 expression below cut-off) ends of the spectrum. Genes are labeled with the gene symbols. For unnamed genes the IMAGE clone numbers (IM) are given. The upper half contains genes more highly expressed in Ig-unmutated CLL and the lower half contains genes more highly expressed in Ig-mutated CLL. In each group, genes are arranged from top to bottom in descending order of statistical significance

From: Wiestner A, *et al.* ZAP-70 expression identifies a chronic lymphocytic leukemia subtype with unmutated immunoglobulin genes, inferior clinical outcome, and distinct gene expression profile. Blood 2003;101:4944–51. © 2003 by The American Society of Hematology, used with permission

ranging from being similar to normal plasma cells (MM1) to being similar to MM cell lines (MM4)[337]. Clinical parameters linked to poor prognosis (abnormal karyotype and high serum β_2-microglobulin levels) were most prevalent in the MM4 subtype[337]. Fonseca *et al.* identified several genetic markers associated with a shortened survival, chromosome 13 monosomy and hypodiploidy[338]. Genes participating as

immunoglobulin heavy chain (*IgH*) translocation partners include *CCND1* (*cyclin D1, BCL1, PRAD1*) (11q13), *CCND3* (*cyclin D3*) (6p21), *FGFR3–MMSET* (4p16.3) and *MAFB* (20q11)[339,340]. *IgH* translocation simultaneously deregulates two genes with oncogenic potential: *FGFR3* on der(14) and *MMSET* on der(4). In addition to determining the expression level of *CCND1, CCND2* and *CCND3* (*cyclin D1, D2* and *D3*) gene expression profiling can effectively identify MM tumors that overexpress the oncogenes dysregulated by the five recurrent *IgH* translocations: 11q13 (*CCND1*); 6p21 (*CCND3*); 4p16 (*MMSET* and usually *FGFR3*); 16q23 (c-*maf*); and 20q11 (*mafB*). Hideshima *et al.* proposed five TC (translocation/ cyclin D) groups that can be distinguished based on the five recurrent *Ig* translocations (T) and *cyclin D* expression (C): TC1 tumors (high levels of *CCND1* (*cyclin D1*) or *CCND3* (*cyclin D3*) as a result of an *Ig* translocation); TC2 tumors (low to moderate levels of *CCND1* despite the absence of a t(11;14) translocation); TC3 tumors (a mixture of tumors that do not fall into one of the other groups, with most expressing *CCND2* (*cyclin D2*)); TC4 tumors (high levels of *CCND2*, and also *MMSET*); and TC5 tumors (highest levels of *CCND2*, and also high levels of either c-*maf* or *mafB*)[341]. Patients with tumors that have a t(4;14) translocation (TC4) have a substantially shortened survival with either standard or high-dose therapy (median overall survival 26 months and 33 months, respectively), and patients with a t(14;16) (TC5) have a similarly poor prognosis (median overall survival, 16 months with conventional therapy). By contrast, patients with tumors that have a t(11;14) translocation (TC1) appear to have a marginally better survival following conventional chemotherapy (median overall survival, 50 months), but apparently a remarkably better survival following intense therapy (predicted 88% overall survival at 80 months). Using gene expression profiling to identify five recurrent translocations, specific trisomies and expression of *cyclin D* genes, Bergsagel *et al.* divided MM tumors into eight TC (translocation/cyclin D) groups: 11q13, 6p21, 4p16, maf, D1, D1+D2, D2 and none[342].

Acute leukemia and myelodysplastic syndrome

Acute myeloid leukemia (AML) is a heterogeneous group of hematopoietic tumors currently classified by morphology (FAB subtypes), immunophenotyping (flow cytometry) and chromosomal/genetic analysis (cytogenetics/FISH/PCR). Most patients enter complete remission after treatment with chemotherapy, but a large number relapse with resistant disease. Gene expression profiling allows a comprehensive classification of AML that includes previously identified genetically defined subgroups and a novel cluster with an adverse prognosis. The study by Galub *et al.* demonstrated that both acute lymphoblastic leukemia (ALL) and AML have specific gene expression profiles allowing subclassification of acute leukemia based on molecular parameters only[320]. Schoch *et al.*, using two different strategies for microarray data in AML with reciprocal rearrangementst [t(8;21), t(15;17), and inv(16)], revealed a unique correlation between AML-specific cytogenetic aberrations and gene expression profiles[343]; a minimum set of 13 genes was sufficient to predict the karyotypes of AML accurately. Gene expression profiling with DNA microarray technology identified 35 genes associated with prognosis in pediatric AML (Figure 2.4)[344]. Several genes are associated with the outcome of AML, including drug resistance-associated genes (*MDR1, BCRP, NT5C2*) and the *BCL2* family of genes[114,258,301,345]. Most of these genes had not previously been reported to be associated with prognosis and were not correlated with morphologically classified FAB subtypes or with karyotypes. Valk *et al.*, using unsupervised cluster analyses, identified 16 groups of patients with AML on the basis of molecular signatures[346]. Guterrez *et al.* showed that a set of only 21 genes was able to assign AML to one of three classes: acute promyelocytic leukemia (APL), AML with inv(16) and AML without a specific translocation. APL expressed high levels of *FGF13* and *FGFR1* as well as two potent angiogenic factors, *HGF* and *VEGF*. AML with inv(16) showed an upregulation of *MYH11* and a downregulation of a gene encoding a core binding factor protein, *RUNX3*[347]. Genes involved in cell adhesion represented the most altered functional category in monocytic leukemias[347]. Using DNA microarray, the *HOXA9* gene was identified as a predictive marker for the diagnosis of AML[320]; *HOXA9* expression was the only single gene among 6817 tested that showed a strong correlation with clinical outcome; its expression was also correlated

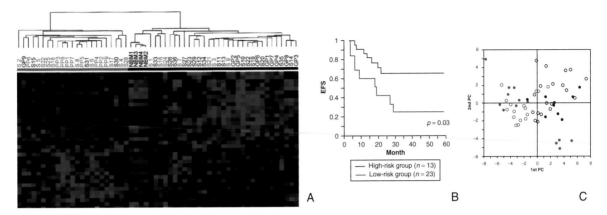

Figure 2.4 Pediatric acute myeloid leukemia. Separation of patients based on their expression of the 35 prognosis-associated genes. (A) Hierarchical clustering of 54 patients and four NBM controls based on the expression of 35 prognosis-associated genes. Patients were divided into two major clusters indicated by red and blue bars (high-risk and low-risk groups, respectively). (B) Kaplan–Meier plots of event-free survival (EFS) of patients divided into high-risk and low-risk groups based on the expression of the 35 prognosis-associated genes (good-prognosis (GP) and poor-prognosis (PP) patients were excluded). EFS differed significantly between the two groups ($p=0.03$ in log-rank test). (C) PCA of 54 patients and four NBM controls based on the expression of 35 prognosis-associated genes. The first and second components, which represent 31.8% and 12.5%, respectively, are shown. Red and blue closed circles indicate the PP and GP patients, respectively. Red and blue open circles indicate other patients who experienced relapse and those who did not experience relapse, respectively. Green closed circles indicate NBM controls. Patients who had relapses, including PP patients, those who did not have relapses, including GP patients, and NBM controls were clustered separately

From: Yagi T, *et al.* Identification of a gene expression signature associated with pediatric AML prognosis. Blood 2003;102:1849–56. © 2003 by The American Society of Hematology, used with permission

with treatment failure in patients with AML. Also, Drabkin *et al.* found that multiple *HOX* genes were overexpressed in AML patients with a poor prognosis compared with those with a favorable prognosis[348]. Low *HOX* gene expression is associated with favorable outcome in APL and AML[349–351]. Comparison between flow cytometry and microarray analysis showed a significant correlation between protein expression and mRNA abundance for genes essential for diagnosing and subclassifying AML and ALL with regard to positivity and expression[352].

ALL has a distinct gene expression profile that allows its distinction from AML and subclassification into a T- and a B-lineage[320,353,354]. Microarray analysis identified *MLL*-positive ALL as a distinct entity with a characteristic gene expression profile[353]. Yeoh *et al.* showed that microarray analysis (Affymetrix U95A) could not only discriminate each of the prognostically

important pediatric ALL subtypes, including T-ALL, ALL with *E2A–PBX1*, *BCR–ABL*, *TEL–AML1 (RUNX1)* and *MLL* rearrangements, and hyperdiploid (>50 chromosomes) ALL, but also identify new subgroups of ALL with a unique expression profile[355]. In addition, gene profiling could predict therapeutic outcome and identify genes associated with increased risk of secondary leukemia (therapy-induced AML)[355]. Holleman *et al.* identified sets of differently expressed genes in B-ALL that correlated with sensitivity or resistance to prednisone (33 genes), vincristine (40 genes), asparaginase (35 genes), or daunorubicin (20 genes)[307]. In that study, a combined gene-expression score of resistance to the four drugs was significantly and independently related to treatment outcome in multivariate analysis[307]. Microarray gene expression analyses of T-ALL revealed clinically relevant molecular subtypes[356,357]. Five different multistep molecular pathways have been identified that lead to T-ALL, involving activation of different T-ALL oncogenes: (1) *HOX11*; (2) *HOX11L2*; (3) *TAL1* plus *LMO1/2*; (4) *LYL1* plus *LMO2*; and (5) *MLL–ENL*[357]. Gene expression studies indicated that activation of a subset of these genes (*HOX11, TAL1, LYL1, LMO1* and *LMO2*) in a much larger fraction of T-ALL cases than those harboring activating chromosomal transloca-tions. Among these molecular subtypes, overexpression of the *HOX11* orphan homeobox gene occurs in approximately 5–10% of childhood and 30% of adult T-ALL cases. Patients with *HOX11*⁺ lymphoblasts have an excellent prognosis when treated with modern combination chemotherapy, while cases at high risk of early failure are included largely in the *TAL1*- and *LYL1*-positive groups[357].

The gene expression data from MDS patients show a high level of heterogeneity between patients. Several genes are commonly upregulated (*RAB20, ZNF183, ARG1* and *ACPL*) and downregulated (*COX2, CD18, KIA0001, FOS, IL7R, ACT2* and *IFI56*)[358]. *RAB20*, which encodes a small GTP-binding protein and is a member of the *RAS* super-family, was upregulated in 50% of MDS patients[358]. Miyazato *et al.* identified several genes, including delta-like protein 1 (*DLK1*), that were differentially expressed between AML and MDS patients[359].

HEMATOPOIETIC CHIMERISM AFTER ALLOGENEIC TRANSPLANTATION

Bone marrow transplantation is frequently being used for both malignant and non-malignant hematologic diseases. Hematopoietic chimerism is a measure of the number of donor and recipient cells in the host fol-lowing stem cell transplantation. Chimerism analysis has become an important tool for the peri-transplant surveillance of engraftment of donor hematopoietic cells in the recipient's bone marrow to assess the bone marrow transplantation outcome. Novel transplant procedures, for example dose-reduced conditioning protocols, rely on chimerism analysis to guide inter-vention (manipulate engraftment), i.e. the reduction of immunosuppression or infusion of donor lymphocytes.

Bone marrow engraftment analysis (chimerism analysis), which measures the recipient cells after allo-geneic stem cell transplantation (allo-SCT), offers the possibility of identifying impending graft rejection and can serve as an indicator for the recurrence of the underlying malignant or non-malignant disease. Most recently, these investigations have become the basis for treatment intervention – for example, to avoid graft rejection, to maintain engraftment and to treat immi-nent relapse by pre-emptive immunotherapy[360]. FISH and PCR-based molecular methods enable a rapid and accurate detection of post-hematopoietic stem cell transplantation chimerism with similar results[361]. Currently, XY-FISH analysis of sex chromosomes after transplantation from a sex-mismatched donor or analysis of polymorphic DNA sequences, i.e. short tan-dem repeats (STR) or variable number of tandem repeats (VNTR), are the most widely used procedures used in the assessment of chimerism[37]. The use of PCR of STR using fluorescent amplification permits quan-tification using Genescan analysis. Alizadeh *et al.* proposed a real-time quantitative PCR assay using TaqMan technology[362].

Presence of hematopoietic cells of recipient origin after successful clinical engraftment is known as mixed chimerism (MC). A patient with stable MC indicates immunologic tolerance between donor and recipient[363]. These patients are less likely to develop graft-versus-host disease but may be at risk for relapse[364,365]. The simple demonstration of MC has little clinical significance. Conversely, increase in the proportion of host cells after allo-SCT (increas-ing mixed chimerism) has been associated with a high risk of disease recurrence[366,367]. Non-relapsed patients show a progressive decrease in peripheral blood chimerism to values below 0.01% (complete chimerism, CC)[368]. The serial and quantitative chimerism analysis at short time intervals by PCR provides a reliable and rapid screening method for the early detection of recurrence of underlying disease and is therefore a prognostic tool to identify patients at highest risk of relapse. The probability of relapse-free survival for patients with CC is 0.67, for patients with decreasing MC 1.0 and for patients with increasing MC 0.1[366]. Bader *et al.* reported that virtually all children with acute leukemia and MDS who develop the phenotype of increasing MC after allo-SCT will relapse[369,370]. Pre-emptive immunotherapy performed on pediatric patients with MDS after allo-SCT that showed increasing MC improved event-free survival from 0% to 50%[371]. The 3-year event-free survival of patients with increasing MC without immunotherapy was 0%[372]. In a series published by Michallet *et al.* (mean follow-up of 39.4 months) the 5-year probabilities of overall survival and event-free survival were 69.5% and 61% for full donor chimerism, 35.4% and 25% for regressive MC, 42.6% and 28.6% for stable MC, and 21% and 10.4% for progressive MC[373]. Jimenez-Velasco *et al.* reported that chimerism determination by RQ-PCR amplification of null alleles and indels constituted a useful tool for the follow-up of patients with acute leukemia after SCT, showing better results than those obtained with conventional PCR[368]. Formankova *et al.* showed that increasing MC in CML patients after bone marrow transplantation correlated with increasing signal of MRD[374]. Several studies showed that chimerism status is closely associated with disease progression and can be used as a prognostic parameter[364,372,375,376].

DNA PLOIDY

The ploidy can be evaluated by flow cytometry (DNA content per cell; Figure 2.5) or by conventional cytogenetics, which give concordance results in most cases. FISH centromeric probes for the chromosomes most frequently involved in aneuploidy can also be used. DNA ploidy bears prognostic implications in many solid and some hematopoietic tumors[377,378]. Although high-grade lymphomas are more often aneuploid than are low-grade lymphomas, there is no evidence that DNA ploidy is an independent prognostic factor in lymphomas. Blastoid MCL subtypes show a tendency to harbor chromosome numbers in the tetraploid range (36% of lymphoblastoid and 80% of pleomorphic types vs. 8% of common variants, a feature clearly separating

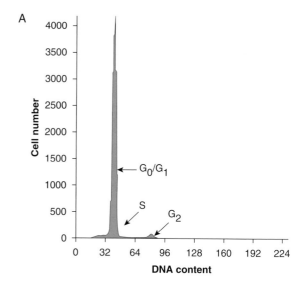

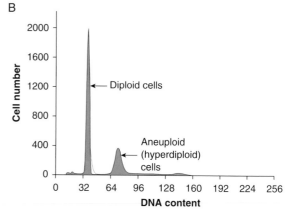

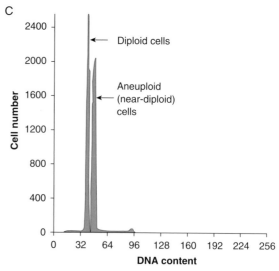

Figure 2.5 DNA ploidy. A, diploid population; B–C, aneuploid cells (B, hyperdiploid, C, near diploid)

these neoplasms from other types of B-cell NHL and possibly being related to cyclin D1 overexpression[379].

Ploidy is an important parameter in both the biology and the clinical evolution of MM. Hypodiploidy in MM is associated with poor prognosis[380,381]. The majority of patients with hypodiploid MM display aberrations of chromosome 13[381,382]. Most recurrent 14q32 translocations occur in non-hyperdiploidy clones. Hypodiploidy and several monosomies (deletions 2, 3, 13, 14 and 19) are independent poor prognostic indicators in myeloma associated with shorter survival[380,381]. Over 50% of MM patients are aneuploid, almost all of them being hyperdiploid. Overall survival is significantly longer in hyperdiploid compared with diploid tumors[383]. The majority of patients with plasma cell leukemia, an aggressive form of plasma cell neoplasm, are diploid[384].

In cutaneous T-cell lymphoma, detection of aneuploid neoplastic T cells in peripheral blood samples of patients is associated with large cell transformation in skin, lymph node, or other tissues[385].

Ploidy is recognized as a prognostic factor in childhood ALL[386–389]. DNA hyperdiploidy (number of chromosomes > 50) confers the most favorable prognostic factor in childhood ALL[387,390–393]. Hypodiploidy (number of chromosomes below 46) and near-triploidy is associated with poor prognosis[394,395]. In the series reported by Zemanova et al., the presence of structural chromosomal rearrangements in a patient with hyperdiploid ALL indicated poor prognosis[396]. Patients with 45 chromosomes (near-diploidy) have a better prognosis than patients with hypodiploidy of fewer than 45 chromosomes[397,398]. Patients with near-haploidy (fewer than 30 chromosomes) have the poorest response to therapy.

In adult patients with ALL, hypodiploidy with fewer than 46 chromosomes confers a poor prognosis, whereas high hyperdiploidy (> 50 chromosomes) is associated with a favorable outcome[399,400]. Patients with hypodiploidy of 30–39 chromosomes are generally older than 40 years, are mainly men and have a common B-cell phenotype[401]. Hypodiploidy with 30–39 chromosomes is characterized by recurrent losses of chromosomes 2, 3, 4, 7, 12, 13, 15, 16 and 17, and the DNA content histograms display two aneuploidy peaks: the hypodiploid peak and the hyperdiploid peak[402]. No patients with near-triploidy have a standard triploidy (three copies of all chromosomes). Charrin et al. suggested that near-triploidy derives from the duplication of hypodiploidy with 30 to 39 chromosomes and that both aneuploidy groups (hypodiploidy with 30–39 chromosomes and near-triploidy) are two expressions of the same disease[402]. The prognosis of patients with hypodiploidy with 30–39 chromosomes and near-triploidy is poor, with median disease-free survival of 8 months and median survival of 10 months[402], which is comparable to patients with $t(9;22)^+$ ALL. The distinction of near-triploidy from hyperdiploidy with more than 50 chromosomes is important, since the latter group have a favorable outcome. DNA aneuploidy is less common in AML than in ALL. There are no data to support that the DNA index in AML is of prognostic value.

CHROMOSOMAL ABERRATIONS

Chromosomal aberrations include numerical and structural abnormalities (Figure 2.6). A cell with 46 chromosomes is called diploid, and a cell with an abnormal number of chromosomes is called aneuploid (< 46, hypodiploid; > 46, hyperdiploid). Monosomy refers to a single chromosome and trisomy to three chromosomes. The chromosomes that are most commonly lost (−) include −5, −7, −X and −Y and those most commonly duplicated (+, trisomy) include +4, +6, +8, +9, +10, +11, +12, +13, +14, +19, +20 and +21. Deletion (del) is a loss of a portion of a chromosome. Common chromosomal deletions include del(5q), del(6q), del(7q), del(13q) and del(20q). Isochromosome (i) is an abnormal chromosome with two chromosome arms positioned as mirror images of each other. The most common isochromosomes include i(1q), i(7q), i(9q), i(11q), i(17q), i(21q) and i(22q). A chromosomal inversion (inv) is a 180° rotation of a chromosome segment. The common inversions include inv(3) and inv(16). A chromosomal translocation (t) is a relocation

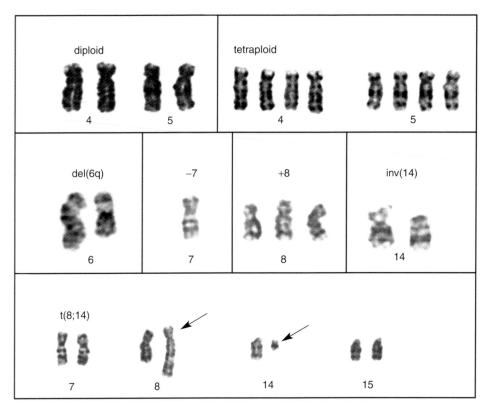

Figure 2.6 Examples of chromosomal abnormalities (see text for details)

of material from one chromosome to a different chromosome. Most translocations are reciprocal and result in either synthesis of a novel fusion protein or relocation of an oncogene to a locus that is highly transcribed. The common translocations include t(9;22), t(15;17), t(14;18) t(11;14), t(8;14) and t(8;21). Many chromosomal abnormalities have a significant influence on prognosis in hematopoietic malignancies. For example, AML patients with t(15;17), t(8;21) or inv(16) comprise the favorable risk group, whereas complex karyotype predicts an extremely poor prognosis (normal karyotype and other non-complex abnormalities comprise the inter-mediate group), isolated del(5q) in MDS is associ-ated with low risk of transformation into AML, hypodiploidy in childhood ALL is associated

with poor prognosis and presence of t(2;5) in T-cell lymphoma defines a subset of anaplastic large cell lymphoma associated with a good prognosis and chemosensitivity (details are presented in the following chapters devoted to specific hematologic malignancies).

del(5q)

The (5q)⁻ syndrome is a distinct category of MDS defined by less than 5% blasts, isolated deletion of the long arm of chromosome 5 (Figures 2.7 and 2.8) and low probability of transformation to AML[225,403]. The molecular mechanisms associated with del(5q) are still unknown. The (5q)⁻ syndrome occurs in elderly patients (median age 67 years), more often in women

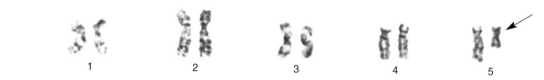

Figure 2.7   Deletion of the long arm of chromosome 5 [del(5q) syndrome]

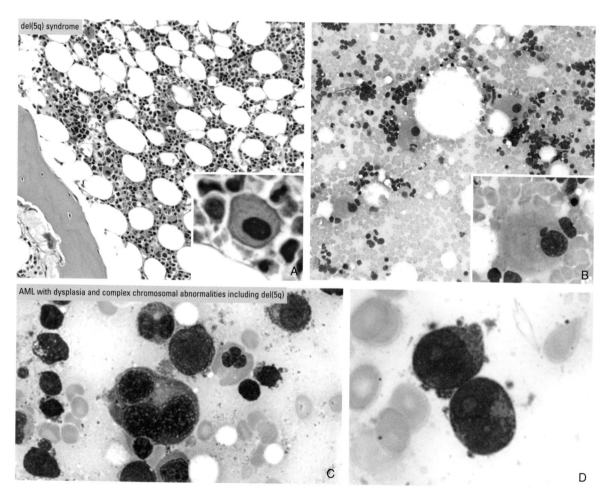

Figure 2.8   Myeloid stem cell disorders associated with del(5q). A–B, Myelodysplastic syndrome with isolated 5q deletion: histologic (A) and cytomorphologic (B) features with characteristic hypolobated micromegakaryocytes (*inset: high magnification*). C–D, Acute myeloid leukemia with dyspoiesis and complex chromosomal abnormalities including del(5q). C, prominent dyserythropoiesis; D, blasts with prominent nucleoli (C–D, aspirate smear, Wright–Giemsa)

than men, and is associated with macrocytic anemia with low reticulocyte counts and high erythropoietin levels[403]. The projected median survival of patients with isolated del(5q) is 107–146 months[403,404].

Deletions of 5q are not limited to (5q)⁻ syndrome. They are present in other types of MDS (both *de novo* and therapy-related) as well as AML. Monosomy 5/del(5q) and monosomy 7/del(7q) represent

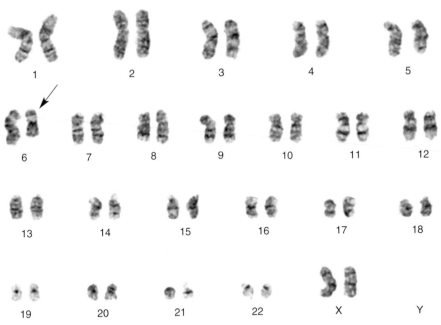

Figure 2.9 B-chronic lymphocytic leukemia/small lymphocytic lymphoma with deletion of the long arm of chromosome 6 (arrow)

the most common cytogenetic abnormalities in therapy-related MDS and AML (t-MDS/t-AML) and are strongly associated with prior exposure to alkylating agents[405]. AML with deletion of (5q) or monosomy 5 (−5) is associated with a very poor prognosis, similarly to AML with complex chromosomal abnormalities, monosomy 7 (−7) and t(9;22).

del(6q21)

Aberrations of the long arm of chromosome 6 (Figure 2.9) are among the most common chromosomal abnormalities in lymphoid neoplasms[406]. In patients with follicular lymphoma (FL), del(6q) has been identified as a negative prognostic factor[407]. In a series by Viardot et al. the loss of material on chromosomal bands 6q25–q27 was the strongest predictor of a shorter survival in FL patients, followed by elevated LDH, presence of more than one extranodal manifestation, and age greater than 60 years[408]. Stilgenbauer et al. did not observe an adverse prognostic impact of 6q deletion in B-CLL[409]. In a more recent report by Cuneo et al., B-CLL with del(6q) was

characterized by a high incidence of atypical morphology, classical immunophenotype with CD38 positivity and intermediate incidence of IgV_H somatic hypermutation[410]. Clinicobiological features and outcome showed that CLL with del(6q) should be allocated to an intermediate-risk category[410].

In cutaneous T-cell lymphomas, loss of 6q is associated with significantly shorter survival[411]. The del(6)(q21–q25) is a recurrent chromosomal abnormality in NK-cell lymphoma/leukemia, a highly aggressive process[412,413].

In pediatric acute lymphoblastic leukemia (ALL) cytogenetically detectable del(6q) is not associated with adverse risk[414]. In adult ALL 6% of cases have long arm deletion of chromosome 6 (6q)[415]. A T-cell phenotype was more frequently associated with del(6q) cases in general and particularly with cases presenting del(6q) as the isolated abnormality. Patients with ALL and del(6q) had a high complete remission rate (83%); however, they had a lower 18-month event-free survival (31% vs. 41%) and a higher relapse rate (70% vs. 37%) compared with patients without del(6q). Overall, del(6q), as an

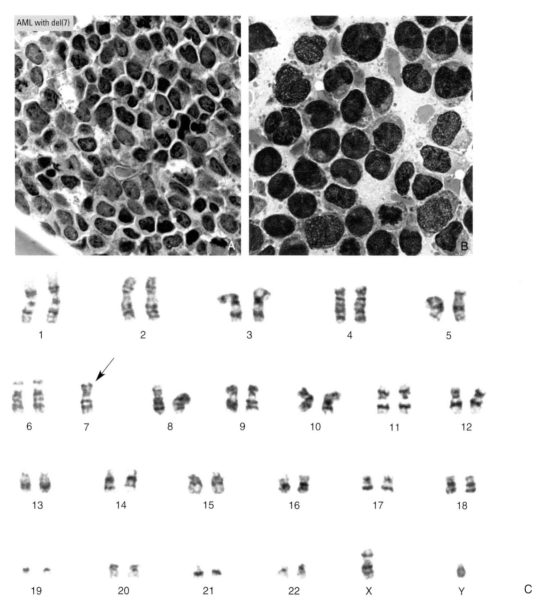

Figure 2.10 Deletion of chromosome 7 in acute myeloid leukemia. A, histology; B, cytology; C, monosomy 7 (arrow)

isolated change, identifies a subset of cases with hyperleukocytosis and a T-cell phenotype and seems to be associated with an unfavorable clinical outcome[415].

del(7q32)

Loss of chromosomal material due to deletion of the long arm of chromosome 7 [del(7q)], or loss of one homolog (−7), is a common finding in all types of myeloid disorder (Figure 2.10), especially in patients with AML and MDS, and is invariably associated with a worse response to treatment and a poor prognosis[416–419]. Primary MDS occurring in adults under 50 years often display abnormalities involving chromosome 7 (31%) and almost half of the patients progressed to AML with an overall median time to progression of 2 months (range 3 weeks to 3 years)[228]. Monosomy 7/del(7q), and, similarly, monosomy 5/del(5q), represent the most common cytogenetic abnormalities in therapy-related MDS and AML and are strongly associated with exposure to alkylating agents.

Monosomy 7 is also reported in myeloid proliferations in children[420] (monosomy 7 being the most common cytogenetic abnormality in pediatric MDS[421]). Pediatric AML, MDS and other myeloproliferations associated with monosomy 7 have a poor prognosis[422]. Children with AML and monosomy 7 have poor disease-free survival when treated by conventional chemotherapy, immunosuppression or supportive measures[423,424]. Allogeneic stem cell transplantation improves outcomes in these patients[425].

del(9p)

The transcription factor CCAAT/enhancer binding protein alpha (CEBPα), encoded by *CEBPA*, is crucial for the differentiation of immature granulocytes. Mutation of *CEBPA* may play an important role in leukemogenesis and prognosis in patients with myeloid stem cell disorders. The overall prevalence of *CEBPA* loss-of-function mutations in AML cases with del(9q) in a non-complex karyotype is 41%, whereas none of the patients who had a del(9q) in a complex karyotype or together with t(8;21) demonstrated mutant *CEBPA*[426]. *CEBPA* mutations were reported exclusively in AML and mutated patients preferentially belonged to M1, M2 and M4 FAB subtypes[427]. In the absence of poor prognostic factors, patients with a *CEBPA* mutation had a favorable outcome, very similar to that of the t(8;21), inv(16) and t(15;17) subgroup[427]. *CEBPA* mutations play a role in a subset of patients with MDS, especially in chronic myelomonocytic leukemia (CMML). Mutations of the *CEBPA* gene, similarly to the internal tandem duplication and point mutations in the *FLT3* gene, partial tandem duplication of the *MLL* gene and overexpression of the *BAALC* gene, have been found to predict outcome in patients with AML and normal cytogenetics[428].

The del(9p) commonly occurs in ALL in children[429].

del(11q)

Translocations or deletions involving the 11q23 region have been observed in ALL, AML, MDS and B-CLL. The 11q deletions identify a new clinical subset of B-CLL characterized by younger age, extensive peripheral, abdominal and mediastinal lymphadenopathy, more advanced clinical stages, more rapid disease progression and a shorter treatment-free interval[430]. The prognostic effect of 11q deletion on survival strongly depended on age: in patients less than 55 years old, the median survival time was significantly shorter in the deletion group (64 months vs. 209 months), whereas in patients ≥55 years old there was no significant difference (94 months vs. 111 months)[430]. The cDNA array confirmed the prognostic impact of 11q23 deletion in B-CLL[431]. The 11q23 deletion is associated with a unique gene expression pattern involving cell signaling and apoptosis genes, including the overexpression of CDC2, a serine/threonine kinase. The 11q23 amplification led to *MLL* gene overexpression, providing evidence for an etiologic role for *MLL* gain of function in myeloid malignancies (*see MLL, below*).

del(13q) and monosomy 13

The 13q deletion occurs in different types of non-Hodgkin's lymphomas (NHL), e.g. B-CLL (Figure 2.11), MCL, a subset of high-grade lymphomas and plasma cell neoplasms[432]. Loss of 13q in cutaneous T-cell lymphomas is associated with significantly shorter survival[411].

In B-CLL, deletion of 13q is the most common abnormality (by FISH studies) followed by deletions of 11q, trisomy 12 and deletions of 17p[433]. The 13q deletions in B-CLL are associated with the longest (92 months) survival[434]. Coexistence of trisomy 12 and 13q14 deletion was found in 17.5% of patients[435]. In this group, del(13q14) was the prevalent clone, with percentages 25–35% higher than those observed for trisomy 12, suggesting clonal evolution[435].

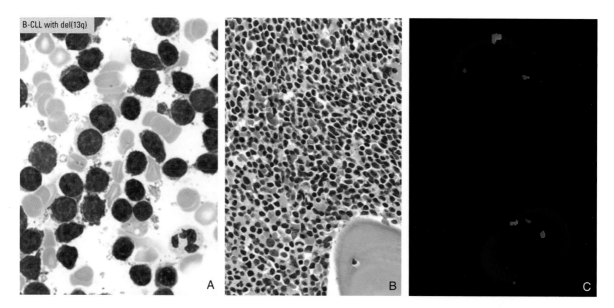

Figure 2.11 B-CLL with a deletion of the long arm of chromosome 13 at q14.3, including D13S19 (FISH). This abnormality is associated with a better prognosis in CLL patients. A, cytology; B, histology (bone marrow core biopsy); C, FISH

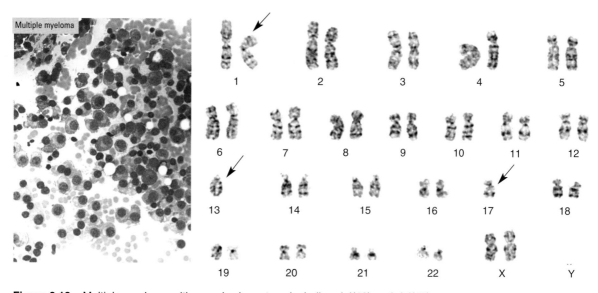

Figure 2.12 Multiple myeloma with complex karyotype including del(13) and del(17)

Monosomy 13 is one of the most frequent chromosomal abnormalities in MM (Figure 2.12)[436]. The complete or partial deletion of chromosome 13 or translocations involving 13q by conventional cytogenetics in MM is associated with a poor outcome, even with high-dose treatment and autologous stem cell transplantation[381,437–439]. The del(13q) is detected more frequently by FISH than by metaphase cytogenetics. The overall survival of patients with monosomy 13/del(13q) by cytogenetics (median 35.2 months) and del(13q) by FISH only (median 33.2 months) is not

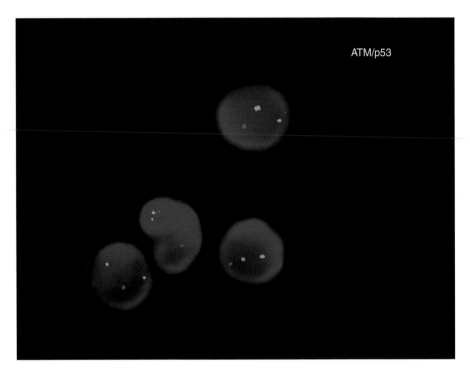

ATM/p53

Figure 2.13   Deletion of chromosome 17 (by FISH analysis)

significantly different and is shorter than in patients with diploid chromosome 13 by either technique[440]. The latter is associated with prolonged survival (65.6 months)[440].

del(17p)

Figure 2.13 presents the deletion of chromosome 17 by FISH analysis. Chromosome 17p is the site for *p53* (*TP53; see below*). Loss of the short arm of chromosome 17 is associated with a *p53* mutation on the remaining allele in several hematopoietic malignancies.

Deletion of 17p is associated with a poorer prognosis in many hematopoietic malignancies (Figure 2.14). The deletion of the short arm of chromosome 17 is usually associated with other chromosomal rearrangements[441]. MDS with del(17p) is associated with dysgranulopoiesis (pseudo-Pelger–Huët nuclei), small vacuoles in the cytoplasm of neutrophils and poor prognosis[442]. *p53* mutations are

found in the majority of patients with 17p deletion and MDS. Deletion of the short arm of chromosome 17 confers a poor prognosis in AML.

The del(17p) has an adverse clinical outcome in FL[443]. In B-CLL, 17p deletion is associated with lack of *Ig*V$_{H}$ mutations and poor prognosis[444]. Abnormal p53 predicts shorter survival, is more common in refractory B-CLL and correlates with an aggressive disease and transformation. B-CLL patients with del(17p) do not respond to rituximab[445]. Patients with MM with deletions of chromosome 17 (Figure 2.15) have a poor prognosis (in contrast, trisomy 17 is associated with prolonged survival in MM). Chromosome 17p13.1 deletions are frequent in MM involving the central nervous system.

del(20q)

Deletions of the long arm of chromosome 20, del(20q), occur in AML, MDS, chronic myeloproliferative disorders and occasional cases of

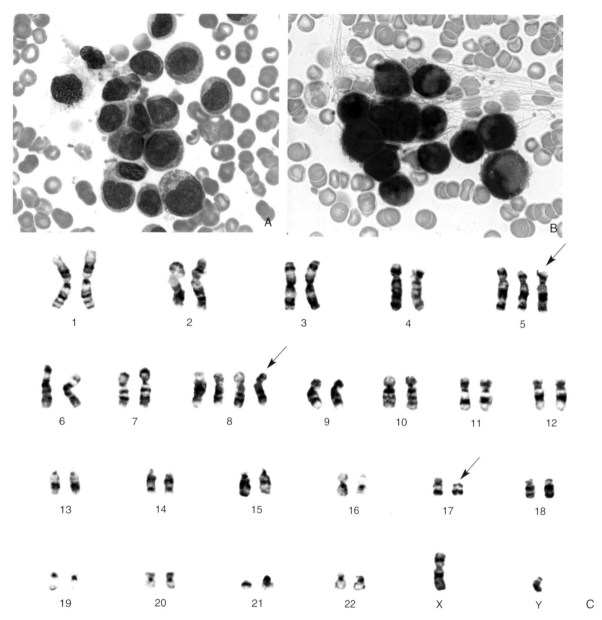

Figure 2.14 Acute monocytic leukemia (AML-M5) with complex chromosomal abnormalities (+5, +8, +8, del17p). A, aspirate smear with numerous monoblasts; B, positive cytochemical staining with NSE; C, routine cytogenetic analysis. Deletion of the short arm of chromosome 17 is associated with a poor prognosis in AML. Trisomy 5 and trisomy or tetrasomy 8 are often associated with monocytic differentiation of AML

angioimmunoblastic T-cell lymphoma. In a subset of patients, del(20q) is accompanied by other chromosomal abnormalities. Morphologically, myeloid disorders with del(20q) are characterized by prominent dyserythropoiesis and dysmegakaryopoiesis[446].

i(7q)

Isochromosome 7q is frequently found in hepatosplenic γδ T-cell lymphoma[447]. The prognosis of this lymphoma is poor, with median survival time of 16 months[447].

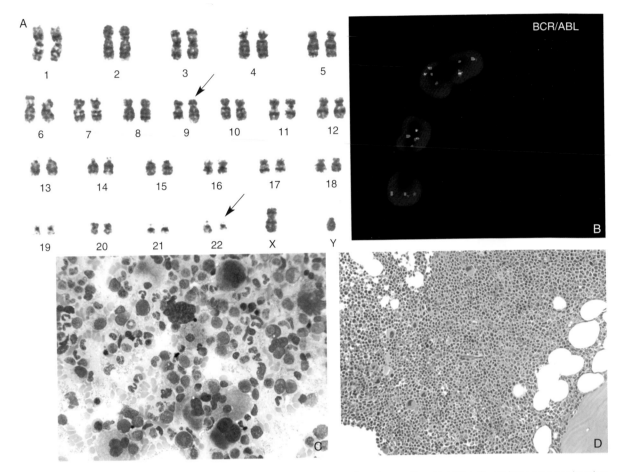

Figure 2.32   The t(9;22) translocation in chronic myeloid leukemia. A, cytogenetics; B, FISH; C, aspirate smear showing myeloid hyperplasia with leftward shift, blue-sea histiocytes and atypical megakaryocytes; D, histology (core biopsy) showing hypercellular marrow

observed in a subset of MM (3–14% by conventional cytogenetics)[502,503]. In MM (Figure 2.35), cyclin D1/Bcl-1 upregulation is detected more often than t(11;14)(q13;q32), suggesting that other chromosome 11 abnormalities, as well as additional mechanisms, must be responsible for the cyclin D1 overexpression. Panani *et al.* showed that t(11;14) had a worse impact on disease outcome as compared with t(14q32) with an unidentified partner chromosome[504]. Cyclin D1 expression is also frequently found in hairy cell leukemia (HCL), where it appears to be unrelated to translocations or amplification of the *cyclin D1/BCL1/CCND1* gene[505].

t(11;17)

The t(11;17)(q23;q21) is present in a subset of patients with APL. This translocation results in fusion of the *RARα* gene (17q21) with the *PLZF* gene (11q23). t(11;17)/*PLZF–RARα* APL differs from classic APL with t(15;17) by its poor response to chemotherapy, resistance to ATRA and poorer prognosis when treated with ATRA alone[506,507]. Patients treated with combination chemotherapy can achieve a complete remission, however[508]. Another translocation of the *RARα* gene involves the *STAT5b* gene on chromosome 17q11 and the *NuMa* gene on chromosome

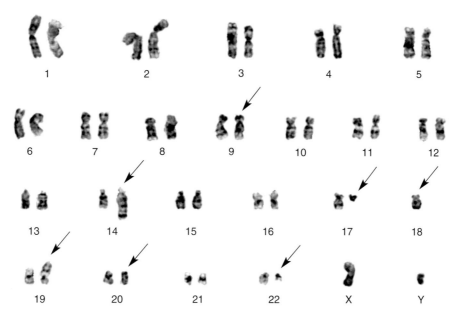

Figure 2.33 Acute lymphoblastic leukemia with complex chromosomal abnormalities, including t(9;22)

11q13. APL with either t(11;17)(q13;q21)/ *NuMA–RARα* and t(17;17)(q11;q21)/*STAT5b–RARα* present with morphologic and clinical features similar to classic type [t(15;17)].

t(11;18)(q21;q21)

The t(11;18)(q21;q21) resulting in the *API2–MALT1* fusion transcript is an exclusive finding in extranodal marginal zone B-cell lymphoma of the MALT type[509]. Within the gastrointestinal tract, extranodal MALT lymphoma occurs most often in the stomach and rarely in the small and large intestine and esophagus. Gastric MALT lymphoma is associated with *Helicobacter pylori* infection. Apart from t(11;18)(q21;q21), other chromosomal aberrations in MALT lymphoma include t(1;14)(p22;q32), t(14;18)(q32;q21), trisomies 3, 12 and 18; *p53* loss of heterozygosity (LOH)/mutation and *fas* gene mutation. The cases with t(11;18) usually do not show other genetic aberrations[510]. Gastric MALT lymphomas positive for t(11;18) (approximately 30% of cases) are more often associated with

involvement of the lymph node and distal sites than t(11;18)-negative cases[467]. The presence of the t(11;18) translocation is a negative predictor for gastric MALT lymphoma to respond to *Helicobacter pylori* eradication therapy[511]. Gastric MALT with the t(11;18)(q21;q21), however, does not adversely affect the response of gastric MALT lymphoma to chemotherapy with cladribine (2CdA)[512]. This makes cladribine an attractive agent for treatment of gastric MALT lymphoma unresponsive to *Helicobacter pylori* eradication. (*See also: API2–MALT1* fusion gene, Chapter 3; below.)

t(11;19)(q23;p13.1)

Patients with AML and t(11;19)(q23;p13.1) and associated abnormalities of chromosome 11q23 have an intermediate survival[225].

t(12;12)

The t(12;21)(p13;q22) is a cryptic abnormality observed in 25% of children with B-lineage ALL,

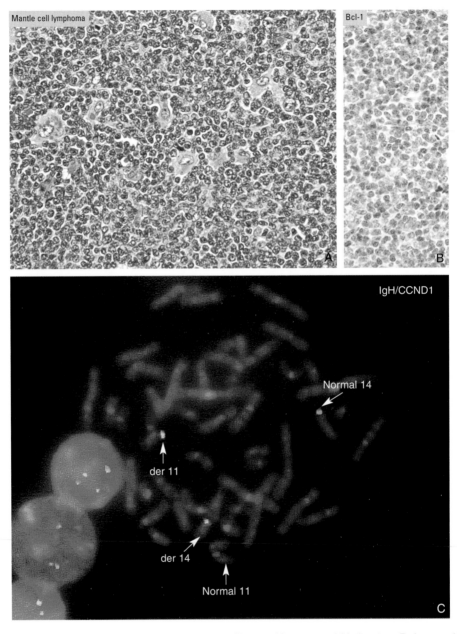

Figure 2.34   Mantle cell lymphoma. A, diffuse lymphoid infiltrate with scattered histiocytes; B, immunohistochemical staining for cyclin D1 (Bcl-1); C, t(11;14) by FISH analysis

and is associated with a favorable prognosis. The t(12;21) in most cases is not associated with hyperdiploidy or with the t(1;19), t(4;11) or t(9;22) ALL[513].

t(12;21)

The t(12;21)(p12;q22) is commonly found in pediatric ALL[429]. This translocation generates the

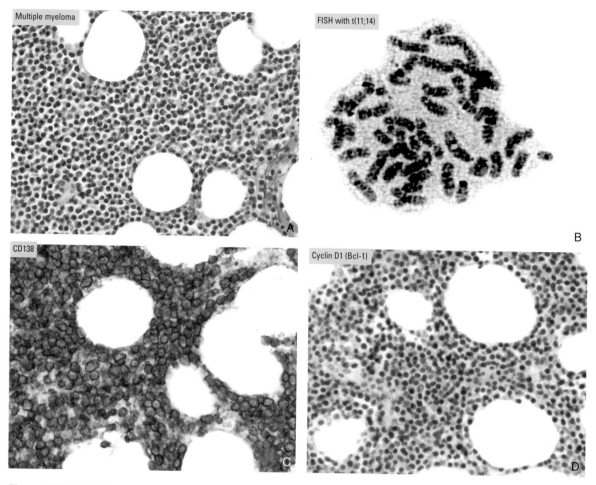

Figure 2.35 Multiple myeloma, bone marrow. A, histology section shows diffuse plasma cell infiltrate in the bone marrow; B, t(11;14) by FISH analysis (yellow dots); C–D, immunohistochemistry shows expression of CD138 (C) and cyclin D1/Bcl-1 (D) by plasma cells

TEL–AML1 (RUNX1) chimeric gene. TEL–AML1–(RUNX1)-positive ALL has a favorable prognosis.

t(14;18)(q32;q21)

The t(14;18)(q32;q21) is characteristic of FL (Figure 2.36), but overexpression of Bcl-2 is also observed in other lymphomas, including B-CLL and MALT lymphoma. Translocation involving *BCL2* at 18q21 is rare in B-CLL.

In FL breakpoints of t(14;18) occur in the major breakpoint region (mbr) or in the minor cluster region (mcr) at the 3′ end of *BCL2* and bring *BCL2* at 18q21 into the Ig heavy chain locus.

The same breakpoint on chromosome 18, involving the *MALT1* gene (not the *BCL2* gene) is seen in marginal zone lymphomas of the MALT type. In MALT lymphomas with t(14;18) there appears to be interaction between the *MALT1* gene and the *BCL10* gene. Both genes and their products can be detected by FISH and/or immunohistochemistry. The t(14;18)/*IgH–MALT1* cases typically involve ocular adnexae and lung and are not reported in the gastric location.

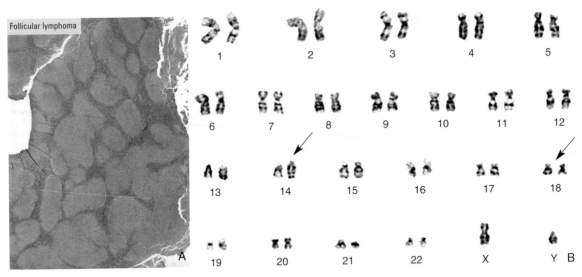

Figure 2.36 Follicular lymphoma with t(14;18). A, histologic section with typical nodular architecture; B, classic cytogenetics with t(14;18) (arrows)

t(15;17)

The reciprocal translocation t(15;17)(q22;q21) is the diagnostic hallmark of APL (AML-M3; Figure 2.37)[506]. The t(15;17) translocation creates two chimeric genes: the *PML–RARα* gene is formed on the derivative 15, whereas the reciprocal *RARα–PML* fusion is located on the derivative 17. The PML gene product possesses growth suppressor and proapoptotic activity[514,515]. RARα is a transcription factor that mediates the effect of retinoic acid. The *PML–RARα* plays an important role in leukemogenesis by impairing the growth suppressor and proapoptotic activities of *PML*. It is also important in mediating the differentiation response to ATRA treatment[506,516,517]. The introduction of novel targeted therapies in the form of ATRA and arsenic trioxide has changed the clinical course of APL over the past 25 years from one that was fatal for the majority of patients to one that represents one of the most curable subtypes of AML. Reciprocal translocation of 17q21 is found in more than 95% of cases of APL. The remaining APL cases show complex or variant translocations involving chromosomes 15 or 17 and other chromosomes as well as masked

insertions. To date, five different fusion partners of *RARα* have been identified. The vast majority of cases are characterized by the presence of the t(15;17)(q22;q12–21), which involves the *PML* gene. The other chromosomal aberrations include t(11;17)(q23;q21), t(5;17) (q35;q12–21), t(11;17) (q13;q21) and der(17). APL associated with t(15;17), t(5;17) and t(11;17)(q13;q21) (which involves the *NPM* and *NuMA* genes, respectively) appears to be sensitive to ATRA. In contrast, APL associated with t(11;17)(q23;q21) leading to *PLZF/RARα* rearrangement is typified by a lack of differentiation response to retinoids, and patients treated with ATRA alone have a poor prognosis[507]. In *PML/RARα*-positive APL about 70% of patients are expected to be cured with a combination of ATRA and anthracycline-based chemotherapy. Additional chemotherapy at the time of molecular relapse improves survival of patients compared with those whose treatment is delayed at the point of hematological relapse. Quantitative RT-PCR technology is expected to improve the predictive value of MRD monitoring and therefore to guide therapy in order to reduce the rate of relapses and to increase rates of cure in high-risk patients[517].

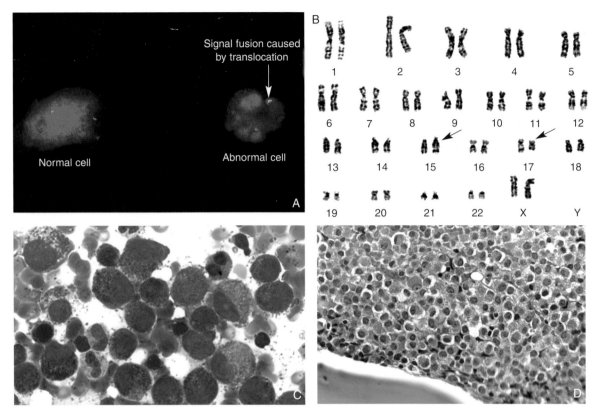

Figure 2.37 Acute promyelocytic leukemia. A, FISH analysis showing fusion resulting from t(15;17) translocation; B, standard cytogenetics with t(15;17); C, aspirate smear showing hypergranular promyelocytes; D, histology with replacement of the normal marrow elements by atypical promyelocytes

Additional chromosomal changes have been reported in 25–40% of APL[455]. The prognostic significance of chromosomal abnormalities in addition to t(15;17) in APL is uncertain. De Botton *et al.* reported a lack of prognostic significance of secondary chromosomal changes in APL patients treated with ATRA and chemotherapy[455].

GENETIC MARKERS

For *AML1*, *see ETO* and *RUNX1*, *below*. The *AML1* gene is now termed the *RUNX1* gene.

API2–MALT1

The t(11;18)(q21;q21) is a characteristic chromosomal translocation in extranodal marginal zone B-cell lymphoma (mucosa-associated lymphoid tissue (MALT) lymphoma). The t(11;18) translocation results in fusion between *API2* (also known as c-*IAP2*) on 11q21 (a member of the *IAP* family with caspase-inhibitory functions) and *MALT1* on 18q21, encoding the paracaspase. The API2–MALT1 fusion protein has been shown to enforce activation of NF-κB signaling and increase inhibition of apoptosis[283], partially by neutralizing apoptosis promoted by Smac[285]. There also appears to be interaction of some of the product of *API2–MALT1* fusion and *BCL10*, involving NF-κB-mediated inhibition of apoptosis, and hence promotion of MALT lymphomas[464,465]. Figure 2.38 presents typical morphologic features of MALT lymphoma.

ATM

The *ATM* gene (ataxia telangiectasia mutated) located on chromosome 11q22-23 participates in activation

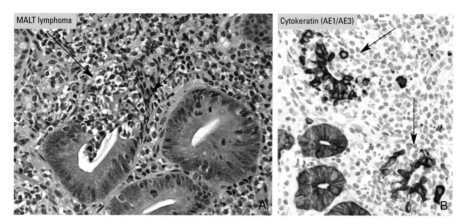

Figure 2.38   Gastric marginal zone lymphoma (MALT type). A, histology section with atypical lymphoid infiltrate and lymphoepithelial lesions (arrows); B, the lymphoepithelial lesions easily visualized with cytokeratin staining

of *p53* (*TP53*) after DNA damage. The *ATM* gene encodes a large protein that belongs to a family of kinases that function in DNA repair and cell cycle checkpoint control (mainly intra-S phase) following DNA damage. The *ATM*/*p53*-dependent DNA damage response pathway plays an important role in the progression of lymphoid tumors. Frequent inactivating mutations of the *ATM* gene have been reported in patients with rare sporadic T-cell prolymphocytic leukemia (T-PLL), B-CLL and MCL. Inactivation of the *ATM* or *p53* gene in B-CLL leads to aggressive disease[336]. The *p53* dysfunction in B-CLL can occur in the absence of the *p53* mutation and that dysfunction is associated with mutation of the gene encoding ATM, a kinase implicated in *p53* activation[518,519]. B-CLL patients with *ATM* deficiency have significantly shorter survival times (35 vs. 97 months) and more aggressive disease, suggesting that *ATM* is involved in the leukemogenesis of B-CLL[336,520,521]. In occasional patients, the deletions of *ATM* can extend to the *MLL* gene locus. *ATM* gene mutations do not play a pivotal role either in the pathogenesis of FL or in its transformation to DLBCL[522].

BCL1/cyclin D1 (CCND1)

The *BCL1* locus (major genomic breakpoint cluster region designated as *BCL1* for *B*-cell lymphoma/leukemia 1) on chromosome 11 (including the *CCND1* gene coding for cyclin D1) is activated by its juxtaposition near the enhancer region of the Ig heavy chain locus on chromosome 14. This phenomenon is caused by the t(11;14)(q13;q32) translocation, and occurs in MCL. The *CCND1* transcript or its encoded protein (cyclin D1/Bcl-1) can be detected by PCR, cytogenetics/FISH (Figure 2.39) or immunohistochemical staining. Cyclin D1 forms a complex with cell cycle-dependent kinase (CDK) 4 (and CDK6), which inactivates the retinoblastoma protein (pRb) via phosphorylation. Cyclin D1 (previously PRAD1) is overexpressed in MCL and only rarely in other hematopoietic malignancies.

All cases of MCL (both typical and blastoid) contain t(11;14)(q13;q32). Other hematopoietic tumors with this translocation include MM. Hairy cell leukemia rarely may express cyclin D1/Bcl-1 at mRNA or protein level, but the levels of expression are lower than in MCL and the expression is not associated with t(11;14), *BCL1* rearrangements or *CCND1* gene amplification. Cyclin D1 expression is also found in MM patients and is associated either with a t(11;14)(q13;q32) or extra copies of chromosome 11. Myeloma patients with the t(11;14) or trisomy 11 significantly overexpressed cyclin D1 in comparison with patients without 11q abnormalities, who have cyclin D1 mRNA levels similar to those of healthy donors.

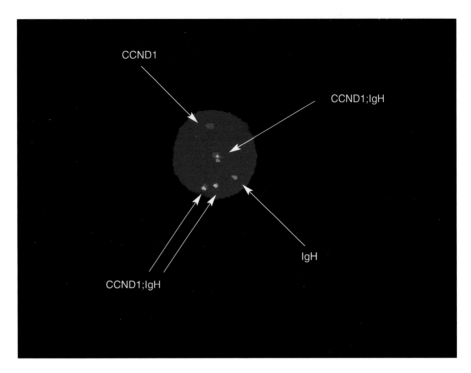

Figure 2.39   CCND1/IgH fusion as a result of t(11;14)(q13;q32.3) in multiple myeloma (FISH analysis)

Cyclin D1 overexpression is closely associated with 11q abnormalities and identifies a subset of MM patients who are more likely to have prolonged duration of remission and event-free survival following autologous transplantation[523]. Most authors have reported no significant difference regarding overall survival between cyclin D1+ and cyclin D1− patients[524,525]. In the series by Hoechtlen-Vollmar *et al.*, however, the amplification of the *CCND1* gene in MM was a significantly unfavorable parameter with regard to overall survival and progression-free survival by univariate analysis[526]. In multivariate analysis, cyclin D1 amplification and serum β_2-microglobulin were independent and well-suited parameters for predicting survival[526]. The relatively high frequency of cyclin D1 expression, compared with the chromosome 11 abnormalities, suggests that upregulation of cyclin D1 protein might be the result of other mechanisms as well[527,528]. *De novo* CD5+ DLBCL do not express cyclin D1/Bcl-1.

BCL2

The *BCL2* family of proto-oncogenes is a critical regulator of apoptosis whose expression frequently becomes altered in human cancers, including some of the most common types of lymphomas and leukemias[529]. The *BCL2* gene encodes a 26-kDa protein that inhibits apoptosis through the mitochondrial pathway (*see* Apoptosis, above). Apart from Bcl-2, antiapoptotic proteins include Bcl-X$_L$ and Mcl-1, and proapoptotic proteins include BAX, Bak, Bcl-X$_S$, Bid and Bik. The *BCL2* gene was originally discovered in FL (Figure 2.40) with t(14;18)(q32;q21) translocation[279]. The t(14;18) translocation places *BCL2* under the control of the immunoglobulin heavy chain (*IgH*) Eµ enhancer, which induces production of high levels of Bcl-2 protein. Bcl-2 can easily be detected by routine immunohistochemistry. The Bcl-2 protein is located in the mitochondrial inner membrane, where it functions as a major negative regulator of apoptosis. Bcl-2 is widely expressed in normal lymphoid tissues, but is absent in germinal center B cells. Overexpression of Bcl-2 due to the t(14;18) represents an example of oncogenesis mediated by decreased cell death. Bcl-2 expression has been detected frequently in aggressive NHL, regardless of t(14;18), and is associated with an unfavorable prognosis[257,272,530,531]. *BCL2* gene amplification is another important mechanism for Bcl-2 protein overexpression in DLBCL[274,532,533].

High Bcl-2 expression is more frequent in B-cell NHL (51%) than in T-cell NHL (17%) and is heterogeneously distributed among the different histological subtypes[257]. DLBCL display Bcl-2 expression in 30–60% of cases, more frequently in nodal than in extranodal tumors[532,534–536]. Bcl-2+ DLBCL with t(14;18) probably represent a progression from FL. In DLBCL, Bcl-2 protein-positive cases significantly outnumber cases with t(14;18), suggesting that mechanisms other than translocation are operative in DLBCL[272]. Alternative mechanisms for Bcl-2 protein expression include, among others, increased *BCL2* copy number (e.g. 18q+), or transcriptional deregulation by NFκB[327]. The presence of a *BCL2* translocation at diagnosis has no impact on prognosis in patients with DLBCL[272,537,538], but the Bcl-2 protein expression (>50% positive tumor cells) is associated with decreased disease-free or overall survival[272,531,538–541]. Cases with t(14;18) and additional chromosomal aberrations have a worse prognosis than DLBCL with t(14;18) only. Hermine *et al.* reported the independent effect of Bcl-2 protein expression to be predictive of poor disease-free survival, in agreement with the role of Bcl-2 in chemotherapy-induced apoptosis[257]. Multivariate analysis confirmed the significant benefit for survival and event-free survival when rituximab was added to the standard chemotherapy regimen in Bcl-2+ DLBCL, suggesting that rituximab is able to prevent chemotherapy failure in patients with Bcl-2 protein overexpression[5]. Maartense *et al.* reported a difference in the impact of Bcl-2 overexpression on prognosis between elderly patients (>65 years) and younger patients (<65 years) with DLBCL; a negative prognostic value of overexpression of Bcl-2 and *p*53 is not of concern for patients older than 65 years[542]. Some FL do not express Bcl-2, suggesting inhibition of apoptosis due to other factors (e.g. Bcl-X$_L$) rather than Bcl-2 overexpression[543].

Bcl-2 family proteins are expressed in a subset of peripheral T-cell lymphomas, and the level of expression correlates with some histologic types, apoptotic rate and proliferation[544]. In anaplastic large cell lymphoma (ALCL) Bcl-2 and ALK expression are mutually exclusive[545]. ALK+ ALCL are sensitive to chemotherapy, therefore it is suggested that Bcl-2 expression may be associated with chemoresistance. In systemic ALCL the expression of apoptosis-regulating proteins, Bcl-2 and *p*19, and activation of caspase 3 are strongly related to ALK status[287]. Ten Berge *et al.* suggested that the difference in clinical outcome between ALK+ and ALK− cases may be due to differences in levels of apoptosis inhibition[287]. A high number of Bcl-2+ tumor cells in ALCL carries an unfavorable prognosis.

Bcl-2 is expressed in about 60% of cases of classical Hodgkin's lymphoma (HL), more often in the nodular sclerosis type than in the mixed cellularity type[546]. Although simultaneous expression of Bcl-2, Mcl-1 and LMP-1 in classical HL was reported to correlate with an excellent survival[547], the expression of Bcl-2 in patients with HL treated with doxorubicin, bleomycin, vinblastine and dacarbazine is associated with inferior failure-free survival and overall survival[546].

Among AML, the percentage of Bcl-2+ cells is higher in M4 and M5 types, according to FAB classification, and in cases with high white blood cell counts[258]. High expression of Bcl-2 is associated with a low complete remission rate after intensive chemotherapy (29% in cases with ≥20% positive cells vs. 85% in cases with <20% positive cells) and with a significantly shorter survival. In multivariate analysis, the percentage of Bcl-2+ cells, age, and the percentage of CD34+ cells are independently associated with poor survival in AML patients[258].

Increased Bcl-2 expression in childhood ALL is inversely related to the presence of chromosomal translocations. However, it does not reflect increased disease aggressiveness or resistance to chemotherapy[548].

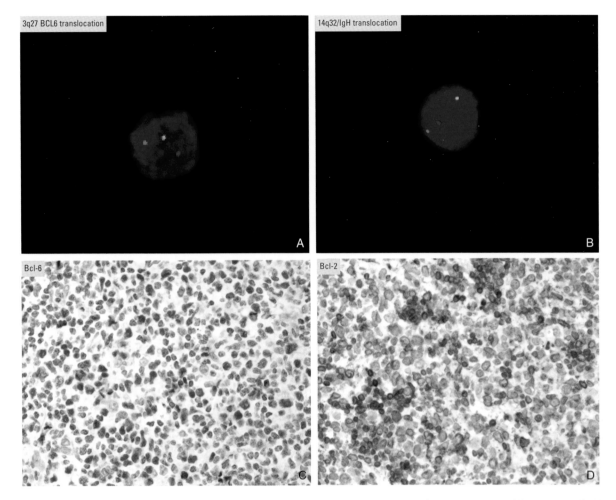

Figure 2.40   Follicular lymphoma with *BCL2* and *BCL6* expression due to 3q27/BCL6 translocation (A) and 14q32/IgH translocation (B); A–B, FISH analysis; C–D, immunohistochemistry

BCL6

BCL6 (on 3q27) is a proto-oncogene involved in cell cycle control, lymphocyte differentiation and immunologic response. It encodes a transcription protein, with a POZ/zinc finger motif that is required for germinal center formation, antibody-affinity maturation, and T-helper-2-mediated responses[549]. The 3q27 can be translocated to a number of alternative chromosomes, but most commonly include immunoglobulin heavy (14q32) and light chain (2p12;22q11) loci. *BCL6* gene rearrangement is more common than the occurrence of 3q27 translocations, suggesting

alternative ways of gene rearrangement. *BCL6* represses genes involved in lymphocyte activation and differentiation, in cell cycle control and inflammation[549,550]. Bcl-6 protein is selectively expressed by germinal center B cells in normal lymphoid tissues. In lymphomas, *BCL6* is expressed in those tumors arising from follicular center cells, including FL (approximately 100%; Figure 2.40), Burkitt's lymphoma (100%), the majority of DLBCL (>80%) and nodular lymphocyte-predominant HL (>80%)[551–554]. Biological consequences of Bcl-6 expression in DLBCL might vary according to the presence or absence and the nature of the underlying alteration of the *BCL6* gene (the partner involved in the translocation)[555]. Mutations within the 5′ non-coding domain of the BCL6 gene occur frequently in germinal center and post-germinal center lymphomas, including DLBCL, FL and Burkitt's lymphoma and can contribute to the deregulation of BCL6 expression[549,555]. The altered expression of BCL6 represses genes involved in apoptosis. The BCL6 proto-oncogene suppresses the expression of the p53 (TP53) tumor suppressor gene (by binding two specific DNA sites within the p53 promoter region) and modulates DNA damage-induced apoptotic responses in germinal center B-cells[556].

Most studies show a favorable prognostic impact of a high level of BCL6 expression (either by RT-PCR or immunohistochemistry). BCL6 rearrangement has been described as an independent factor of favorable clinical outcome in DLBCL[557]. Also, high BCL6 mRNA expression appears to be a favorable prognostic factor in DLBCL[558]. As mentioned above, the predictive value of BCL6 translocation on survival depends on the partner in BCL6 translocation. Non-Ig/BCL6 translocations are an indicator of poor prognosis in DLBCL when compared with translocations involving immunoglobulin genes[559]. Colomo et al. showed lack of correlation between the immunophenotyping profile of DLBCL (germinal center-CD10+/Bcl-6+/MUM1−/CD138−; germinal center-CD10−/Bcl-6+/MUM1−/CD138−; post-germinal center-CD10−/Bcl-6+/−/MUM1+/CD138− and plasmablastic-CD10−/Bcl-6/MUM1+/CD138+) and clinical outcome[541]. Through the use of gene expression profiling, DLBCLs have been recently subdivided into three distinct categories: germinal center B-cell-like (GCB), activated B-cell-like (ABC) and type 3 DLBCL[199,325,326]. DLBCLs with the GCB profile express genes restricted to the germinal center such as BCL6, whereas DLBCLs with the ABC profile express plasma cell genes such as XBP1, IL4, IRF and caspase 8[326]. GCB-type lymphomas are positive for CD10 and/or Bcl-6, and are negative for post-germinal center cell markers typical of plasma cells, such as MUM1 or CD138. Patients

with GCB DLBCL had a significantly better overall survival than those with ABC DLBCL[199]. Based on a central role of BCL6 in the pathogenesis of DLBCL, Melnick et al. predicts that targeting BCL6 transcriptional repression complexes in malignant B cells may constitute a novel form of transcription therapy for lymphomas and possibly other tumors[560,561].

Although BCL6 translocation is not necessary for large cell transformation of FL, the translocation may constitute a subgroup with a higher risk of transformation into aggressive lymphoma[562]. Mutations of the BCL6 gene are also observed in a subset of B-CLL, typically in cases harboring mutated IgV_H[563]. In B-CLL, BCL6 mutations did not appear to correlate with prognosis in the series by Sahota et al.[564]. However, in a study reported by Sarsotti et al., coexistence of IgV_H and BCL6 mutations was correlated with a shorter treatment-free interval compared to cases harboring only the IgV_H mutation (median, 55 months vs. not reached), resembling the clinical course of unmutated IgV_H cases (median treatment-free interval, 44 months), indicating that BCL6 mutations identify a subgroup of Binet stage A B-CLL patients with a high risk of progression despite the presence of the mutated IgV_H gene[563]. As expected, in the same series, deletions of 17p13 (p53 locus) and 11q22 (ATM locus) were observed in cases with unmutated IgV_H[563].

BCL10

At least three distinct chromosomal translocations, t(11;18)(q21;q21), t(1;14)(p22;q32) and t(14;18)(q32;q21), involving API2 (also known as c-IAP2), BCL10 and MALT1, have been implicated in the molecular pathogenesis of MALT lymphoma. The t(11;18)(q21;q21) fuses the N-terminus of the API2 gene to the C-terminus of the MALT1 gene and generates a functional API2–MALT1 product. The t(1;14)(p22;q32) and t(14;18)(q32;q21) bring the BCL10 and MALT1 genes respectively to the IgH locus and deregulate their expression. In normal

B-cell follicles, both *MALT1* and *BCL10* are expressed predominantly in the cytoplasm of centroblasts (high expression), centrocytes (moderate) and B-cell of mantle zone (weak). In MALT lymphoma, *MALT1* and *BCL10* expression varied among cases with different chromosomal translocations. In MALT lymphomas with t(14;18)(q32;q21), tumor cells showed strong homogeneous cytoplasmic expression of both *MALT1* and *BCL10*. In cases with evidence of t(1;14)(p22;q32) or variants, tumor cells expressed *MALT1* weakly in the cytoplasm but *BCL10* strongly in the nuclei. In all MALT lymphomas with t(11;18)(q21;q21), tumor cells expressed weak cytoplasmic *MALT1* and moderate nuclear *BCL10*[565]. The *BCL10* gene encodes an N-terminal caspase recruitment domain (CARD) – an NF-κB-activating protein. The *BCL10* mutation may play a pathogenic role in B-cell MALT lymphoma development, particularly in aggressive and antibiotic unresponsive tumors.

BCR–ABL

See t(9;22), above.

BCRP

Breast cancer resistance protein (*BCRP*) expression in AML is associated with poor clinical outcome. The expression of the *BCRP* gene reduces the response to chemotherapy in AML, and *BCRP* expression is higher at the time of relapse[345].

ETO

RUNX1–ETO is generated by the t(8;21) translocation found in approximately 10–15% of AML. Those AMLs usually represent FAB M2 morphology, often express CD19 and CD56 and are characterized by good response to chemotherapy and high remission rate. AML with t(8;21) belongs to a good prognostic group, similarly to those associated with t(15;17)/APL and inv(16). The ETO gene (*for* eight twenty-one) is a transcription factor at chromosome 8q22, and *RUNX1–ETO* fusion acts as an inhibitor of transcription involving core-binding factor DNA-binding sites. The *ETO* is a co-repressor that links the transcriptional pathogenesis of acute leukemias and B-cell lymphomas and offers a compelling target for transcriptional therapy of hematologic malignancies[566,567].

Fibronectin 1 (*FN-1*)

Fibronectin-1, an extracellular glycoprotein, is a ligand for the integrin family of cell-adhesion receptors that regulate cytoskeletal organization. The presence of the *FN-1* gene in DLBCL was reported to be associated with a better prognosis[568].

FLT3 (13q12)

FMS-like tyrosine kinase 3 (Flt3) is a member of the class 3 receptor tyrosine kinase family that is preferentially expressed on hematopoietic progenitor cells and mediates stem cell differentiation and proliferation. *FLT3* is expressed at high levels in 70–100% of AML and in a high percentage of ALL, and is almost universally expressed in childhood B-ALL[569–574]. Mutations of *FLT3* have been detected in about 30% of patients with AML and a small number of patients with ALL or MDS[575]. Cases of B-ALL with *MLL* gene rearrangements and those with high hyperdiploidy (>50 chromosomes) express the highest level of *FLT3*, with activating mutations of *FLT3* in 18% of *MLL*-rearranged and 28% of hyperdiploid cases[574]. The *FLT3* inhibitor CEP-701 selectively induces apoptosis *in vitro* in leukemic cells expressing high levels of *FLT3*[574]. In AML, there is a statistically significant coincidence of invaginated nuclear morphology, loss of HLA-DR and presence of the *FLT3* internal tandem duplication (ITD), suggesting that AML with these three features may represent a distinct AML subset[576]. Two types of activating *FLT3* mutations have been described in AML: small ITD (20% of AML) and mutations in the critical

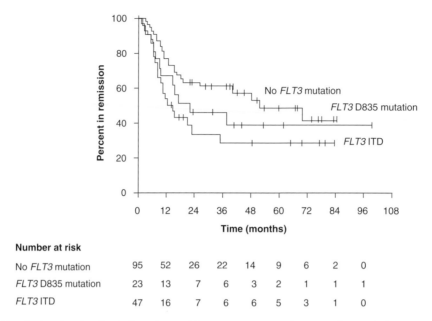

Number at risk									
No *FLT3* mutation	95	52	26	22	14	9	6	2	0
FLT3 D835 mutation	23	13	7	6	3	2	1	1	1
FLT3 ITD	47	16	7	6	6	5	3	1	0

Figure 2.41   Remission duration for AML patients with normal cytogenetics according to *FLT3* mutation status

From: Frohling S, *et al.* Prognostic significance of activating *FLT3* mutation in younger adults (16 to 60 years) with acute myeloid leukemia and normal cytogenetic. Blood 2002;100:4372–80. © 2002 by The American Society of Hematology, used with permission

Asp835 residue in the activation loop of *FLT3*. *FLT3* mutations are indicative of a poor prognosis, independent of other risk parameters. Patients with *FLT3* mutations (especially ITD) have significantly shorter overall survival (Figures 2.41 and 2.42) when compared with patients without mutations of *FLT3*[120]. The 5-year event-free survival rate for patients with an *FLT3*/ITD was 14%, significantly lower than that for patients without mutations (69%)[577]. Chillon *et al.* confirmed a high frequency of *FLT3* mutations in APL and in adult AML without recurrent cytogenetic translocations; *FLT3* was never altered in patients with inv(16), t(8;21) or 11q23 abnormalities[578]. In the same series, the *FLT3* mutations were associated with some negative prognostic features at diagnosis (leukocytosis, high blast cell percentage and elevated LDH values), but were not found to be an independent prognostic factor[578]. In a study by Schnittger *et al.*, patients with *FLT3* length mutations had a significantly shorter event-free survival (7.4 vs. 12.6

months) because of a higher relapse rate, but overall survival for patients with or without *FLT3* length mutations was similar[319]. Overexpression of *FLT3* ($> 2 \times 10^5$ copies/μg RNA) is an unfavorable prognostic factor for overall survival in AML without *FLT3*/ITD[579]. A high mutant/wild-type *FLT3* ratio enhances the predictive value of *FLT3* for survival[580]. Patients with a high mutant/wild-type ratio (i.e. greater than 0.78) had significantly shorter overall and disease-free survival, whereas survival in patients with a ratio below 0.78 did not differ from those without *FLT3* aberrations[580]. Whitman *et al.* identified three genotypic groups of AML: (1) normal *FLT3*(wild-type/wild-type); heterozygous *FLT3*(ITD/wild-type); and hemizygous *FLT3*(ITD/−). Disease-free survival and overall survival were significantly inferior for patients with *FLT3*(ITD/−)[581]. Although disease-free survival and overall survival for *FLT3* (wild-type/wild-type) and *FLT3*(ITD/wild-type) groups did not differ, overall survival of the

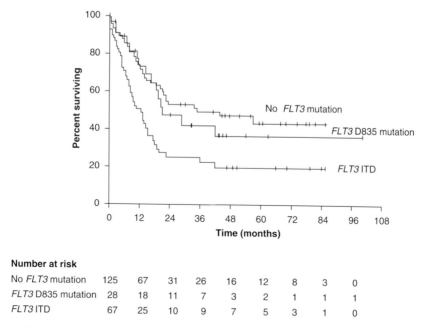

Figure 2.42 Overall survival for patients with normal cytogenetics according to *FLT3* mutation status

From: Frohling S, *et al*. Prognostic significance of activating *FLT3* mutations in younger adults (16 to 60 years) with acute myeloid leukemia and normal cytogenetics. Blood 2002;100:4372–80. © 2002 by The American Society of Hematology, used with permission

FLT3(ITD/–) group was worse than in the other groups[581]. In pediatric AML the presence of the *FLT3* mutations (ITD) is the single most significant, independent prognostic factor for poor outcome[569,582]. *FLT3*/ITD predicts a poor outcome in MDS[583,584]. Shih *et al.* showed that one-third of MDS patients acquire activating mutations of *FLT3* or the N-*RAS* gene during AML evolution[583].

FOXP1

The human Forkhead-box (*FOX*) gene family consists of at least 43 members[585]. *FOXO3* and *FOXO4* genes are fused to the *MLL* gene in hematological malignancies[585]. *FOXP1* (Forkhead box-P1) is a transcription factor gene that is differentially expressed in resting and activated B cells. *FOXP1* gene has been mapped to chromosome 3p14.1. *FOXP1* expression has been demonstrated in a subset of DLBCL and is more common in the ABC type with non-germinal center phenotype (MUM1[+]/ Bcl-2[+]) in the absence of t(14;18). Barrans *et al.* showed that high FOXP1 expression was almost exclusively confined to patients who lacked the germinal center phenotype, who expressed MUM1 and Bcl-2 in the absence of t(14;18), and who were identified as a subgroup of patients with particularly poor outcomes in a group with already poor prognoses[586]. The series reported by Banham *et al.* showed that FOXP1 protein expression has prognostic significance in patients with *de novo* DLBCL, treated at a single institution[587]. The overall survival curves showed that patients grouped as FOXP1[+] (40%) had a significantly decreased overall survival (median overall survival of 1.6 and 12.2 years in FOXP1[+] and FOXP1[–] cases, respectively). In addition, FOXP1-positive patients showed a clear trend towards earlier progression in comparison to the FOXP1[–] patients. The analysis of FOXP1 expression with low, intermediate and high IPI showed that FOXP1[-] patients had better overall survival within each group, indicating that FOXP1 expression has predictive value independent of the IPI[587].

JAK2

The Janus family of cytosolic tyrosine kinases (JAK) plays an essential role in development and normal hematopoiesis[588]. *JAK2* plays a central role in non-protein tyrosine kinase receptor signaling pathways, which could explain its involvement in malignancies of different hematologic lineages[588,589]. The fusion of *TEL* to *JAK2* has been reported in acute leukemia and blast phase of CML. Mutations of *JAK2* have been reported in a subset of chronic myeloproliferative disorders such as polycythemia vera and essential thrombocythemia[590].

LMO-2

LMO-2 plays an important role in erythropoiesis and angiogenesis and is the most frequent site of chromosomal translocation in childhood precursor T-ALL. It is not expressed in normal T lymphocytes but is present at high levels in germinal center B cells. The expression of *LMO-2* in DLBCL is associated with prolonged survival[568].

MDR genes

Resistance to chemotherapy is a poor prognostic factor. The failure of treatment may be due to rapid efflux of the chemotherapeutic agents from the intracellular environment or the inability of cancer cells to undergo apoptosis. The expression of multidrug resistance (MDR)-related proteins and/or *MDR* genes has been correlated with tumor sensitivity to treatment and clinical outcome in many hematologic malignancies, including AML, ALL, B-CLL and NHL. The best known *MDR* gene – *MDR1* – encodes P-glycoprotein, a 170-kDa membrane protein acting as a multispecific drug efflux pump. P-glycoprotein belongs to the adenosine triphosphate (ATP)-binding transporter family. P-glycoprotein confers long-term resistance to caspase-dependent (but not to caspase-independent) apoptotic stimuli[591]. The methods for identification of MDR include molecular tests (e.g. PCR) for gene expression and immunophenotyping. P-glycoprotein can be detected by flow cytometry and/or immunohistochemistry using monoclonal antibodies (e.g. MRK16, C219 and JSB-1). The MDR phenotype is often associated with an increased expression of P-glycoprotein at the plasma membrane[592]. MDR-related proteins, including P-glycoprotein, may be activated in association with overexpression of mutant or inactivated *p53* (*TP53*). Other proteins that may confer drug resistance include multidrug resistance-associated protein 1 (MRP1), lung resistance protein (LRP) and breast cancer resistance protein (BCRP). Although the status of P-glycoprotein expression correlates with relapse rate and overall survival, some patients relapse in spite of low levels of *MDR1* or *MRP1*. Phosphorylation of P-glycoprotein, mutations of *MDR* genes and cell cycle stage can influence the functional status of the efflux pump.

MDR is frequently expressed in AML and is associated with a lower complete remission rate and, in some studies, with lower overall survival for patients on standard chemotherapy[113,114,593-596]. The three major candidates accounting for the development of MDR in AML are the *MDR1*, *MRP1* and *LRP* genes. AML in the elderly is associated with an increased frequency of unfavorable cytogenetics and *MDR1* expression, both of which independently contribute to poor outcome[113,114]. Approximately 70% of elderly patients with AML express *MDR1*[113]. Complete remission in elderly AML patients ranges from 81% in MDR1[-] *de novo* AML and favorable to intermediate cytogenetics, to 13% in MDR1[+] secondary AML with unfavorable cytogenetics. *MDR1*/P-glycoprotein expression is less common in younger patients with AML (35%) and is also associated with resistance disease and lower complete remission rate[114]. However, contrary to adult patients, expression of *MDR1* fails to define a poor prognostic group

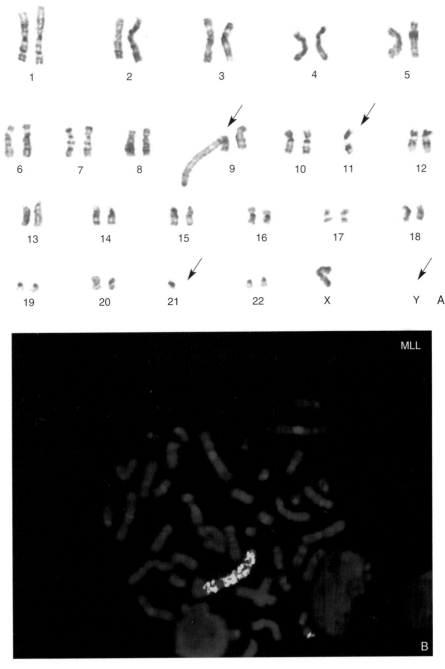

Figure 2.43 *MLL* amplification. Amplification of *MLL* and translocation of chromosome 11 to chromosome 9 and −21, −Y in acute leukemia. A, cytogenetic studies showing abnormal chromosome 9 with additional material from chromosome 11 with amplified *MLL*; B, FISH analysis showing numerous copies of *MLL*

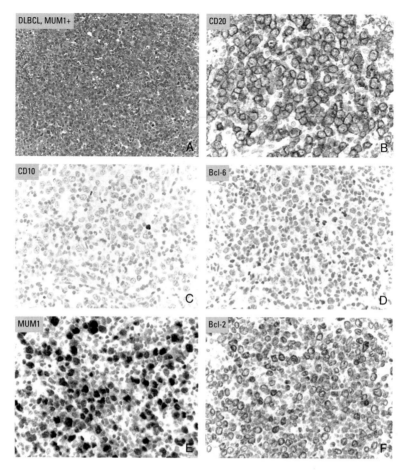

Figure 2.44 Diffuse large B-cell lymphoma with MUM1 expression. A, histology; B–F, immunohistochemistry. Lymphomatous cells express CD20 (B), MUM1 (E) and Bcl-2 (F) and are negative for CD10 (C) and Bcl-6 (D)

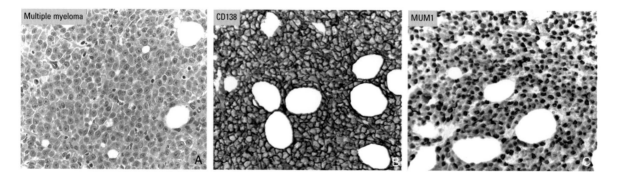

Figure 2.45 MUM1 expression in multiple myeloma. A, histology; B–C, immunohistochemistry. Myeloma cells are positive for CD138 (B) and MUM1 (C)

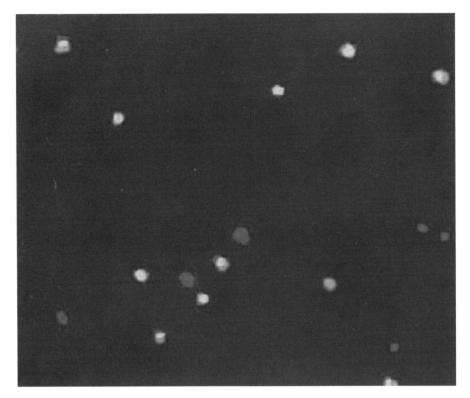

Figure 2.46 c-*MYC* expression due to t(8;14) in Burkitt's lymphoma (FISH analysis)

a role in B-cell differentiation[624,625]. PAX5 is expressed in precursor and mature B-cell lymphoproliferations, HL and a small subset of plasma cell neoplasms (Figure 2.48). The t(9;14) results in the juxtaposition of the *PAX5* gene with the *Ig* heavy chain locus of chromosome 14. The t(9;14)(p13;q32) translocation is associated with approximately 50% of lymphoplasmacytic lymphoma[626,627]. A number of other reciprocal translocations involving 9p13 have been identified (1p25, 3q27, 7q11, 10p13, 12q13). Deregulation of *PAX5* expression has been reported in splenic marginal zone B-cell lymphoma[628].

PML–RARα

See also t(15;17) above. The *PML* (promyelocytic leukemia) tumor suppressor gene is involved in the pathogenesis of APL, in which it is fused to the *RARα* gene as a consequence of the t(15;17) chromosomal translocation[506]. Inactivation or loss of *PML* leads to a proliferative advantage of cells, impairs cellular senescence in response to oncogenic stimuli and impairs cellular differentiation after exposure to differentiating agents such as retinoic acid and vitamin D. Mutations of the *PML* gene in APL are associated with resistance to retinoic acid and a very poor prognosis[629]. Mutations of the *PML* gene can also be found in non-APL AML, MDS, MM and occasional lymphomas[629].

RAS

Four alleles of *RAS* have been identified: H-*RAS* (Harvey), Ki-*RAS* (Kirsten; A and B) and N-*RAS* (neuroblastoma). Activation of the Ras protein participates in the control of cell proliferation, survival and differentiation. Point mutations of *RAS* (codons 12, 13 and 61) are present in AML and

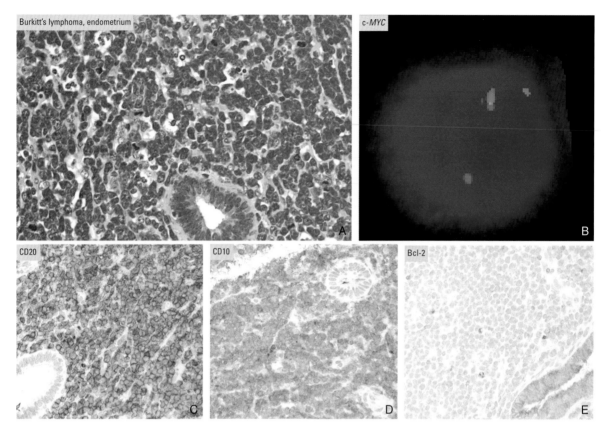

Figure 2.47   Burkitt's lymphoma, endometrium. A, histology with diffuse high-grade lymphoid infiltrate; B, FISH with c-*MYC* expression; C–E, immunohistochemistry. Lymphomatous cells are positive for CD20 (C) and CD10 (D), and are negative for Bcl-2 (E)

in MDS, especially CMML, and usually involve N-*RAS* and less commonly Ki-*RAS*. Point mutations of *RAS* occur in about 20% of *de novo* AML patients[569,630–632]. Published data did not reveal the association of activating *RAS* mutations with adverse prognosis[569,630–632]. In contrast to *p53*, *RAS* mutations are less common in therapy-related MDS or AML than in *de novo* disease[405]. In a study reported by Stirewalt *et al.*, AML patients with *RAS* mutations had higher white blood cell (WBC) counts, a lower percentage of CD34+ blasts and less resistant disease[569]. In a report by Shih *et al.*, N-*RAS* mutations had no prognostic impact at either the MDS or the AML stage but N-*RAS* mutations were more frequent in MDS progressing to AML than in MDS at

the time of diagnosis[583]. *RAS* mutations may play a role in progression of MGUS to MM[633].

RB1 (retinoblastoma gene)

The retinoblastoma (pRb) protein is encoded by the *RB1* tumor suppressor gene and plays a critical role in cell cycle control. pRb regulates the G_1/S transition of the cell cycle[239,539]. Abnormalities in the *RB1* gene are responsible for retinoblastoma[634]. pRb inactivation is a frequent phenomenon in tumors of different cell lineages, including hematologic malignancies[635–638]. Loss of pRb is seen in adult precursor lymphoblastic leukemia (ALL), but pRb or p53 alterations alone are not strong independent predictors of outcome[639]. Concurrent expression of pRb and p53 may predict a poor response to therapy in ALL[639].

In reactive lymphoid tissues, pRb is expressed by proliferating cells such as germinal center B cells. In DLBCL, loss of pRb expression is an adverse prognostic factor, whereas high pRb expression (>80%) is associated with extended survival[539]. In HL, high expression of pRb correlates with better survival, and loss of pRb expression is associated with adverse outcome[254,637].

pRb is frequently absent or phosphorylated in anaplastic large cell lymphoma (ALCL) and the absence of pRb expression is associated with better clinical outcome in patients with ALCL[640]. In a study by Rassidakis *et al.*, 5-year progression-free survival for patients with pRb-negative ALCL was 89.4% compared with 47.7% for patients with total pRb-positive ALCL[640].

In AML the prognostic value of low *RB1* expression is controversial, but the majority of published studies found low *RB1* expression to be a negative prognostic indicator[641]. Jamal *et al.* reported no significant differences in the frequency of complete remission or length of survival between AML patients with normal and those with abnormal pRb[636]. No mutation of *RB1* has been reported in AML or MDS. However, *RB1* mutations occur in accelerated phase and blast crisis of CML. Figure 2.49 presents pRb expression in Burkitt's lymphoma.

RUNX1 (AML1)

RUNX1 (AML1), located on chromosome 21q22, is one of the most important hematopoietic transcription factors. *RUNX1* is frequently affected in leukemia and MDS with 21q22 translocations. It is involved in a number of different chromosomal translocations, including t(8;21) (q22;q22), t(X;21)(p22;q22) and t(19;21)(q13;q22) in AML[642–644], t(3;21)(q26;q22) in MDS and blast crisis of CML[645], and t(12;21) (p13;q22) in B-ALL[646]. The t(8;21)(q22;q22) translocation, present in 10–15% of AML, results in the production of the RUNX1–ETO fusion protein.

This translocation is most often associated with FAB M2 morphology and co-expression of CD19 and CD56 by CD13⁺/CD33⁺ myeloblasts. *RUNX1* point mutations are common in high-risk MDS, but not in chronic idiopathic myelofibrosis[647]. *RUNX1* mutations in pediatric hematologic malignancies are infrequent, but are possibly related to AML-M0, acquired trisomy 21 and leukemic transformation. These patients may have a poor clinical outcome[648].

TEL–RUNX1(AML1)

ALL with *TEL–RUNX1* fusion resulting from t(12;21) have a very good outcome with standard chemotherapy. This in part may be due to TEL–AML1/RUNX1 protein activity as a transcriptional repressor of multidrug resistance gene (*MDR1*) expression[649]. *TEL* deletions, trisomy 21 and an additional der(21)t(12;21) are seen in 55%, 14% and 15% of *TEL–RUNX1*⁺ ALL, respectively[650]. The t(12;21) translocation resulting in *TEL–RUNX1* gene fusion is present in approximately 25% of patients with precursor B-lineage pediatric ALL. The 12p aberrations and near-tetraploidy are more common in *TEL–RUNX1*⁺ patients, whereas the incidence of diploidy, pseudodiploidy, hypodiploidy, low hyperdiploidy, near-triploidy, del(6q), chromosome 9 and 11q23 abnormalities is similar among *TEL–RUNX1*⁺ and *TEL–RUNX1*⁻ patients[650]. None of the *TEL–RUNX1*⁺ patients had a high hyperdiploid karyotype. Univariate analysis indicated that among *TEL–RUNX1*⁺ patients those with a deletion of the non-translocated *TEL* allele had a worse prognosis than those without this abnormality[650]. The presence of *TEL–RUNX1* gene fusion in childhood B-ALL does not seem to be associated with high *in vitro* drug sensitivity, except for L-asparaginase[651].

TP53 (p53)

p53 (TP53) is a tumor suppressor gene that codes for a multifunctional DNA-binding protein (transcription factor) involved in cell cycle arrest, DNA repair, differentiation and apoptosis. *p53* accumulates in

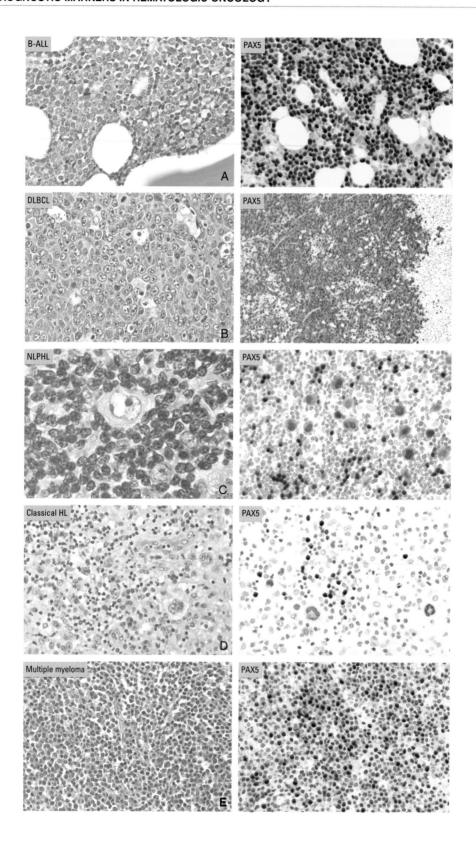

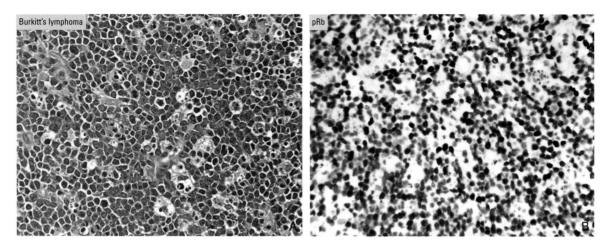

Figure 2.49   Burkitt's lymphoma with expression of retinoblastoma protein (A, histology; B, immunohistochemical staining for pRb)

response to DNA damage and coordinates the cellular response to such damage by inducing apoptosis or cell cycle arrest[652]. Inactivation of *p53* by mutation or deletion occurs in approximately 50% of cancers and is associated with genomic instability[652] and resistance to chemotherapy[653]. The negative regulation of cell cycle progression by *p53* is in part regulated by induction of *p21CIP1*. *p53* is one of the most frequently mutated genes in human cancer, mainly in solid tumors[654]. Based on the published data, Imamura *et al.* reported *p53* abnormalities in hematopoietic malignancies with the following frequencies: B-CLL, 15%; Richter's syndrome, 40%; low-grade B-cell lymphoma, rare; high-grade B-cell lymphoma, 30%; Burkitt's lymphoma, 40%; HL, 70%; MM, 5%; HCL, 10%; CML (chronic phase), rare; CML (blast crisis), 20–30%; MDS, 5%; AML, 15%; common ALL, 3%; mature B-ALL, 50%; and adult T-cell lymphoma/leukemia, 40%[256]. Deletions of one allele and mutations of *p53* are reported in 5% of AML and MDS. The wild-type p53 protein has a short half-life (6–20 minutes) and therefore

does not accumulate in tissue in amounts allowing for immunohistochemical detection[256]. Missense mutations of *p53* result in stabilization of the p53 protein and therefore increased levels of p53 usually reflect *p53* mutations[655]. However, since only a fraction of lymphomas with p53 overexpression have *p53* mutations, other mechanisms may also play a role in stabilization of the p53 protein.

p53 gene mutations in lymphoid neoplasms have been detected mainly in high-grade lymphomas and have been associated with tumor progression in follicular and small lymphocytic lymphomas. B-cell lymphomas with *p53* mutations often have c-*MYC* activation. Deletions of *p53* in B-CLL (Figure 2.50) are associated with disease progression and atypical morphologic and immunophenotypic features[656]. In B-CLL the presence of *p53* mutation or deletion is strongly associated with adverse clinical outcome and predicts a poor response to conventional therapy (drug resistance)[518,657–660]. *p53* mutations occur in only 10–15% of B-CLL patients[657,659]. However, *p53* dysfunction in B-CLL can occur in the absence of

Figure 2.48   PAX5 expression in hematolymphoid neoplasms: precursor B-lymphoblastic leukemia (B-ALL; A), diffuse large B-cell lymphoma (DLBCL; B), nodular lymphocyte predominant Hodgkin's lymphoma (NLPHL; C), classical Hodgkin's lymphoma (HL; D) and multiple myeloma (E)

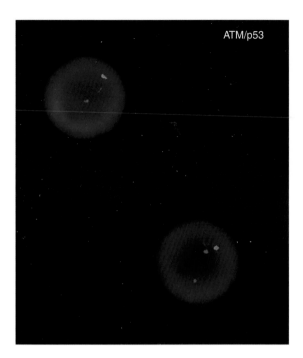

Figure 2.50 ATM/p53 aberrations in B-chronic lymphocytic leukemia

mutation and may be associated with mutation of the gene encoding ATM, a kinase implicated in *p53* activation[518,520,521]. Deletions affecting chromosome bands 11q22–q23 and 17p13 led to a reduced expression of the corresponding genes, *ATM* and *p53*. Inactivation of the *ATM* or *p53* gene is frequent in B-CLL and leads to aggressive disease. Patients with ATM deficiency had significantly shorter survival times (35.66 vs. 97.3 months) and more aggressive disease, suggesting that *ATM* is involved in the leukemogenesis of B-CLL. The *ATM* gene may also play a role in the reported 11q23 abnormality in B-CLL, which also characterizes an aggressive disease[520]. Approximately 14% of B-CLL carry deletions of the long arm of chromosome 11 at 11q22–23. Loss of heterozygosity at 11q22-23 and, more recently, absence of ATM protein, have been associated with a poor prognosis in B-CLL[521]. Functional impairment of the p53 pathway because of the inactivation of *p53* or *ATM* can be detected by exposing leukemic cells to ionizing radiation, culturing them overnight and examining them by western blotting for levels of p53 and p21 (a transcriptional target of *p53*)[518]. In type A defect (associated with *p53* mutation) baseline p53 levels are increased, reflecting the prolonged half-life of mutant p53 as compared with the wild-type protein. In contrast, in the type B defect (associated with the *ATM* mutation) baseline p53 levels are not increased, but there is impaired accumulation of p53 in response to radiation[518]. Recently, Carter *et al.* proposed flow cytometry assay to analyze p53 dysfunction in B-CLL[661]. Figure 2.51 presents immunohistochemical detection of p53 in B-CLL.

p53 mutations are associated with an aggressive clinical course of splenic marginal zone B-cell lymphoma[662]. A subset of patients with MCL has *p53* mutations/overexpression, which confer a poorer prognosis[663]. *p53* mutations occur more often in MCL with atypical/blastic cytology, and p53 mutations preceded the development of variant cytology in some patients. Overexpression of *p53* protein was observed in 75% with *p53* mutations and in none of the wild-type cases. The median survival of the cases with mutant *p53* was only 1.3 years, whereas the median survival of cases with germline (wild-type) *p53* was 5.1 years[663]. The *p53* mutation has a limited role in the transformation of FL into higher-grade neoplasms.

Mutations of *p53* are detected in up to 30% of DLBCL and Burkitt's lymphoma[664–667]. Overexpression of *p53* has been shown to have prognostic significance in DLBCL and is associated with chemotherapy refractoriness. The presence of *p53* gene mutations has a negative impact on overall survival in DLBCL. Cox's regression model showed that the high-risk IPI and *p53* gene mutations had an independent negative impact on overall survival in DLBCL[668].

In patients with MM, *p53* deletions are associated with higher serum calcium and creatinine levels, but there is no association with patient age, gender, levels of β_2-microglobulin, C-reactive protein, hemoglobin and albumin, or lytic bone lesions. There is no associations of *p53* deletions with 13q deletions or translocations t(11;14) or t(4;14). Patients with *p53* deletions had significantly shorter progression-free (median, 7.9 vs. 25.7 months) and overall survival (median,

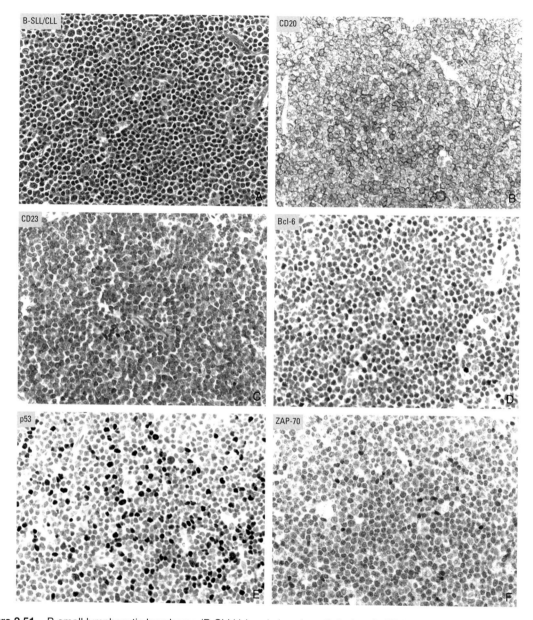

Figure 2.51 B-small lymphocytic lymphoma (B-SLL)/chronic lymphocytic leukemia (CLL) with phenotypic expression of p53, ZAP70 and Bcl-6. A, histology; B–F, immunohistochemistry. Tumor cells are positive for CD20 (B), CD23 (C), Bcl-6 (D), p53 (subset; E) and ZAP-70 (F)

14.7 vs. 48.1 months) than patients without a *p53* deletion. A multivariate analysis confirmed *p53* deletion as an independent prognostic factor predicting shortened progression-free or overall survival in patients with MM after high-dose chemotherapy and autologous stem cell transplantation[669].

Neoplastic cells in classical HL (but not NLPHL) frequently express p53. In peripheral T-cell lymphoma, p53-positive cases (by immunohistochemistry) show significantly higher proliferative activity, more frequent expression of Bcl-2 and less frequent expression of p21/WAF1 than p53-negative cases[670]. Analysis of the survival curves showed that p53 expression was an independent prognostic variable associated with a significantly poorer clinical outcome, in terms of both overall survival and event-free survival[670].

p53 mutations are present in 15% AML, and 11% MDS[659]. In AML, 33% of mutated cases and 81% of non-mutated cases treated with intensive chemotherapy achieved complete remission. Median survival is shorter in patients with mutated p53 when compared with unmutated p53 (2.5 months vs. 15 months). In the MDS patients who received chemotherapy, 8% of mutated cases and 60% of non-mutated cases achieved complete remission or partial remission, and median survival was 2.5 and 13.5 months, respectively[659]. In all MDS cases (treated and untreated), the survival difference between mutated cases and non-mutated cases was also highly significant. The p53 mutation is a strong prognostic indicator of response to chemotherapy and survival in AML and MDS[659].

IgV_H gene mutations

Based on IgV_H mutations, B-cell lymphoproliferative disorders can be classified into three categories: (1) those with unmutated IgV_H genes, in which it was postulated that the cell of origin had not entered the germinal center; (2) tumors with ongoing IgV_H gene mutations, such as follicle center lymphomas, in which malignant cells remain under the influence of the germinal center reaction; and (3) B-cell tumors with mutated stable IgV_H genes, such as MM, which were postulated to have irreversibly traversed through the germinal center[671].

In B-CLL (see Chapter 4), an unmutated IgV_H gene is a poor prognostic factor[672,673]. In MCL mutated IgV_H was associated with a higher rate of complete remission, but there was no correlation between IgV_H mutation status and other clinical characteristics or overall survival[674].

WT1

The transcription factor Wilms' tumor gene (WT1) is an important prognostic marker in AML and MDS and may be useful for disease detection and monitoring. WT1 overexpression may be due to mutations (10% AML) or upregulation of other transcription factors (e.g. PAX2, PAX8 and GATA). A high expression of Wilms' tumor gene (WT1) in AML seems to correlate with a poor outcome, and its increased levels can be predictive of an impending relapse. Higher levels of WT1 expression are associated with a shorter overall survival and event-free survival. The WT1 gene has been shown to interact with the promoter of the multidrug resistance gene (MDR1). Galimberti et al. found that high levels of WT1 were significantly correlated with high levels of the MDR1 gene[675].

CHAPTER 3

Phenotypic markers

ALK1

Anaplastic lymphoma kinase 1 (ALK1) is expressed in anaplastic large cell lymphoma (ALCL), which is a T-cell lymphoma composed of large pleomorphic cells, which have irregular kidney-shaped nuclei ('hallmark cells') expressing CD30, and often pan-T antigens and epithelial membrane antigen (EMA). The most frequent chromosomal abnormality in ALCL is t(2;5)(p23;35), which involves the *ALK* gene on chromosome 2 and the nucleophosmin gene (*NPM*) on chromosome 5. Variant translocations involving *ALK* and other partner genes can also be detected in ALCL. In contrast to t(2;5) associated with both nuclear and cytoplasmic staining for ALK1 protein, the variant translocations are associated with cytoplasm-only staining with ALK1 by immunohistochemistry (Figure 3.1). The prognosis of ALK⁺ ALCL is favorable, except for cases with peripheral blood involvement, which are aggressive. Patients with ALK⁻ tumors have a poor prognosis, similar to peripheral T-cell lymphoma, unspecified. It is therefore suggested that ALK⁻ lymphomas with anaplastic features represent a variant of CD30⁺ peripheral T-cell lymphoma.

A rare variant of diffuse large B-cell lymphoma (DLBCL) may express ALK without the t(2;5) translocation. This protein appears to be a full-length ALK receptor (and not a chimeric molecule characteristic for ALCL)[472,473]. The majority of ALK⁺ DLBCL display a complex t(2;17)(p23;q23) involving the clatherin gene[473].

Bcl-1 (cyclin D1)

Cyclin D1 (Bcl-1) can be detected by immunohistochemistry on tissue sections, where it presents with nuclear staining. The expression of cyclin D1 is most often associated with t(11;14) and is seen in mantle cell lymphoma (MCL) and some multiple myelomas (MM). Cyclin D1 can be expressed without the translocation, e.g. in a small subset of MM patients and in hairy cell leukemia (HCL). *See also molecular markers above (Chapter 2).*

Bcl-2

Expression of Bcl-2 protein can be visualized by immunohistochemistry on a routinely formalin-fixed and paraffin-embedded tissue section and by flow cytometry on fresh specimens. Bcl-2 is a mitochondrial membrane-associated protein, which acts as an inhibitor of apoptosis. Bcl-2 interacts with other proteins involved in the control of apoptosis, including the apoptosis-promoting BAX, and the Bcl-2/BAX ratio determines the susceptibility of the cell towards undergoing apoptosis. *See also molecular markers (BCL2), above (Chapter 2).*

Bcl-10

Strong nuclear expression of Bcl-10 is typical for lymphomas with t(1;14)(p22;q32); *see above (Chapter 2)*. It is characteristic for MALT (mucosa-associated

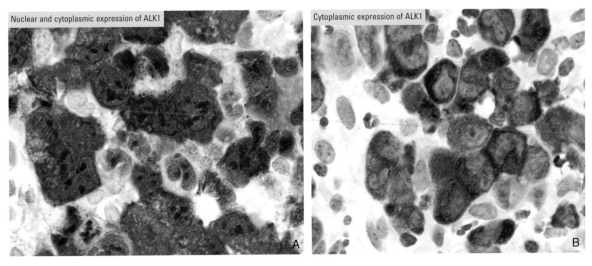

Figure 3.1 Pattern of ALK1 expression in anaplastic large cell lymphoma. A, nuclear, nucleolar and cytoplasmic; B, cytoplasmic only

lymphoid tissue) lymphoma, usually in the lung or stomach. The presence of t(1;14), similarly to t(11;18), contributes to the *Helicobacter pylori*-independent growth of gastric lymphoma and unresponsiveness of the tumors to *Helicobacter pylori* eradication therapy. The t(1;14) rearrangement produces a fusion of a novel gene, *BCL10*, which encodes an NK-κB-activating protein at 1p22 to an *IgH* enhancer at 14q32. The Bcl-10 protein is normally localized in the cytoplasm, but in MALT lymphomas with t(1;14) as well as with t(11;18)/*API2–MALT1* the protein is expressed in nuclei. MALT lymphomas with Bcl-10 expression have a more aggressive clinical course and often disseminated disease.

CD5

CD5, a 67-kDa pan-T-cell antigen, is also expressed by a subset of normal B cells and is typically present in B-chronic lymphocytic leukemia/small lymphocytic lymphoma (B-CLL/SLL) and MCL. Only a small proportion of diffuse large B-cell lymphomas express CD5 (Figure 3.2). Lack of cyclin D1 (Bcl-1) expression and lack of a history of B-CLL/SLL distinguishes CD5+ DLBCL from MCL and Richter's syndrome. The prognosis of *de novo* CD5+ DLBCL is markedly worse than that for CD5− DLBCL[676].

CD7

CD7+ acute myeloid leukemia (AML) patients showed a significantly lower response to treatment than CD7− AML patients, and had a poorer prognosis[677,678]. Figure 3.3 presents AML with CD7 expression.

CD10

CD10 protein (common acute lymphoblastic leukemia (ALL) antigen, CALLA) is a cell surface metalloproteinase that reduces the cellular response to peptide hormones. Among hematopoietic cells, CD10 is expressed by immature B and T cells, germinal center B cells, granulocytes and several neoplasms. CD10 expression does not have independent prognostic significance in either the larger subgroup of B-ALL patients or in T-ALL[679]. CD10 is expressed by Burkitt's lymphoma, the majority of follicular lymphomas (FL; Figure 3.4), a subset of DLBCL and a subset of angioimmunoblastic T-cell lymphomas. CD10 expression is associated with a better prognosis in follicular lymphoma and DLBCL[680–682]. It is suggested that CD10 expression may potentiate apoptotic activity of B and T cells, and, as a consequence, those tumors are more sensitive to treatment. Comparative genomic hybridization revealed

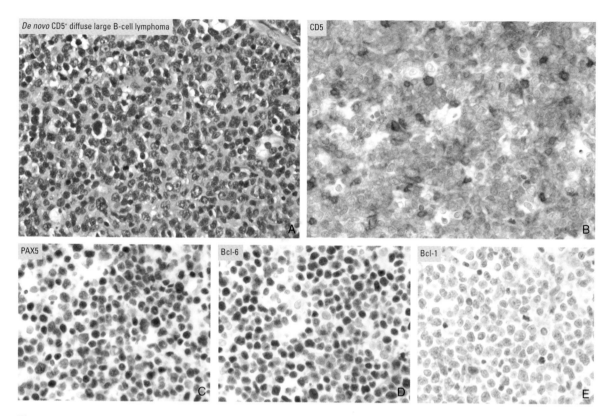

Figure 3.2 *De novo* CD5⁺ diffuse large B-cell lymphoma. A, histology: diffuse large cell infiltrate. B–E, immunohistochemistry: lymphomatous cells are positive for CD5 (B), PAX5 (C) and Bcl-6 (D). Bcl-1 is not expressed (E), which excludes the blastoid variant of mantle cell lymphoma

significant differences in chromosomal aberrations between FL and CD10⁺ DLBCL[683]. Chromosomal imbalances were observed in 60% of FL and in 100% of CD10⁺ DLBCL. The t(14;18) was present in only 31% of CD10⁺ DLBCL and the pattern of comparative genomic hybridization was different from that observed in FL with t(14;18), suggesting that CD10⁺ DLBCL may form a unique subtype of DLBCL[683]. On the other hand, FL without t(14;18) and with *BCL6* rearrangement defines a subtype of FL that is often CD10-negative and has distinct clinicopathologic features[684].

CD13 and CD33

The pan-myeloid antigens CD13 and CD33 are expressed by AML (Figure 3.5) and 10–20% of ALL[685–687]. The relations of myeloid-antigen expression to other features of ALL and to prognosis have been controversial. Initial multivariate data showed that myeloid-antigen expression was an important predictor of relapse in childhood ALL and that the presence of pan-myeloid antigens (CD13/CD33) in ALL was associated with a poor prognosis[685,687]. In subsequent clinical trials, however, myeloid-antigen expression was not found to have an adverse prognostic significance for childhood ALL, probably owing to contemporary intensive chemotherapy[686,688,689].

The CD33 molecule is a cell-surface differentiation protein that is expressed on normal progenitor and myeloid cells, as well as on more than 80% of AML blasts. It belongs to the family of the sialic acid-binding immunoglobulin-like lectin (Siglec). CD33 antigen is rapidly internalized upon binding to

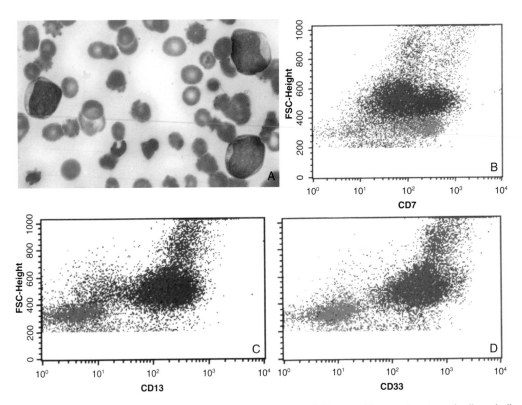

Figure 3.3 Acute myeloid leukemia with CD7 expression. A, myeloblasts with prominent nucleoli and dispersed chromatin; B–D, flow cytometry. Blasts are positive for CD7 (B), CD13 (C) and CD33 (D)

gemtuzumab ozogamicin (Mylotarg), an anti-CD33 antibody–drug conjugate, delivering the drug (calicheamicin) into the cell, with subsequent double-stranded DNA breaks[690]. Gemtuzumab ozogamicin is currently approved for relapsed AML in patients older than 65 years, but is being evaluated in combination with chemotherapy[691]. It is highly effective as a single treatment for patients with molecularly relapsed APL, including those with very advanced disease[692].

CD20

CD20 is present on pre-B cells and mature B cells, but not on precursor cells or terminally differentiated plasma cells. The function of CD20 remains poorly understood, although it has been implicated in B-cell activation, regulation of B-cell growth and regulation of transmembrane calcium

flux. Figure 3.6 shows the expression of CD20 analyzed by flow cytometry in B-CLL with large cell transformation.

Rituximab (Rituxan), a monoclonal antibody directed against the CD20 antigen, is widely used for the treatment of B-cell non-Hodgkin's lymphoma (NHL). Recent randomized trials have shown an advantage of rituximab-containing regimens over chemotherapy alone[4,693,694]. The addition of rituximab to CHOP chemotherapy results in a significant improvement in clinical outcome of aggressive lymphoma, except for patients with HIV-associated lymphomas. Rituximab shows high single-agent activity in both previously untreated and relapsed or refractory indolent NHL. B-cell lymphomas with expression of CD20 may lose the CD20 positivity after anti-CD20 immunotherapy (Figure 3.7). Rituximab was shown to mediate antibody-dependent cellular cytotoxicity (ADCC) and complement-dependent

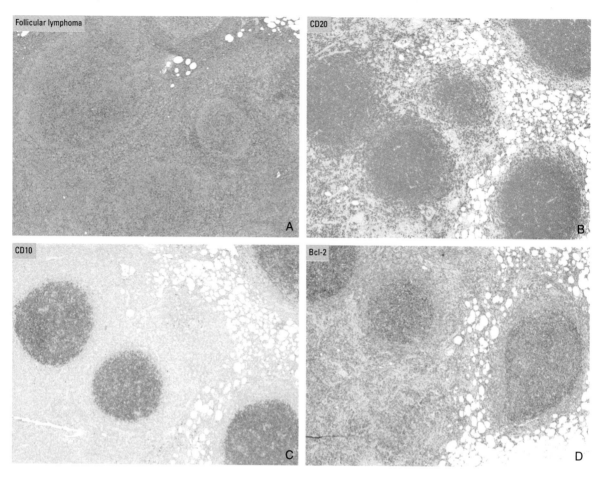

Figure 3.4   Follicular lymphoma with CD10 expression. A, histology; B–D, immunocytochemistry: neoplastic follicles are positive for CD20 (B), CD10 (C) and Bcl-2 (D)

cellular cytotoxicity, and to induce non-classic (caspase-independent) apoptosis of lymphoma cells *in vitro*[695–698]. In B-CLL, B-prolymphocytic leukemia (B-PLL) and MCL, the levels of CD20, measured by standard immunofluorescence or using calibrated beads, correlated linearly with the lytic response to rituximab regardless of diagnostic group[699]. Patients most likely to respond to rituximab can be predicated by overexpression of Bcl-2, Ki-67 expression, polymorphism for FcR-γ III (binding site for rituximab) and DNA microarray [5,246,700,701]. Gene expression patterns in the tumors that subsequently failed to respond to rituximab appeared more similar to those of normal lymphoid tissues than to gene expression patterns of tumors from rituximab responders[701]. In B-CLL, the

response to rituximab varies by cytogenetic groups: del(17), 0% response; del(11), 66%; del(13), 86%; +12, 25%; and normal, 0%[445]. A high serum lactate dehydrogenase (LDH) level, high or high–intermediate International Prognostic Index (IPI), and high Ki-67 expression are associated with a decreased response in the case of FL.

Among patients with CD20+ post-transplant lymphoproliferative disorders, rituximab therapy and low IPI are associated with improved overall survival[702]. Expression of CD20 in classical Hodgkin's lymphoma (HL) appears to be a poor prognostic factor for time-to-treatment failure and overall survival[703]. CD20 is expressed in a subset of B-ALL. Favorable results were observed in treatment of B-ALL with

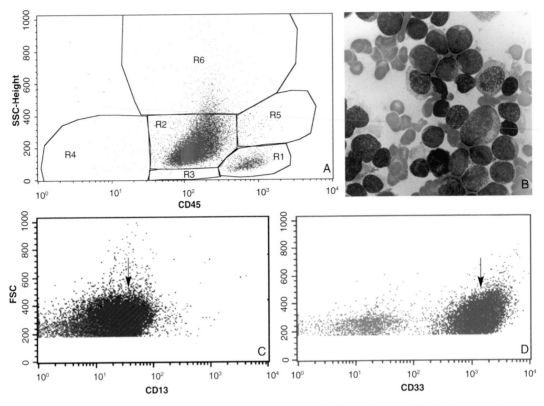

Figure 3.5 Expression of CD13 and CD33 in acute myeloid leukemia. A, blasts (green dots) display moderate expression of CD45 and low side scatter; B, cytology; C, expression of CD13 (arrow); D, expression of CD33 (arrow)

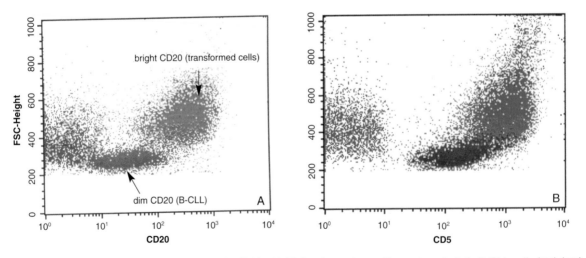

Figure 3.6 B-chronic lymphocytic leukemia (B-CLL) with Richter's syndrome (flow cytometry). A, B-CLL cells (red dots) display dim expression of CD20, and transformed cells (blue dots) show bright expression of CD20; B, CD5 expression

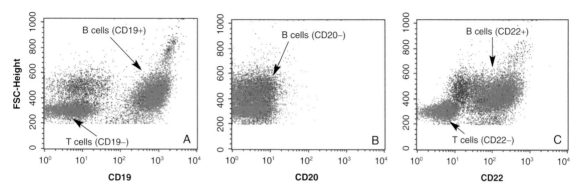

Figure 3.7 Loss of CD20 expression by lymphoma cells after rituximab treatment. Lymphomatous cells are positive for CD19 (A) and CD22 (C), but display negative staining with CD20 (B; arrow)

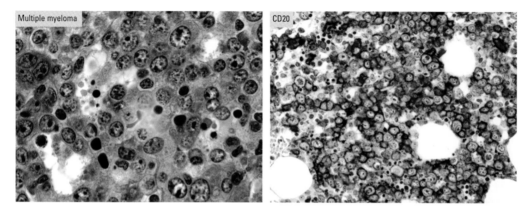

Figure 3.8 Multiple myeloma expressing CD20

rituximab in combination with routine chemotherapy, especially those with a mature phenotype.

In MM (Figure 3.8), CD20 expression was reported to be associated with small mature plasma cell morphology and with t(11;14)[704]. MM cases expressing CD20 showed a tendency towards a poorer prognosis with lower survival[705,706].

CD25

The CD25 (interleukin-2 receptor; IL-2R) is expressed by adult T-cell leukemia/lymphoma (ATCL), HCL and a subset of other T- and B-cell lymphoproliferative disorders. The expression of CD25 in cutaneous T-cell lymphoma may identify a subset of patients at risk of undergoing large cell transformation[707]. Markedly elevated serum soluble IL-2R levels are a particularly prominent feature of certain hematologic malignancies, such as human T-lymphotropic retrovirus type I-associated ATCL and HCL, reflecting tumor burden and response to therapy. Figure 3.9 presents T-cell lymphoma with CD25 expression.

The IL-2R has proved an attractive target for T cell-directed therapies. Denileukin diftitox is the first of a novel class of fusion toxin proteins and is selective for IL-2R/CD25+ T cells, targeting the malignant T-cell clones in cutaneous T-cell lymphoma. Jones *et al.* demonstrated *in vivo* that decreased levels of CD25 expression occurred in T-cell lymphoma when it involved lymph nodes, similar to

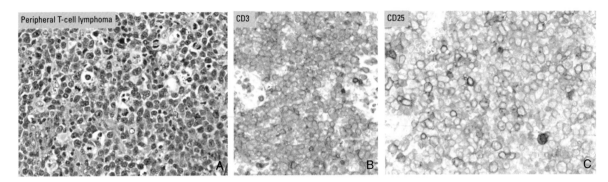

Figure 3.9   Peripheral T-cell lymphoma with CD25 expression. A, histology; B–C, immunohistochemistry (B, CD3 expression; C, CD25 expression)

what is seen with cutaneous lymphocyte antigen (CLA), a mediator of skin homing, and this demonstrable variation related to anatomical localization has implications for IL-2R-targeted immunotherapy[708].

HCL is generally indolent in its natural course; the majority of patients require treatment for life-threatening infections due to pancytopenia or symptomatic splenomegaly. The introduction of interferon-α replaced splenectomy (which was formerly the standard therapy). The purine analogs cladribine and pentostatin give better response rates than with interferon-α and with this treatment long-lasting remissions can be achieved in most patients[709]. Monoclonal antibodies targeting CD20, CD22 and CD25 antigens have shown responses for resistant or relapsing disease[709,710]. The CD25-negative HCL variant is an extremely rare chronic B-cell lymphoproliferative disorder clinically and morphologically distinct from classic HCL. It is thought to represent a hybrid between PLL and HCL with an aggressive clinical course and short survival.

CD30

CD30 is a transmembrane glycoprotein and is a member of the tumor necrosis factor (TNF) super-family[711]. CD30 protein is expressed in activated B and T lymphocytes (with immunoblastic cytomorphology), classical HL and ALCL, and in a subset of B-cell lymphomas (DLBCL, thymic large B-cell lymphoma and occasional FL)[22,712–714]. The effect of CD30 expression on behavior or response to treatment of B-cell lymphoma has not been well investigated. Overexpression of CD30 in HL is thought to result in ligand-independent signaling, leading to activation of NF-κB and survival of malignant cells[715]. Increased levels of serum CD30 are observed in HL patients and are a good marker for predicting a poor prognosis and a poor response to therapy. CD30 is a promising target for antibody-based therapy in HL and ALCL[716,717].

CD34

CD34 is a small peptide attached to the cell membrane of a hematopoietic cell. It is a marker of myeloid immaturity. The circulating myeloid progenitor cells can be easily assessed by flow cytometry. The expression of the CD34 antigen on the blast cells of AML has been regarded as an unfavorable prognostic factor for the achievement of complete remission. However, clinical reports on this issue still remain controversial. No differences were found in complete remission rate, remission duration or survival. Excluding induction deaths from the analysis, the complete remission rate is slightly lower in CD34+ AML (55% vs. 65%), without any impact on survival[718].

The degree of circulating progenitor cell expansion in chronic idiopathic myelofibrosis corresponds to the proliferative activity of the disorder. Recent studies

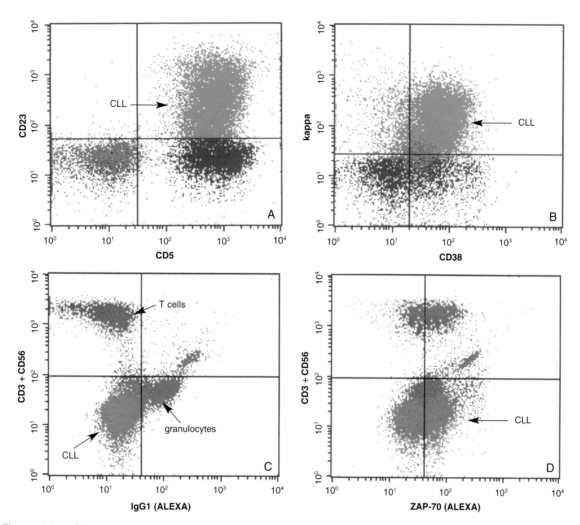

Figure 3.10   CD38 and ZAP-70 expression in B-chronic lymphocytic leukemia (B-CLL) (flow cytometry; B-CLL cells, red dots; T cells, green dots). A, CD5 and CD23 expression; B, CD38 expression; C–D, ZAP-70 expression

suggest that the number of circulating CD34$^+$ cells in peripheral blood is associated with prognosis. The number of CD34$^+$ cells correlates with both leukocyte count and degree of myeloid immaturity, as well as palpable spleen size.

CD38

CD38 is a transmembrane glycoprotein with a widespread cellular expression and functional activity. Based on the percentage of clonal cells expressing

CD38 (Figure 3.10), B-CLL could be divided into two categories: one with <30% CD38$^+$ leukemic cells and another with ≥30% cells[719]. B-CLL with CD38 expression in more than 30% cells contained unmutated IgV_H genes, whereas samples expressing less than 30% CD38$^+$ contained mostly mutated cases indicating a strong inverse relationship between IgV_H gene mutation and CD38 expression[719]. The level of CD38$^+$ cells correlates with clinical stage, response to treatment and overall survival (Figures 3.11 and 3.12): higher CD38 percentages

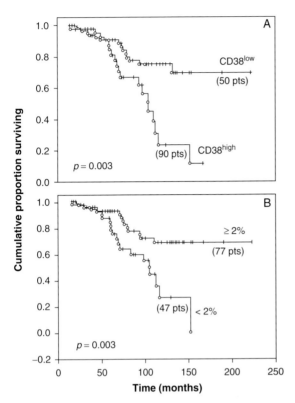

Figure 3.11 Survival of B-cell chronic lymphocytic leukemia (B-CLL) patients based on CD38 expression and IgV_H mutational status. A, Kaplan–Meier curves comparing survival based on the detection of CD38 in < 30% (CD38^{low}) or in ≥ 30% (CD38^{high}; 90 patients (pts)); log-rank test, $p = 0.003$. B, Kaplan–Meier curves comparing survival in B-CLL cases with a mutated (≥ 2% mutations) or unmutated (< 2% mutations) configuration of IgV_H genes

From: Degan M, *et al.* Analysis of IgV_H gene mutations in B cell chronic lymphocytic leukemia according to antigen-driven selection identifies subgroups with different prognosis and usage of the canonical somatic hypermutation machinery. Br J Haematol 2004;126:29–42, used with permission

correlate with more advanced stages, diffuse bone marrow involvement, atypical morphology, trisomy 12, poorer chemosensitivity and significantly shorter survival[720]. CD38$^+$ patients respond poorly to continuous multiregimen chemotherapy and have significantly shorter survival[719,721]. The level of expression of CD38 can be determined easily and rapidly by flow cytometry. In approximately 30% of patients with B-CLL the levels of CD38 expression and IgV_H mutational status are discordant[722,723]. Multivariate analysis demonstrated that Binet stage, IgV_H mutations and CD38 expression are independent prognostic indicators[722]. Median survival time in patients whose cells had unmutated IgV_H genes and expressed CD38 was 8 years; in those with mutated IgV_H genes not expressing CD38, it was 26 years; and for those with discordant results, median survival time was 15 years[722]. Thus, although CD38 expression does not identify the same two subsets as IgV_H mutations in B-CLL, it is an independent risk factor that can be used with IgV_H mutations and clinical stage to select patients with the worst prognoses. CD38$^+$ B-CLL patients are characterized by advanced stage, inferior responsiveness to therapy and a shorter survival (Figures 3.11 and 3.12).

CD44

CD44 is the lymphocyte homing receptor (a putative determinant of lymphoma dissemination). Expression of the standard form of CD44 (CD44s) and CD44 isoforms containing exon v6 (CD44v6) on tumor cells correlate with tumor dissemination in patients with primary nodal DLBCL. In patients with localized nodal disease, CD44s is a strong predictor of tumor-related death independent of the other parameters of the IPI[724].

CD52

Monoclonal antibody therapy has emerged in the past decade as a promising approach in treating B- and T-cell malignancies. Alemtuzumab (Campath-1H) is a humanized monoclonal antibody directed against the CD52 antigen. Similarly to rituximab, alemtuzumab eliminates cells through ADCC, complement activation and apoptosis[725]. CD52 is expressed on all normal and most malignant T lymphocytes. Alemtuzumab has been used in B-CLL, T-PLL and low-grade NHL[726–728]. Alemtuzumab has activity in T-cell malignancies, particularly in T-PLL

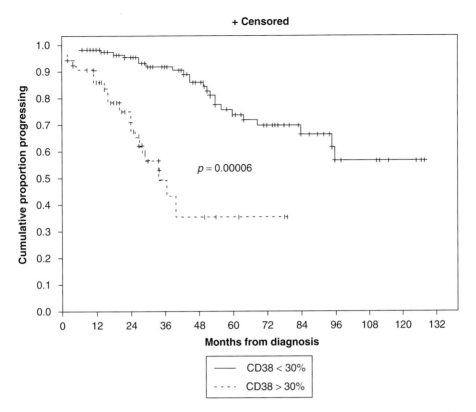

+ Censored

Figure 3.12   Progression-free survival curves based on CD38 expression. Kaplan–Meier plot comparing progression-free survival (from low to intermediate/high-modified Rai stage) based on the detection of more than 30% or less than 30% CD38⁺ B-CLL cells (>30%, 50 cases; <30%, 118 cases). As shown, CD38 patients experienced a highly significant longer progression-free survival ($p = 0.00006$)

From: Del Poeta G, *et al*. Clinical significance of CD38 expression in chronic lymphocytic leukemia. Blood 2001;98:2633–9. © 2001 by The American Society of Hematology, used with permission

and in patients with predominantly blood and bone marrow disease. Overall response is observed in 76% of patients with T-PLL and in 100% of patients with cutaneous T-cell lymphoma[726]. Durable remissions have been seen in heavily pretreated patients and in up to two-thirds of patients who had T-PLL. In T-PLL the response to alemtuzumab is significantly better than that reported with other therapies, suggesting that the drug can be used as a first-line therapy in this aggressive disease[729,730]. Alemtuzumab may also have a role in purging minimal residual disease following other chemotherapy and prior to transplantation[726]. In B-CLL patients who relapsed

after fludarabine, alemtuzumab can induce responses leading to MRD⁻ remission[35,53]. Treatment with Alemtuzumab may be associated with significant hematologic toxicity and infectious complications[731].

CD56

CD56, a neural cell-adhesion molecule (N-CAM) is expressed by natural killer (NK) cells and a subset of T cells and monocytes. Its expression is well recognized in hematolymphoid malignancies of NK-cell lineage, but also in MM, AML, especially with monocytic differentiation, acute DC2 leukemia

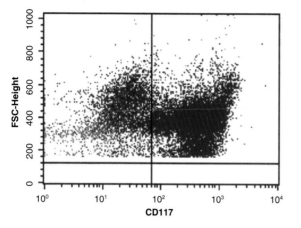
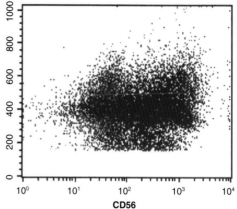

Figure 3.13 CD56+ acute myeloid leukemia

(blastic NK-cell lymphoma/leukemia) and rare cases of DLBCL. CD56 expression has been found to be a risk factor for AML with t(8;21) and t(15;17)[732,733]. CD56 expression in AML with t(8;21) is associated with significantly shorter complete remission duration and survival[732]. Figure 3.13 presents CD56+ AML. Positive expression of CD56 is an unfavorable factor in ALCL[734]. CD56 is positive in 17% of ALCL (Figure 3.14). There are no significant differences in clinical and immunophenotypic characteristics in CD56+ and CD56− ALCL. CD56 expression in subcutaneous panniculitis-like T-cell lymphoma is associated with aggressive clinical course[735,736]. The prognostic significance of CD56 expression in MM is controversial[737,738].

Epstein–Barr virus

There is significant difference in prognosis between the group of polymorphic Epstein–Barr virus (EBV)-associated lymphoproliferative disorders and the group of large cell lymphomas[739]. Evidence for EBV infection related to Richter's transformation was present in 16% of patients in B-CLL/SLL and appears to be associated with a poorer outcome[740]. Figure 3.15 presents the phenotypic features of post-transplant lymphoproliferative disorder.

FLIP

The FLIP family includes both cellular and viral members. The Kaposi's sarcoma-associated herpesvirus protein (KSHV)-FLIP is expressed by human herpesvirus 8 (HHV-8), which is associated with malignancies such as Kaposi's sarcoma and certain lymphomas. Cellular FLIP (cFLIP) is a close homolog of caspase 8 without caspase activity that inhibits Fas signaling and Fas-mediated apoptosis, and has been shown to be a key factor in germinal center B-cell survival. c-FLIP is constitutively expressed in HL and may therefore be a major mechanism responsible for Fas resistance in HL[297,741]. In nodular lymphocyte-predominant HL (NLPHL) the c-FLIP expression may be associated with transformation to large B-cell lymphoma[742]. The expression of c-FLIP was found to be strongly related to a poor prognosis in Burkitt's lymphoma[743]. The 2-year overall survival with c-FLIP expression was 24% compared with 93% in the absence of this marker[743]. FLIP provides prognostic information in DLBCL[266].

HLA-DR

AML with invaginated nuclear morphology, loss of HLA-DR and presence of *FLT3* internal tandem duplications (ITD) may represent a distinct subset[576].

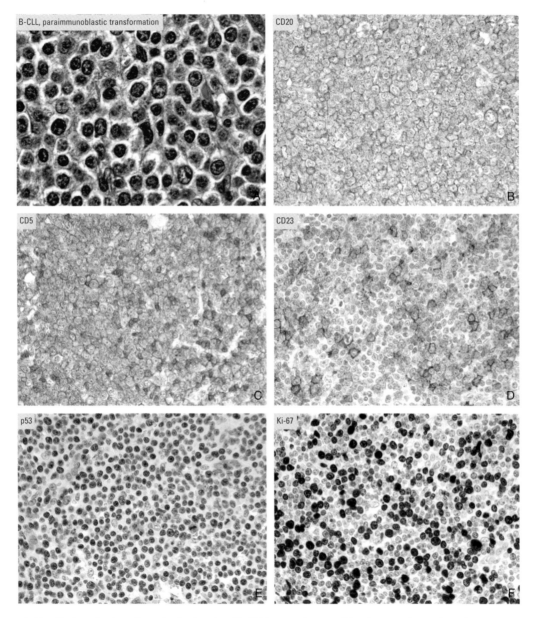

Figure 4.13 B-chronic lymphocytic leukemia (B-CLL), paraimmunoblastic transformation. A, histology; B–F, immunohistochemistry. Large lymphomatous cells with nucleoli are positive for CD20 (B), CD5 (C), CD23 (D), p53 (E) and Ki-67 (F)

deterioration of the patient's performance. The term Richter's transformation (in analogy to the clinical course reported in the original publication) is reserved by some clinicians for the latter[818]. Richter's syndrome occurs in approximately 5% of patients with CLL[212]. The response rates to therapeutic strategies (intensive chemotherapy, monoclonal antibodies and stem cell transplantation) range from 5% to 43% (complete response, 5–38%), and the median survival duration ranges from 5 to 8 months. Despite current aggressive treatments the prognosis is poor[212]. A causal relationship between risk of progression and bone marrow angiogenesis in B-CLL is suggested[236]. The chances of development of Richter's syndrome in

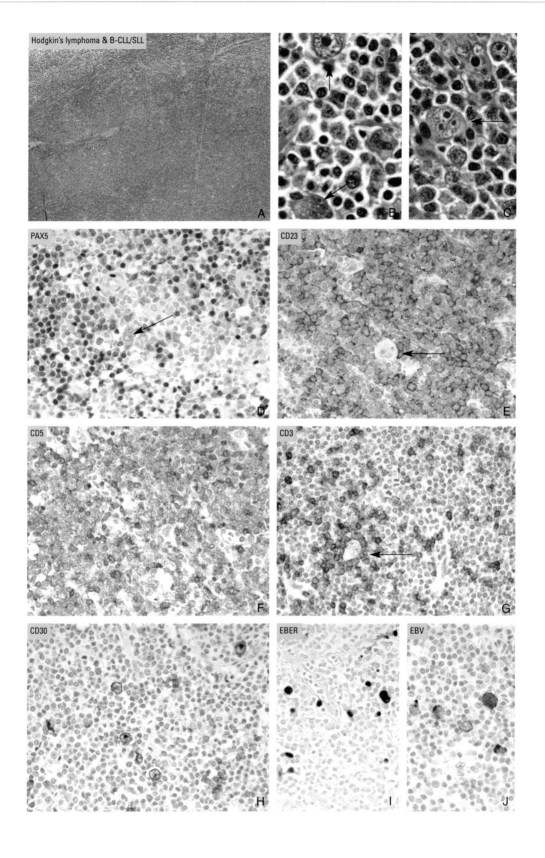

Hodgkin's lymphoma & B-CLL/SLL

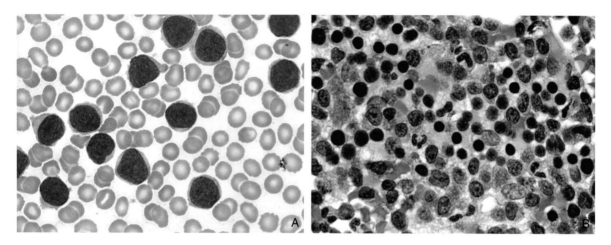

Figure 4.15   B-prolymphocytic leukemia (B-PLL), bone marrow. A, aspirate smear shows medium to large lymphocytes with nucleoli; B, histology with diffuse lymphoid infiltrate composed of atypical lymphoid cells

CLL patients with multiple chromosome changes is higher than in those with either simple trisomy 12 or a normal karyotype[819]. Richter's syndrome can occur in both mutated and unmutated variants of B-CLL. Progression of B-CLL may be associated with del(11q), overexpression of the c-*MYC* gene, deletions of the *RB1* gene and mutations of the *p53* gene[789,813,820,821]. Apart from genetic defects, Richter's syndrome may be triggered by viral infections[813]. Leukemic cells in prolymphocytic/paraimmunoblastic transformation often express p53 (Figure 4.13).

B-small lymphocytic lymphoma

In B-SLL, significant adverse predictors for overall survival are age ≥60 years, B symptoms, elevated serum LDH, low hemoglobin (<11 g/dl), and high IPI score (3–5)[12]. In multivariate analysis, the IPI score was the only significant predictor of overall survival in B-SLL. Anemia and B symptoms were additionally predictive of poor overall survival in patients with low IPI scores[12]. In analysis of cell proliferation, Bcl-2, c-*MYC*, *p53* and apoptosis in B-SLL, Palestro *et al.* showed a trend of association between cell proliferation and c-*MYC* expression with a more aggressive progression of the disease[822].

B-PROLYMPHOCYTIC LEUKEMIA

B-PLL is an infrequent aggressive disorder of mature B cells with distinct clinical and pathologic features most often associated with a poor prognosis. B-PLL (Figure 4.15) is characterized by medium-sized lymphocytes with nucleoli (prolymphocytes, comprising >55% of lymphocytes in blood), very high white blood cell (WBC) count and prominent splenomegaly. The median overall survival time is 5 years and the event-free survival time is 37 months[823,824]. The probability of overall survival for 3, 5 and 10 years is 63%, 56% and 35%, respectively[824]. As detected by univariate and multivariate analysis, advanced age, lymphocytosis (>100×10⁹/l) and

Figure 4.14   B-chronic lymphocytic leukemia/small lymphocytic lymphoma (B-CLL/SLL) and Hodgkin's lymphoma. A–C, histology; D–J, immunohistochemistry. Scattered large cells (B, C; arrows) with prominent nucleoli and often multi-lobed nuclei (Hodgkin cells and Reed–Sternberg cells) are present in the background of small lymphocytic infiltrate (A). Small lymphocytes are positive for PAX5 (D), CD23 (E) and CD5 (F), and large cells are positive for PAX5 (D; arrow) CD30 (H), EBER (I) and Epstein–Barr virus (EBV) (J). Small T cells (CD3⁺) form rosettes around large cells (G; arrow)

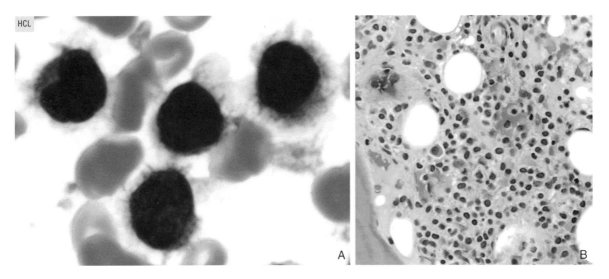

Figure 4.16   Hairy cell leukemia. A, aspirate smear; B, marrow core biopsy

anemia (< 11 g/dl) are associated with a poor prognosis and shorter survival. Patients with *p53* mutations had a worse clinical outcome[823]. The frequency of *p53* mutation (about 50%) in B-PLL is the highest reported in B-cell malignancies and may be responsible for the frequent resistance to therapy of this disease[825]. Gender, B symptoms at presentation, spleen size, thrombocytopenia, low IgG and complement levels, presence of paraproteinemia and the pattern of bone marrow infiltrate do not indicate the prognosis in B-PLL[824].

HAIRY CELL LEUKEMIA

Hairy cell leukemia (HCL) is an indolent chronic B-cell lymphoproliferative disorder characterized by bone marrow involvement, splenomegaly and pancytopenia. The characteristic 'hairy cells', present in the peripheral blood and bone marrow, are the hallmark of this leukemia (Figure 4.16). HCL is an uncommon disease, comprising approximately 2–3% of all adult leukemias in the USA[826]. Leukemic cells express CD11c, CD19, CD20, CD22, CD25 and CD103. Factors associated with a worse prognosis include high WBC count, low hemoglobin levels and prominent splenomegaly. Treatment of HCL is usually considered for symptomatic patients (significant

neutropenia, anemia, thrombocytopenia, symptomatic splenomegaly, constitutional symptoms due to HCL, or recurrent serious infections)[709,826–828]. Interferon-α treatment induces remission in approximately 90% of patients with HCL, but complete remission is obtained in only 5–10%[827]. The prognosis of HCL has improved over the past few years, with 4-year survival at 80%. With the purine analogs cladribine (2-chlorodeoxyadenosine, 2-CdA), and pentostatin, response rates are even better than with interferon-α, and long-lasting remissions can be achieved in most patients[709]. Other new treatment options include rituximab and BL-22 immunotoxin[826]. A striking improvement of survival rates has been observed, from 58.9% survival at 5 years for patients diagnosed before 1985 to 87.5% at 5 years for patients diagnosed after 1985[828,829]. HCL patients treated with cladribine had an overall survival rate of 97% recorded at 108 months[830]. Jehn *et al.* reported an overall survival at 12 years after the start of cladribine treatment as 79%[831].

Late in the course of the disease, patients may display lymphadenopathy, more often mediastinal and retroperitoneal than peripheral[832]. Patients with adenopathy may show good response to interferon-α in spite of persisting bone marrow involvement[833]. Figure 4.17 presents histologic and phenotypic features of HCL involving the lymph node.

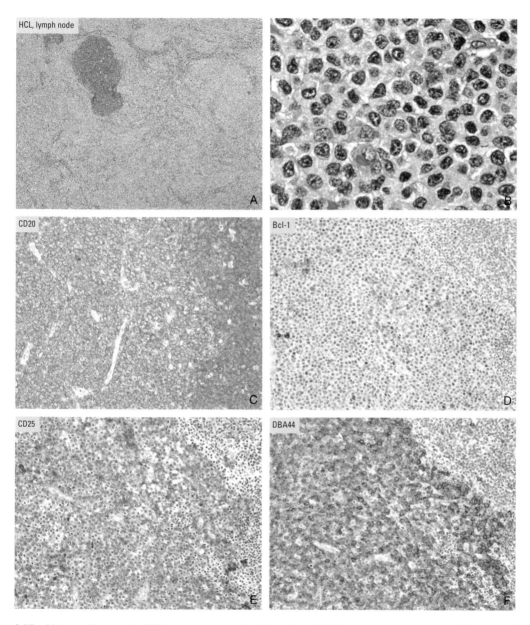

Figure 4.17   Hairy cell leukemia (HCL), lymph node. A–B, histology; C–F, immunohistochemistry. Diffuse interfollicular/paracortical infiltrate of atypical lymphoid cells with irregular nuclei (A–B). Leukemic cells are positive for CD20 (C), Bcl-1 (D), CD25 (E) and DBA44 (F)

Patients with HCL were initially reported to have increased risk of secondary malignant tumors (hematopoietic and non-hematopoietic) and opportunistic infections (*Mycobacterium kansasi*, blastomycosis, coccidioidomycosis)[834–836]. In a series by Goodman *et al.*, 22% of patients developed second malignancies[830]. Frassoldati *et al.* reported a second malignancy in 3.7% of patients, mostly detected several years after the onset of HCL[828]. In a study published by Flinn *et al.*, the survival rates and incidence of subsequent malignancies for patients with HCL treated with pentostatin (either initially or

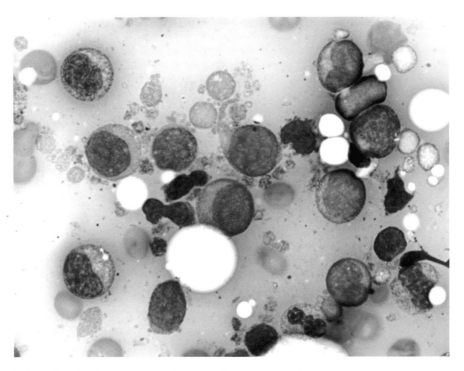

Figure 4.18   Hairy cell leukemia, 'blastic' transformation (aspirate smear)

after interferon-α failure) were not higher than expected in the general population[837]. Blastic transformation of HCL is extremely rare (Figure 4.18).

FOLLICULAR LYMPHOMA

FL is the most frequent subtype of low-grade malignant lymphoma in Western countries, accounting for one-third of NHL. FL are a heterogeneous group of tumors, characterized in the majority of cases by an indolent clinical course, nodular growth pattern (Figure 4.19), t(14;18)(q32;q21) and co-expression of CD10, Bcl-2 and Bcl-6. FL frequently involves the bone marrow with characteristic paratrabecular distribution (Figure 4.20). Clinically, FL is characterized by relatively long median survival, response to initial treatment and a continuous pattern of relapses, sometimes followed by histologic transformation into high-grade lymphoma[838]. Transformation and development of resistance to chemotherapy

in the course of the disease are the main causes of death in patients with FL.

Clinical features

Approximately 65% of patients are in stage III or IV at the time of diagnosis[201]. Bone marrow involvement is found in about 40% of patients and B symptoms in 17% of patients. More than 80% are in the low-risk group with respect to IPI. Long-term survival is relatively high when the disease is diagnosed in stages I or II[197]. With current therapy the expected median survival is approximately 8–10 years[838]. FL shows the most favorable prognosis of all low-grade lymphomas, and patients with FL have relatively long median survival times and exhibit good responses to initial therapy. However, patients with FL should be considered to be affected by a fatal malignancy that tends to relapse over time. They have a shorter response to salvage therapy after every relapse

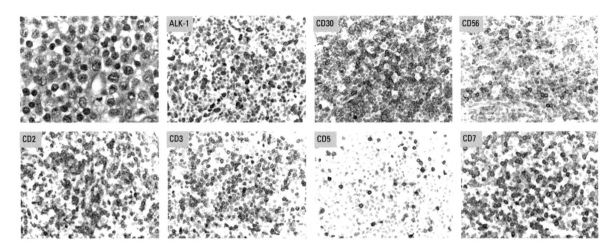

Figure 3.14   CD56⁺ anaplastic large cell lymphoma

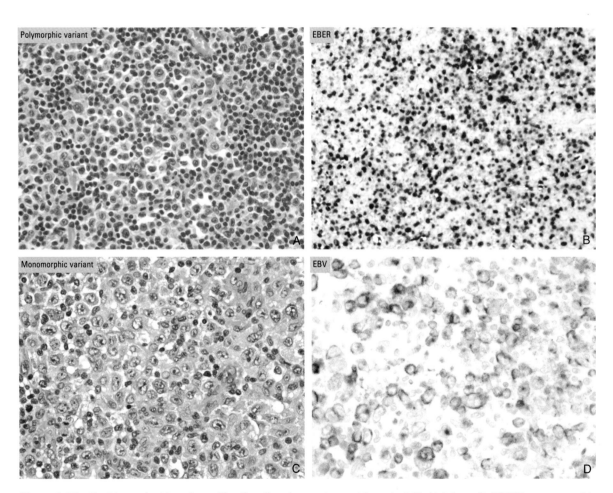

Figure 3.15   Post-transplant lymphoproliferative disorders: polymorphic variant (A, histology; B, EBER); monomorphic variant (C, histology; D, Epstein–Barr virus (EBV) immunohistochemical staining)

HLA-DR is not expressed in acute promyelocytic leukemia (APL). The majority of B-cell lymphoproliferations are HLA-DR[+], whereas most T-cell lymphomas are HLA-DR[−]. In a study by Medeiros *et al.* neither MHC class I (HLA-A, B, C) nor MHC class II (HLA-DR) antigen expression by the lymphomas consistently correlated with patient survival or freedom from relapse[744]. Other studies associate HLA-DR expression with a better prognosis. Darom *et al.* reported that HLA-DR antigen expression was associated with a favorable clinical outcome of gastric large B-cell lymphoma[745]. Miller *et al.*, however, reported that HLA-DR[−] patients with DLBCL had a significantly shorter survival duration compared with HLA-DR[+] patients (0.5 years vs. 2.8 years)[746]. Recent gene profiling studies have suggested that the presence of major histocompatibility complex class II genes (e.g. HLA-DRA) correlates with better survival in DLBCL: the 5-year overall survival was 24% in the lowest 10% of HLA-DRA expression, 37% in the 10–25% group, 50% in the 25–50% group and 55% for patients in the highest 50%[747].

Ki-67 (MIB1)

See Chapter 1 (Cell Proliferation).

Survivin

Survivin is a member of the inhibitor of apoptosis protein (IAP) family. It is expressed in the G_2/M phase, associates with microtubules and is rapidly downregulated after cell cycle arrest. Survivin functions both as an apoptosis inhibitor and as a regulator of cell division, thus linking cell death and cell proliferation. It interferes with the activation of caspases, called the 'cell death executioners'. Survivin is not expressed in mature, fully differentiated tissues, but is expressed in most human cancers (lung, colon, pancreas, prostate and breast)[748]. Survivin is also found in approximately 50% of high-grade NHL, but not in low-grade lymphomas[748]. The overexpression of survivin is associated with an increased recurrence rate and poor prognosis in different human tumors[260,261,305].

Among MCL, survivin is commonly expressed with a nuclear and mitotic pattern, and the level of expression is higher in blastoid MCL variants. Survivin is associated with the proliferative activity, but not with the ploidy status of the tumors[749]. The number of apoptotic cells is independent of survivin or Ki-67 expression. Overall survival was significantly shorter in MCL patients with high survivin expression. However, in a multivariate analysis, the proliferative index was a better predictor of survival than the survivin score. Overexpression of survivin in DLBCL significantly affects prognosis. Immunohistochemistry revealed survivin expression in virtually all tumor cells in 60% of DLBCL[261]. The overall 5-year survival rate was lower in patients with survivin expression than in those without (40% vs. 54%). Multivariate analysis incorporating prognostic factors from the IPI identified survivin expression as an independent predictive parameter on survival in addition to LDH and stage. Survivin expression remained an unfavorable prognostic factor for survival independently of IPI[261]. Survivin is prominently expressed in ATCL[750]. Increased mRNA expression of survivin in ATCL is associated with shorter survival[750]. Survivin is expressed in approximately half the cases of ALCL and independently predicts unfavorable clinical outcome[751].

The prognostic value of survivin expression in AML is not yet well established. Adida *et al.* did not see significant differences in complete remission rates or overall survival between survivin[+] and survivin[−] AML patients using the log-rank test[305]. Also, Carter *et al.* did not identify a correlation between survivin expression, cytogenetics, age, or white blood cell count (WBC), and suggested that levels of survivin expression in AML patients did not have prognostic impact[306].

ZAP-70

ZAP-70 (70-kDa zeta-associated protein), a tyrosine kinase, is a key signaling molecule for T lymphocytes and NK cells. Although it does not normally function in B cells, it is anomalously expressed in CLL cells with unmutated IgV_H genes and may enhance the signaling process when the B-cell receptor is engaged. The expression of ZAP-70 can be effectively measured by flow cytometry assay, in which the intracellular content of ZAP-70 closely correlates with the IgV_H mutational status[752,753].

B-CLL is a heterogeneous disease with a highly variable clinical course. Recent studies have shown that expression of ZAP-70 may serve as a prognostic marker in B-CLL. In aggressive disease, the leukemic cells usually express an unmutated IgV_H gene and ZAP-70, whereas in indolent disease, the leukemic cells usually express mutated IgV_H but lack expression of ZAP-70. Patients positive for ZAP-70 by RT-PCR are characterized by an unfavorable clinical course with a significantly shorter progression-free survival as compared with the ZAP-70-negative patients[754]. Recent comparison between a flow cytometry assay for ZAP-70 and the mutational status of IgV_H genes showed a strong association between the expression of ZAP-70 in B-CLL cells (ZAP-70 level above a defined threshold of 20%) and unmutated IgV_H genes. However, 23% B-CLL shows discordant results (mutated IgV_H and ZAP-70 or unmutated IgV_H and lack of ZAP-70 expression)[755]. The ZAP-70 level as measured by flow cytometry was apparently better than the mutational status at predicting the need for treatment and, in contrast to CD38 level, the ZAP-70 level did not change over time[755]. ZAP-70 is a reliable prognostic marker in B-CLL, similar to that of IgV_H mutational status[753].

ZAP-70 may be positive not only in B-CLL/SLL. Carreras *et al.* reported expression of ZAP-70 in a subset of Burkitt's lymphomas (31%), lymphoblastic lymphoma (29%) as well as rare cases of MCL (8%), marginal zone lymphoma (4%) and DLBCL (2%)[756]. In the same series, immunohistochemistry and flow cytometry gave identical results in 48 of the 52 CLL patients[756].

PART II

Prognostic markers in specific hematologic disorders

CHAPTER 4

Peripheral (mature) B-cell lymphoproliferative disorders

Non-Hodgkin's lymphomas (NHL) are classified into numerous histologic and phenotypic subtypes and generally can be divided into indolent (low grade) and aggressive (high grade). In the B-cell category, low-grade lymphomas include small lymphocytic lymphoma/chronic lymphocytic leukemia (SLL/CLL), follicular lymphoma (FL), marginal zone B-cell lymphoma (MZL) and lymphoplasmacytic lymphoma. High-grade lymphomas comprise diffuse large B-cell lymphoma (DLBCL) and its variants, Burkitt's lymphoma (BL), mediastinal (thymic) large B-cell lymphoma and plasmablastic lymphoma. However, even within the specific category of lymphoma, patients vary considerably with regard to outcome (e.g. in the group of high-grade lymphoma, they can be subdivided further into aggressive, such as DLBCL and very aggressive, such as BL). Some lymphomas, despite lack of cytomorphologic features suggesting high grade, have a particularly poor prognosis when treated with multiagent chemotherapy alone (e.g. B-prolymphocytic leukemia (B-PLL) and mantle cell lymphoma (MCL)). Clinical prognostic factors are mainly a surrogate for disease bulk. Factors that are generally associated with poor prognosis in NHL include (among others) age > 60 years, poor performance status, B symptoms, high stage (bone marrow involvement, three or more extranodal sites), increased levels of serum lactate dehydrogenase (LDH), abdominal mass > 10 cm and transformation from previous low-grade lymphoma. The major prognostic factors in NHL were combined into a prognostic model, the IPI (International Prognostic Index), which recognizes four risk groups with different survival rates (*see* Chapter 1). Although designed for aggressive lymphomas, the IPI proved to be useful for patients with low-grade lymphomas, as well. A separate grading system for follicular lymphoma (FLIPI) was recently proposed[13].

B-CHRONIC LYMPHOCYTIC LEUKEMIA (B-SMALL LYMPHOCYTIC LYMPHOMA)

B-CLL is a low-grade lymphoproliferative disorder of mature (peripheral) lymphoid cells (Figure 4.1). B-CLL is considered a leukemic counterpart of B-SLL, involving lymph nodes. B-CLL shows considerable variations in cytomorphologic, immunophenotypic and prognostic features (Table 4.1). Typical B-CLL, which constitutes approximately 80% of cases, can be defined as having more than 90% small lymphocytes with weak surface immunoglobulin and CD20 expression and co-expression of CD5 and CD23 (Figure 4.1). Atypical B-CLL shows larger lymphocytes with abundant cytoplasm, prolymphocyte-like or cleaved cells and aberrant phenotype. The clinical course of B-CLL is variable and depends on

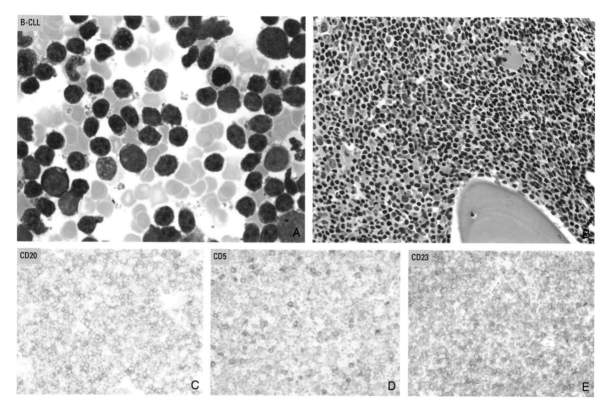

Figure 4.1   B-chronic lymphocytic leukemia, bone marrow. A, aspirate smear; lymphocytosis of small lymphocytes with condensed chromatin; B histology; diffuse small lymphocytic infiltrate; C–E, immunohistochemistry. Leukemic cells express CD20 (C), CD5 (D) and CD23 (E)

Table 4.1   Prognostic factors in B-chronic lymphocytic leukemia

Factor	Prognosis
Binet stage A/Rai stage 0	Favorable
Normal karyotype	Favorable
13q deletion	Favorable
Mutated IgV_H	Favorable
Low levels of IL-6 (<3 pg/ml)	Favorable
Long telomere (Tel-PCR T/S value >0.3)	Favorable
MRD$^-$ status after alemtuzumab or alemtuzumab + fludarabine or stem cell transplantation	Favorable
Binet stage B/Rai stages I–II	Intermediate
Trisomy 12	Intermediate
Discordant ZAP-70 and CD38 results (ZAP-70$^+$/CD38$^-$ or vice versa)	Intermediate
Short lymphocyte doubling time (<12 months)	Poor
CD38 expression ($>30\%$)	Poor
ZAP-70 expression ($>20\%$)	Poor
High β_2-microglobulin levels	Poor
Unmutated IgV_H	Poor
11q deletion	Poor
17p deletion	Very poor
Loss or mutation of the *p53/TP53*	Very poor
Binet stage B-C/Rai stages III–IV	Poor
Diffuse bone marrow involvement	Poor
Atypical cytomorphology/increased prolymphocytes	Poor
Richter's transformation	Poor

IL, interleukin; PCR, polymerase chain reaction

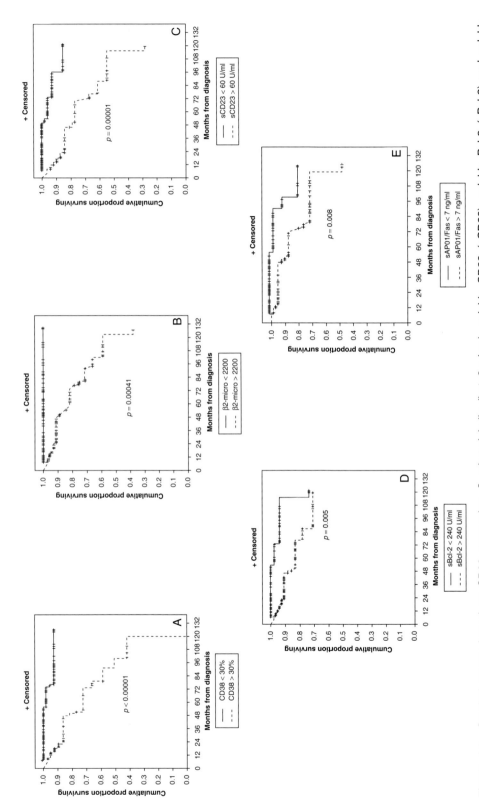

Figure 4.2 Survival curves based on CD38 expression, β_2-microglobulin (beta2-micro), soluble APO1/Fas (sAPO1/Fas) levels. A, Kaplan–Meier plot comparing survival based on the detection of more than 30% CD38$^+$ or less than 30% CD38$^+$ (CD38$^-$) B-CLL cells (>30%, 50 cases; <30%, 118 cases). Less than 30% CD38$^+$ patients experienced a significantly longer survival ($p < 0.00001$). B, B-CLL patients with β_2-microglobulin less than 2200 µg/ml (71 cases) showed a significantly longer survival as compared with patients with β_2-microglobulin more than 2200 µg/ml (94 cases; $p = 0.00041$). None of the patients in the group with β_2-microglobulin less than 2200 µg/ml died during the follow-up period. C, A significantly longer survival ($p = 0.00001$) was found in 83 patients with less than 60 sCD23 U/ml as compared with 84 cases with more than 60 U/ml. D, Seventy-nine patients with more than 240 U/ml sBcl-2 showed a worse outcome ($p = 0.005$) in comparison with 72 cases with less than 240 U/ml sBcl-2. E, Lack of sAPO1/Fas expression identified 93 patients with a longer survival ($p = 0.008$) in comparison with 68 cases with sAPO1/Fas expression

From: Del Poeta G, et al. Clinical significance of CD38 expression in chronic lymphocytic leukemia. Blood 2001;98:2633–9. © 2001 by The American Society of Hematology, used with permission

a number of factors of prognostic relevance; these include clinical factors (age, gender and performance status), laboratory parameters (lymphocyte count, thymidine kinase, soluble CD23, β_2-microglobulin, LDH), morphology (cytologic features, pattern and extent of bone marrow infiltration), genetic markers ($p53$, ATM, IgV_H mutational status) and phenotypic features (surrogate for molecular abnormalities) such as CD38 and ZAP-70 expression. Some patients have aggressive disease and require therapy within a relatively short time after diagnosis, whereas others have indolent, asymptomatic disease and are not likely to benefit from palliative chemotherapy. The median survival of patients with B-CLL is 10 years.

The poor prognostic factors in B-CLL include: an absence of mutations in the variable region of the immunoglobulin heavy-chain gene (unmutated IgV_H gene), ZAP-70 expression, HLA-G expression, 17p deletion, loss or mutation of the $p53$ $(TP53)$ gene, CD38 positivity (in >30% of cells), deletion of chromosome 11q23, increased LDH, high Binet/ Rai stage, advanced age, and atypical morphology[12,434,720,722,757-759]. Figure 4.2 presents survival curves based on CD38 expression, β_2-microglobulin, soluble CD23 (sCD23), soluble Bcl-2 (sBcl-2) and soluble APO1/Fas (sAPO1/Fas) levels. Patients with poor prognostic factors have median survival of approximately 3 years.

Clinical features

Although B-CLL remains incurable with standard treatments, significant improvements in remission rates have been achieved with newer therapeutic approaches, such as the purine analogs (e.g. fludarabine) in combination with monoclonal antibodies and stem cell transplantation[760]. The majority of responses to treatment are partial, and complete responses tend to be transient, with the majority of patients eventually relapsing. The response rate in relapsing or resistant patients is low[761,762]. Achievement of a good quality response to therapy is an independent predictor of prolonged survival. In patients treated with fludarabine, cyclophosphamide and mitoxantrone, parameters associated with a complete response are disease status (e.g. relapsed or resistant), β_2-microglobulin levels and the number of prior treatments[763]. The combination of rituximab and fludarabine or fludarabine-containing regimens has yielded overall response rates of 95%, with complete response rates up to 66% in previously untreated CLL[764].

The duration of survival of patients with B-CLL depends on the stage of the disease at the time of diagnosis. The traditional staging systems for CLL, Rai (0 to IV) and Binet (A–C) (Table 1.2, Chapter 1) are based on anemia and thrombocytopenia and the presence of adenopathy, splenomegaly and hepatomegaly. Both systems divide CLL into low risk (0, A), intermediate risk (I–II, B) and high risk (III–IV, C), with the median survival ranging from 14–15 years for low-risk patients to 2–3 years for high-risk patients. Clinical stage is an important prognostic parameter in B-CLL.

Serum markers (*see also Chapter 1*), reflecting tumor burden (LDH, β_2-microglobulin, CD23) and proliferative potential (thymidine kinase) are important prognostic markers in B-CLL[757,765]. Serum β_2-microglobulin and thymidine kinase independently predict progression-free survival in patients with CLL[766]. The percentage of p53-positive cells and the serum levels of β_2-microglobulin are predictive of survival in CLL patients[758]. The β_2-microglobulin and serum (soluble) CD23 concentrations correlate with CD38+ B-cell percentages[720,767]. In a study by Molica *et al.* the presence of increased serum levels of β_2-microglobulin and CD23, and diffuse bone marrow involvement, were associated with high-risk disease, whereas the absence of any adverse variable was associated with prolonged survival[768]. A high level of soluble CD23 is a strong predictor of progressive disease[769]. Apostolopolous *et al.* reported that the ratio of helper to suppressor T cells (CD4/CD8), the proportion of circulating natural killer (NK) cells and the NK activity were significantly low in clinical stage B and C patients[770]. Among patients presenting with advanced disease, those who subsequently had a more severe course, characterized mainly by frequent respiratory infections, were found to have at presentation a significantly lower CD4/CD8 ratio, a very low proportion of NK cells and decreased amount of gammaglobulins, in comparison with patients with a much milder later course[770].

Recent therapies (stem cell transplantation, purine analogs, immunotherapy with rituximab and alemtuzumab) improved the outcome for patients with B-CLL. In patients treated with fludarabine, the overall response rate was 78% and the median survival was 63 months[771]. More than half the patients who relapsed after fludarabine therapy responded to salvage treatment, usually with fludarabine-based regimens. Patients with B-CLL who have failed to respond to purine analogs have the poorest prognosis, with a median survival of approximately 10 months and

5-year survival of less than 10%[42,771]. Patients who failed on fludarabine can respond to immunotherapy with alemtuzumab (Campath), with some patients achieving minimal residual disease (MRD)-negative remissions[35,53]. In a study by Moreton et al., 50% purine analog-refractory patients responded to alemtuzumab[53]. Detectable CLL was eradicated from the blood and bone marrow in 20% of patients and the median survival was significantly longer in MRD⁻ patients compared with those achieving MRD⁺ complete remission (CR), partial remission or no remission. Overall survival for patients with MRD⁻ remissions was 84% at 60 months[53].

Morphologic features

Patients with atypical B-CLL (Figure 4.3), similarly to B-CLL/PLL have a poorer prognosis, owing to more advanced stage and a higher proliferative fraction[772,773]. In a series published by Matutes et al., CLL with trisomy 12 had a high frequency of either CLL/PLL (31%) or atypical morphology (24%). Atypical morphology and CLL/PLL were even more frequent when trisomy 12 was associated with other chromosomal abnormalities (70% vs. 46%)[772]. Atypical morphology (defined as either >10% prolymphocytes or >15% lymphocytes with cleaved nuclei or lymphoplasmacytoid cells) is an independent poor prognostic factor in B-CLL, especially in Binet stage A disease[774].

Pattern and extent of bone marrow involvement (diffuse vs. non-diffuse; Figure 4.4) have prognostic

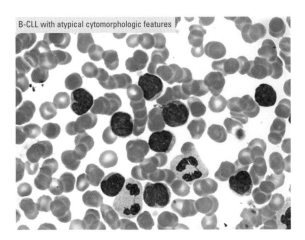

Figure 4.3 B-chronic lymphocytic leukemia (B-CLL) with atypical cytomorphologic features. Note the nuclear irregularities

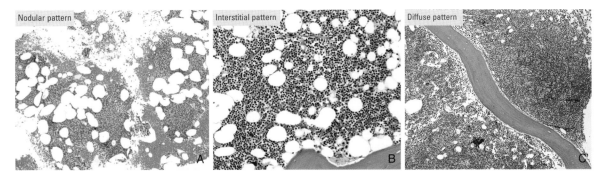

Figure 4.4 B-chronic lymphocytic leukemia (B-CLL), patterns of bone marrow involvement

implications[775], although this is not independent of the staging, and the latter appears to be a better predictive factor of survival probability in B-CLL patients[776]. Patients with >70% marrow involvement before therapy have a significantly shorter time to progression[777]. The extent of bone marrow involvement after chemotherapy does not correlate with the interval between treatment and relapse[777]. B-CLL in CR as defined by National Cancer Institute (NCI) criteria[51] (<30% lymphocytes in the bone marrow with a morphologically normal trephine biopsy) may show up to 5% of leukemic cells persisting in the bone marrow (MRD)[35].

Molecular features

During an immune response, a series of point mutations occurs in the immunoglobulin genes of a B cell. These somatic mutations occur in the germinal centers of the peripheral lymphoid tissue. By sequencing the IgV_H genes, CLL can be divided into two types[719,721]. Approximately 60% of B-CLL can be considered post-germinal center memory B cells with somatically mutated IgV_H, and the remaining cases have IgV_H genes in germline configuration (unmutated IgV_H). In addition, it has been demonstrated that B-CLL having mutated IgV_H genes show a relatively high frequency of BCL6 mutations, further evidence supporting their origin from germinal center-related B cells[778]. Patients with mutated IgV_H genes have a relatively benign condition that is stable or only slowly progressive, with an average survival of 25 years. By contrast, patients with unmutated leukemic cells have aggressive disease and an average survival of 8 years. In pivotal studies, Damle et al.[719] and Hamblin et al.[721] have shown that the presence of unmutated IgV_H genes predicts an inferior survival in CLL. Currently, the unmutated IgV_H gene is one of the strongest predictors of aggressive disease[199,672,719,721,723,779,780]. The median survival of patients with mutated IgV_H genes, unmutated IgV_H genes and loss or mutation of the p53 gene regardless of IgV_H gene status is 310, 119 and 47 months, respectively[672]. Abnormalities of p53 in CLL correlate with aggressive disease and transformation.

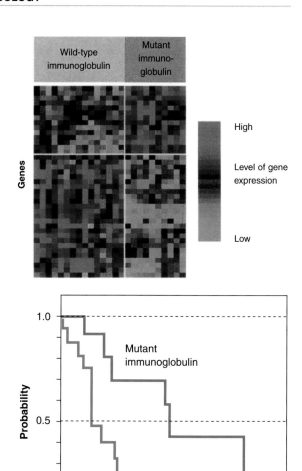

Figure 4.5 B-chronic lymphocytic leukemia. Molecular analysis shows 39 genes differently expressed in two subgroups of B-CLL, one with unmutated (wild-type) immunoglobulin genes (blue) and one with somatically mutated immunoglobulin genes (purple). The Kaplan–Meier curve shows that the two subgroups differ with respect to the time to initial treatment after diagnosis

From: Staudt LM. Molecular diagnosis of the hematologic cancers. NEJM 2003;348:1777–85. © 2003 by Massachusetts Medical Society, used with permission

The incidence of p53 abnormalities in the series published by Thornton et al. was 15%, with a significant difference between untreated patients (7%) and the pretreated/refractory group (50%)[781].

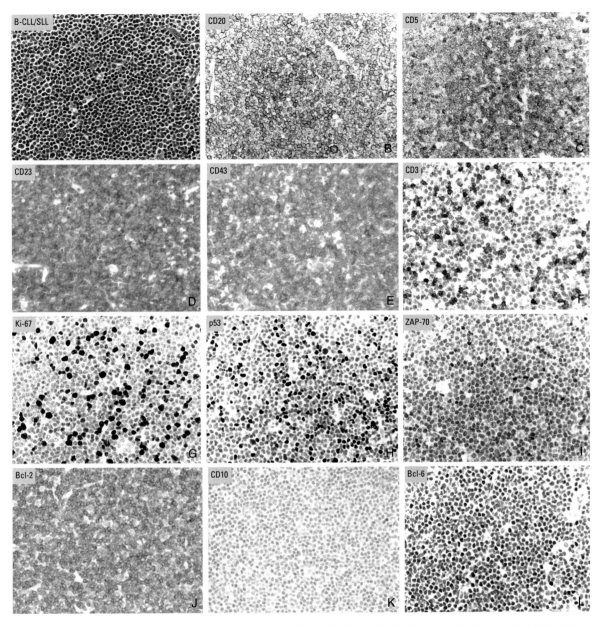

Figure 4.6 Phenotypic features of B-chronic lymphocytic leukemia/small lymphocytic lymphoma (B-CLL/SLL). A, histology; B–L, immunohistochemistry. Leukemic cells are positive for CD20 (B), CD5 (C; compare with CD3 staining, F), CD23 (D), CD43 (E) and Bcl-2 (J). Occasional cases have increased proliferation index determined by Ki-67 (G), over-expression of p53 (H) and aberrant expression of Bcl-6 (L; compare with CD10, K). Expression of ZAP-70 (I) by immuno-histochemistry correlates with that determined by flow cytometry

Abnormal p53 was predicted for shorter survival, regardless of the method used (fluorescence *in situ* hybridization (FISH) or protein expression by flow cytometry). The p53 abnormalities are more common in refractory CLL with mutations occurring at the known 'hot spots'. Testing for *p53* deletions by FISH and flow cytometry is an effective and simple way of screening patients who are likely to have aggressive disease[781]. High-risk genomic aberrations such as 17p– and 11q– occur almost exclusively

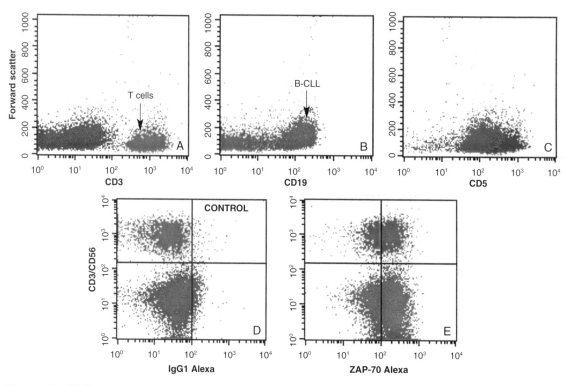

Figure 4.7 ZAP-70 expression (flow cytometry) in B-chronic lymphocytic leukemia (B-CLL) (red, B-CLL; green, T cells)

in the unmutated subgroup, whereas favorable aberrations such as 13q− are overrepresented in the mutated subgroup[723]. Figure 4.5 shows the pattern of expression of 39 genes in two groups of B-CLL (mutated and unmutated IgV_H gene) with their respective Kaplan–Meier survival curves. Quantification of lipoprotein lipase (*LPL*) and metalloproteinase 29 (*ADAM29*) gene expression is a strong (poor) prognostic indicator in CLL, and appears to provide better prognostic assessment than ZAP-70 in advanced stages of disease.

Phenotypic features

Phenotypic feature of B-CLL/SLL are presented in Figure 4.6. Aggressive disease is not always associated with a rearranged IgV_H gene that is unmutated[782,783]. Two subtypes of B-CLL can be distinguished by the differential expression of a small number of genes, one of which encodes ZAP-70, an intracellular tyrosine kinase with a critical role in T-cell receptor

signaling[784]. ZAP-70 is associated with enhanced signaling by the cell-surface immunoglobulin receptor of leukemic B-cells, irrespective of the mutational status of IgV_H[785]. Measurement of ZAP-70 can serve as a surrogate for the mutational status of the IgV_H gene[752,753,755]. ZAP-70 expression correctly predicted IgV_H mutational status in 93% of patients[786]. Quantitative mRNA analysis of ZAP-70 correlates with the results from the DNA microarray analysis, which suggests that the quantitative reverse transcriptase polymerase chain reaction (RT-PCR) assay might be suitable for measuring ZAP-70 expression in a clinical setting[786]. Additionally, ZAP-70 protein expression may be measured by immunohistochemistry (Figure 4.6) and/or flow cytometry (Figure 4.7). The expression of ZAP-70 measured by flow cytometry assay closely correlates with the IgV_H mutational status[752,753,755]. Rassenti *et al.* suggested that the expression of ZAP-70 appeared to be a stronger predictor of the need for treatment in B-CLL than the mutational status of IgV_H[755]. Among the patients with ZAP-70-positive CLL cells, the median time from diagnosis to initial therapy in those who had an unmutated IgV_H gene (2.8 years) was not significantly different from the median time in those who had a mutated IgV_H gene (4.2 years). However, the median time from diagnosis to initial treatment in each of these groups was significantly shorter than the time in patients with ZAP-70-negative CLL cells who had either mutated or unmutated IgV_H genes. The median time from diagnosis to initial therapy among patients who did not have ZAP-70 was 11.0 years in those with a mutated IgV_H gene and 7.1 years in those with an unmutated IgV_H gene[755].

CD38 is a cell-surface enzyme involved in regulating B-cell activation. The percentage of CD38+ B-CLL cells in the unmutated and mutated groups were significantly different[719]. B-CLL with CD38 expression in >30% cells contained unmutated IgV_H genes, whereas samples expressing <30% CD38+ contained mostly mutated genes[719]. The level of CD38+ cells correlates with clinical stage, response to treatment and overall survival; higher CD38 percentages correlate with more advanced Rai stages, poorer chemosensitivity and significantly shorter survival[720]. CD38+ patients respond poorly to continuous multiregimen chemotherapy and have significantly shorter survival[719,721]. The level of expression of CD38 can be determined easily and rapidly by flow cytometry. Despite its correlation with the mutational status of IgV_H, CD38 measurement gives discordant results in about 30% of cases, and its levels may vary during the course of disease; therefore a more specific surrogate marker is needed. Nuckel *et al.* reported that the expression of human leukocyte antigen G (HLA-G) was associated with an unfavorable prognosis and immunodeficiency in B-CLL[787]. Multivariate analyses showed that CD38 expression is an important prognostic factor associated with a high incidence of lymph node involvement, lower hemoglobin level, hepatomegaly, and high β_2-microglobulin and soluble CD23 levels[720,767]. Survival curves for patients with B-CLL in regard to phenotypic markers and mutational status of IgV_H genes are presented in Figures 4.8 and 4.9.

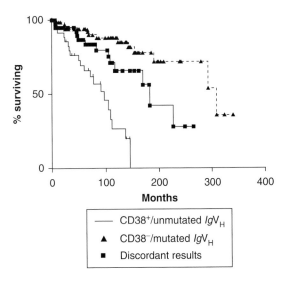

Figure 4.8 Survival curves for 145 patients with B-chronic lymphocytic leukemia (B-CLL) from date of diagnosis, comparing patients whose cells are CD38+ with unmutated IgV_H genes ($n=34$) with those whose cells are CD38− with mutated IgV_H genes ($n=70$) and those whose cells gave discordant results for the two assays ($n=41$)

From: Hamblin TJ, *et al.* CD38 expression and immunoglobulin variable region mutations are independent prognostic variables in chronic lymphocytic leukemia, but CD38 expression may vary during the course of the disease. Blood 2002;99:1023–9. © 2002 by The American Society of Hematology, used with permission

In univariate analysis, age, clinical stage, IgM-fluorescence intensity, CD23 and FMC7 had significant prognostic importance, with high IgM-fluorescence intensity, high FMC7 and low CD23 expression being associated with a short survival and in Cox multiple regression analyses, age, CD23, IgM-fluorescence intensity, and clinical stage had independent prognostic importance[788].

Chromosomal aberrations

Genomic aberrations in CLL are important independent predictors of disease progression and survival. Chromosomal abnormalities are detected in 90% of B-CLL patients using FISH methodology. The most frequent abnormalities include del(13q), trisomy 12, del(11q), del(14q) and del(6q)[458,672,789]. Patients

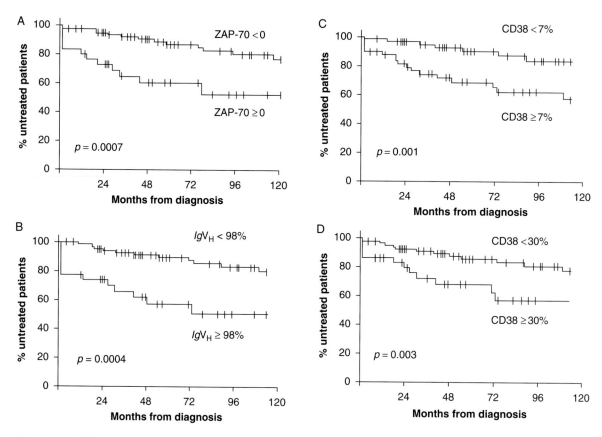

Figure 4.9 Effect of prognostic features on the clinical course of chronic lymphocytic leukemia (CLL). Rate of disease progression as assessed by the treatment-free time interval measured in months from diagnosis for *ZAP-70* mRNA expression (A), *IgV*$_H$ mutation status (B), CD38 protein expression with cut-off of 7%; (C) and CD38 protein expression with cut-off of 30% (D)

From: Wiestner A, *et al.* ZAP-70 expression identifies a chronic lymphocytic leukemia subtype with unmutated immuno-globulin genes, inferior clinical outcome, and distinct gene expression profile. Blood 2003;101:4944–51. © 2003 by The American Society of Hematology, used with permission

with normal karyotype or deletion of 13q14 as the sole genetic abnormality have a better prognosis than those with a complex karyotype or deletion of 11q23 or 17p13. The patients with a deletion of 13q14 (Figure 4.10) as a single aberration have the longest estimated median treatment-free interval and survival time[430,434,790]. The estimated median survival time of this group was longer as compared with the groups without detectable aberrations and the group with trisomy 12. Deletions of 13q are associated with typical morphologic and phenotypic features[791–794].

Deletion of 11q22–q23 and deletion of 17p13 are independent prognostic markers in multivariate

analysis identifying subgroups of patients with rapid disease progression and short survival times[430,672,795–797]. Aberrations of 11q identify a subset of B-CLL with extensive adenopathy, rapid disease progression and inferior survival. The pathogenic role of 17p13 deletions is associated with the location of the tumor suppressor gene *p53 (TP53)*. *p53* abnormalities predict poor survival and treatment resistance[603,657]. Deletions of *p53* have been reported to occur in B-CLL showing disease progression and atypical morphologic and immunophenotypic features[656], although in one series 17p deletions showed an equal distribution between typical

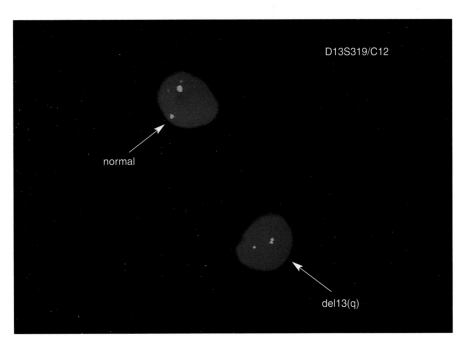

Figure 4.10   B-chronic lymphocytic leukemia with del(13q); FISH analysis

and atypical cases independent of clinical stage[792]. The presence of *p53* mutation or del(17q) (p13.1) predicts a poor response to conventional therapy in chronic lymphocytic leukemia[660]. Alemtuzumab may be an effective initial therapy for patients with *p53* mutations or del(17q)(p13.1) or both, as opposed to fludarabine, chlorambucil or rituximab[660].

FISH studies show a similar pattern of chromosomal gains and losses detected in typical and atypical B-CLL[792], but trisomy 12 was associated with atypical variant of B-CLL[774,798–800]. In most studies, patients with trisomy 12q13 have atypical morphology and immunophenotype, a diffuse bone marrow infiltration pattern and/or lymphocyte doubling time below 12 months, elevated serum β_2-microglobulin levels and shorter survival times than patients with a normal karyotype or 13q deletions[434,790,801]. Geisler *et al.*, however, did not show prognostic significance of an additional copy of chromosome 12 alone or its relationship to atypical morphology[444]. Also, evaluation of the prognostic impact of trisomy 12 by FISH did not reveal a significant difference in survival between patients with or without trisomy 12[434,444,796,802,803].

In patients with an atypical CLL immunophenotype, chromosome abnormalities, including trisomy 12 with complex karyotype, 14q+, del(6q) and chromosome 17 abnormalities, are found in about 50% of the patients, and in particular chromosome 17 abnormalities suggest a poor prognosis[444]. The response rate to chemotherapy is significantly higher in patients with normal karyotypes than in those with abnormal karyotypes, especially with complex changes (Figure 4.11). In a series by Dohner *et al.*, five categories were defined. The median survival times for patients with 17p deletion, 11q deletion, 12q trisomy, normal karyotype and 13q deletion as the sole abnormality were 32, 79, 114, 111 and 133 months, respectively[434]. Patients in the 17p− and 11q− deletion groups had more advanced disease than those in the other three groups. Patients with 17p deletions had the shortest median treatment-free interval (9 months), and those with 13q deletions had the longest (92 months)[434]. The response to rituximab was noted to vary by cytogenetic group: del(17)(p13.1), 0%; del(11)(q22.3), 66%; del(13) (q14.3), 86%; +12, 25%; and normal, 0%[445].

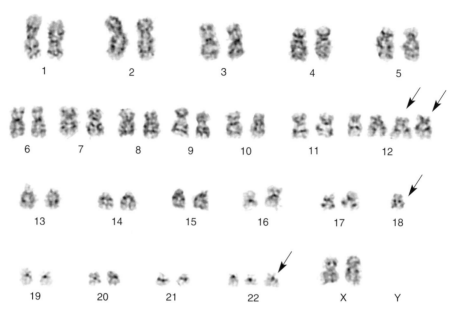

Figure 4.11   B-chronic lymphocytic leukemia with clonal evolution. Complex chromosomal abnormalities: 48,XX, +12, +12, −18, +22

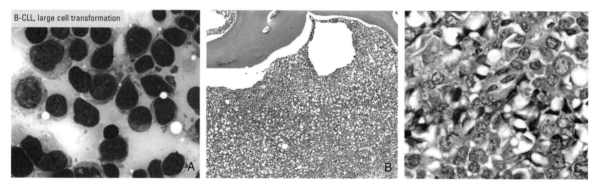

Figure 4.12   B-chronic lymphocytic leukemia (B-CLL) large cell transformation (Richter's syndrome), bone marrow. A, aspirate smear; B–C, histology

Disease progression

Transformation of B-CLL (Figures 4.12, 4.13 and 4.14) to more aggressive disease occurs in 5–10% of patients. Clinical and laboratory features observed in patients with transformation include generalized adenopathy, systemic symptoms (fever, weight loss, worsened performance status), cytopenia (anemia and/or thrombocytopenia), increased LDH level, hypercalcemia and monoclonal gammopathy[804]. Morphological progression of B-CLL/SLL is

represented by prolymphocytic transformation[805,806], paraimmunoblastic variant[807], Hodgkin's lymphoma (HL)[808–812], DLBCL[740,789,813–816] and precursor B-lymphoblastic lymphoma/leukemia (B-ALL)[817]. B-CLL can also be complicated by classical HL, which may be considered a variant of Richter's syndrome. Progression of B-CLL/SLL to DLBCL, which is frequently referred to as Richter's transformation, can present as a localized enlargement of a single lymph node histologically showing DLBCL or increasing generalized adenopathy with rapid

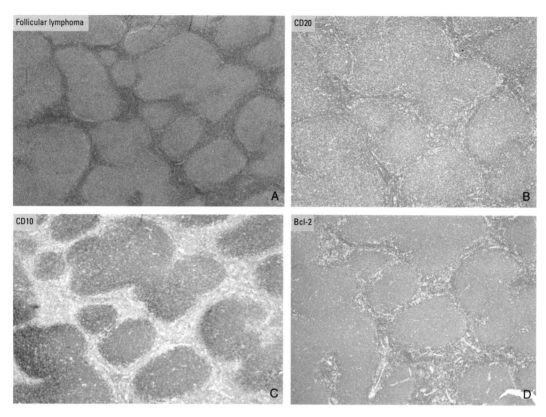

Figure 4.19   Follicular lymphoma, lymph node. A, histology; B–D, immunohistochemistry. Lymph node section shows distinct nodular architecture (A). Lymphomatous cells are positive for CD20 (B), CD10 (C) and Bcl-2 (D)

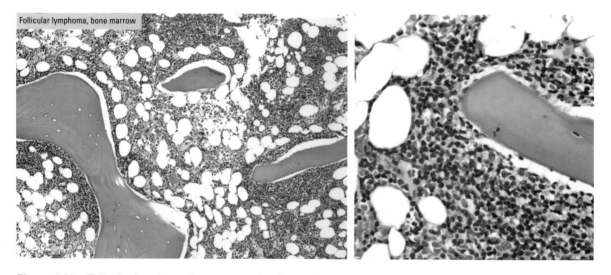

Figure 4.20   Follicular lymphoma, bone marrow involvement

and eventually die of disease-related causes[839,840]. The major independent prognostic factors include age and serum LDH levels. Adverse prognostic factors in FL include age >60 years, Ann Arbor stage III–IV, hemoglobin level <120 g/l, B symptoms, hepatosplenomegaly, bulky disease, number of nodal areas >4, high number of extranodal involvement sites, high serum β_2-microglobulin level, poor performance status, high erythrocyte sedimentation rate and high serum LDH level[6,13,125,181,841–847].

In selected stage I and II follicular NHL patients, deferred therapy is an acceptable approach; more than half of the patients in the series reported by Advani *et al.* remained untreated at a median of 6 or more years, and survival was comparable to that seen in reports with immediate treatment[848]. Allogeneic bone marrow transplant results in long-term disease-free survival for approximately 50% of patients with advanced FL[849]. The influence of bone marrow biopsy histology on prognosis and management of FL remains controversial. Extensive bone marrow involvement, however, is a significant predictor of poor survival in patients with grade 1 and 2 FL[850].

The survival rate is higher in extranodal FL than in nodal FL. Patients with primary cutaneous FL have a more favorable long-term prognosis than those with equivalent nodal disease[851]. FL in non-cutaneous extranodal sites have similarly favorable outcome[852]. The majority of extranodal FL do not harbor t(14;18)[851,852]. In FL of the gastrointestinal tract, the estimated 5-year disease-free survival was 62%, and the median disease-free survival was 69 months[853]. Figure 4.21 presents histomorphologic features of extranodal FL.

Prognostic index

Different prognostic scores have been proposed to predict the outcome of FL patients at diagnosis. The IPI, originally designed for aggressive lymphomas, is an important factor in predicting survival and response to treatment in low-grade lymphomas, including FL[6–11,190]. Because some important prognostic factors applied to low-grade lymphomas are not included in the IPI, and only a few patients with FL are classified in the poor-risk category when using the IPI, a new prognostic index for FL was proposed[13]. The Follicular Lymphoma International Prognostic Index (FLIPI) includes five variables associated with adverse prognosis: age (>60 years vs. ≤60 years); Ann Arbor stage (III–IV vs. I–II); hemoglobin level (<120 g/l vs. ≥120 g/l); number of nodal areas (>4 vs. ≤4); and serum LDH level (above normal vs. normal or below). Three risk groups can be identified based on the FLIPI index: low risk (0–1 adverse factor); intermediate risk (2 factors); and poor risk (≥3 adverse factors). The FLIPI appears more discriminant than the IPI proposed for aggressive NHL[13]. The FLIPI is also useful in patients with FL progression. Five-year survival from progression (SFP) was 55% (95% confidence interval 44–66%). The distribution according to the FLIPI at relapse was 39% good prognosis, 24% intermediate prognosis and 37% poor prognosis. Five-year SFP for these groups was 85%, 79% and 28%, respectively. Other variables at relapse with prognostic significance for SFP were age, presence of B symptoms, performance status, bulky disease and number of involved nodal sites, LDH, hemoglobin level, histological transformation and the IPI for aggressive lymphomas. In the multivariate analysis, bulky disease, B symptoms and FLIPI at relapse were the most important variables for predicting 5-year survival from progression. In patients with FL at first relapse/progression, the FLIPI, along with the presence of bulky disease and B symptoms, are features that predict 5-year survival from progression[14].

Morphologic and phenotypic features

The clinical usefulness of histologic grading in FL is controversial, mostly due to the subjective nature and poor reproducibility of most systems in current use. Based on the absolute number of centroblasts in ten neoplastic follicles evaluated under a 40× high-power microscopic field (hpf), FL is divided into grade 1 (0–5 centroblasts/hpf), grade 2 (6–15 centroblasts/hpf) and grade 3 (>15 centroblasts/hpf)

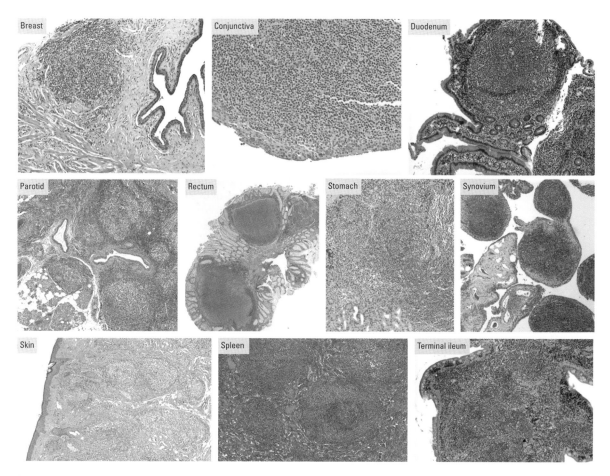

Figure 4.21   Follicular lymphoma, extranodal

(Figures 4.22, 4.23 and 4.24). Based on the presence of centrocytes, grade 3 FL is further subdivided into 3a (centrocytes present) and 3b (no centrocytes). Although the majority of studies show a significantly more aggressive clinical course for FL grade 3[190–192], the survival of patients treated with current protocols as for aggressive lymphoma is similar to that of grade 1 and 2[194,195]. Generally, grades 1, 2 and 3a FL are considered to belong to a spectrum of indolent lymphomas, in contrast to grade 3b FL or FL with extensive diffuse areas of large cells, which behave more like DLBCL. In some reports, however, there were no significant differences in overall survival or event-free survival between FL grades 3a and

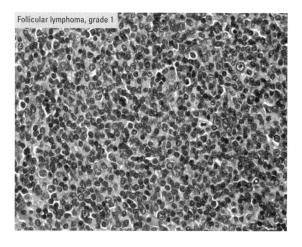

Figure 4.22   Follicular lymphoma, grade 1

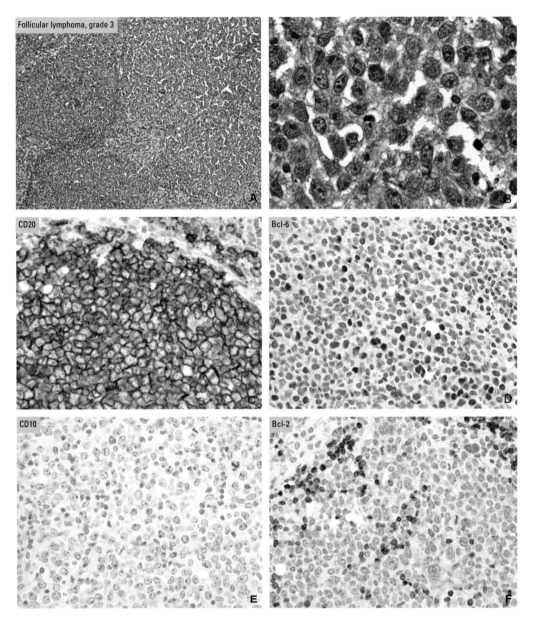

Figure 4.23 Follicular lymphoma, grade 3. A–B, histology; C–F, immunohistochemistry. Lymph node with distinct nodular pattern (A). Lymphomatous cells are large with nucleoli and occasional mitoses (B). They are positive for both CD20 (C) and Bcl-6 (D) and negative for both CD10 (E) and Bcl-2 (F)

3b[194,854,855]. Classical banding cytogenetic studies suggested that follicular lymphomas grade 3 with preserved maturation to centrocytes (FL 3a) are closely related to FL grades 1 and 2 and frequently harbor the t(14;18), whereas FL grade 3b, consisting of centroblasts exclusively, frequently show 3q27 alterations[856]. The measurement of cellular proliferation does not appear to add additional prognostic information in FL[190,857]. However, in more recent studies, proliferation measured by Ki-67 (MIB1)

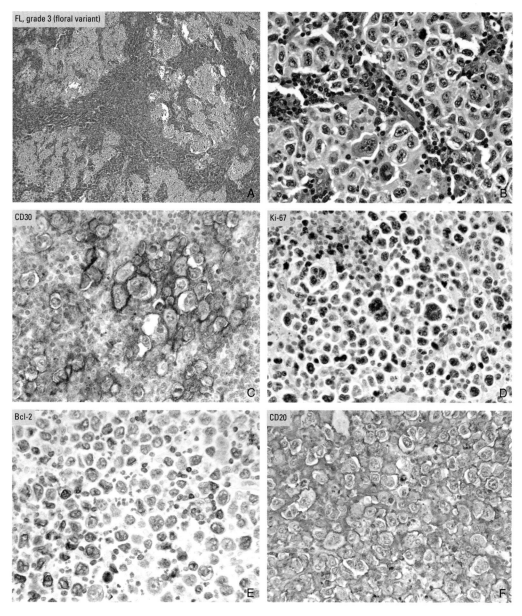

Figure 4.24   Follicular lymphoma, grade 3 (floral variant). A–B, histology; C–F, immunohistochemistry. Lymph node shows irregular nodules composed of large pleomorphic cells (A–B). The lymphomatous cells express CD30 (C), Ki-67 (D), Bcl-2 (E) and CD20 (F)

correlated with disease-free survival in patients treated with chemotherapy and interferon-α or chemotherapy and rituximab[246,327]. The growth pattern has hardly any influence on survival as long as more than 50% of the lymphoma exhibits a follicular pattern[201].

FL cases with a predominant diffuse component (>50% diffuse areas of large cells) have a significantly worse overall survival and event-free survival[854]. Patients with CD10+ tumors and high levels of Bcl-6 expression have favorable overall survival,

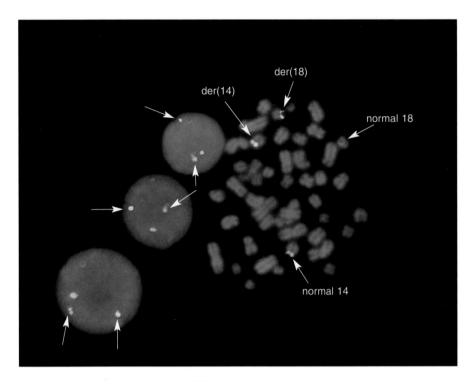

Figure 4.25   Follicular lymphoma with t(14;18); FISH analysis

disease-specific survival and time to treatment failure compared with patients with low levels of Bcl-6 expression and lack of CD10[681].

Chromosomal aberrations

The majority of FL have t(14;18) (q32;q21) translocation (Figures 4.25 and 4.26), which occurs in 80–90% of cases[407,858]. FL without t(14;18) (q32;q21) and with *BCL6* rearrangement are usually characterized by prominent nodal architecture, a monocytoid component and lack of CD10 and Bcl-2 expression, but there are no significant differences regarding age, performance status, bone marrow involvement or overall survival when compared with FL with t(14;18)[684].

The presence of an isolated t(14;18) is uncommon in FL. The majority of cases display evidence of secondary chromosomal alterations at initial diagnosis[859]. Recurrent alterations seen at the 10% or greater level include: +X, +1q21-q44, +7, +12q, +18q, del(1)(p36), del(6q) (Figure 4.27), del(10)(q22–q24), and the development of polyploidy. Changes that correlate with morphologic progression include: del(1)(p36), del(6q), del(10)(q22–q24), +7, and the presence of polyploidy[859]. Patients with abnormalities of chromosome region 1p21–22, 6q23–26 or the short arm of chromosome 17 had a significantly shorter survival in univariate analysis[407]. Multivariate analysis identified a break at 6q23–26 and 17p as independent prognostic factors. The risk of transformation into a DLBCL is significantly higher in patients with either a 6q23–26 or a 17p abnormality. FL with del(17p) and +12 have an adverse clinical outcome[443]. Unfavorable overall survival is associated also with del(1)(p36) and dup(18q)[860]. Chromosomal analysis of FL at the time of diagnosis can provide important information about the risk of transformation and survival[407].

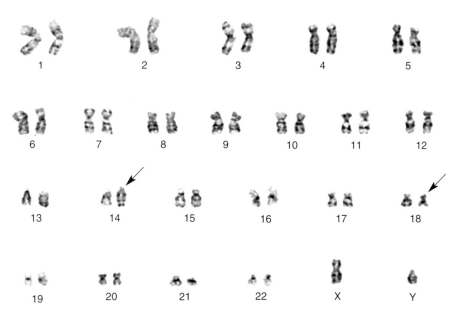

Figure 4.26   Follicular lymphoma with t(14;18), routine cytogenetic analysis

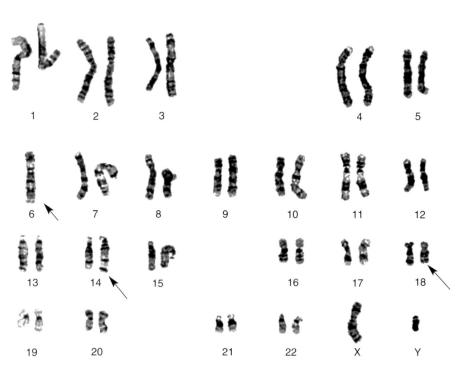

Figure 4.27   Follicular lymphoma with t(14;18) and additional deletion of chromosome 6

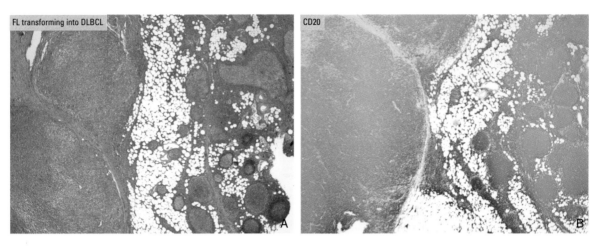

Figure 4.28 Follicular lymphoma (FL) with transformation into diffuse large B-cell lymphoma (DLBCL). A, Nodular and diffuse lymphoid infiltrate. B, Both components are positive for CD20

In a series reported by Zhao *et al.*, the *BCLxL* gene (a member of the *BCL2* family) level correlated with the number of apoptotic lymphoma cells, and high *BCLxL* level was significantly associated with multiple sites of extranodal involvement, elevated LDH level, high-risk IPI and short overall survival times[278]. There is no correlation between numbers of circulating t(14;18)-positive cells and response to first-line treatment in FL[54]. The cellular proliferation index does not appear to influence the survival rate of patients with FL[190].

Transformation

Morphologic progression of FL into higher-grade tumors occurs often (25–80%) and takes the form of increased number of centroblasts (progression from FL grade 1 into FL grade 2 and/or 3), DLBCL (Figure 4.28)[201,861–865] or less often blastic transformation in the form of Burkitt's lymphoma or precursor B-lymphoblastic lymphoma/leukemia (Figure 1.18; Chapter 1) with or without terminal deoxynucleotidyl transferase (TdT) expression[866–869]. Progression of FL is often accompanied by a spectrum of morphologic changes and an aggressive clinical behavior. The transformation is commonly associated with accumulation of secondary genetic alterations, which include wide genetic instability[870], non-random chromosomal

changes[860,871–873], c-*MYC* gene rearrangement[866,874–876], *p53* tumor suppressor gene mutations[209,210], somatic mutations of the translocated *BCL2* gene[203,877] and somatic mutations of the *BCL6* gene[870,875,878]. *BCL6* gene mutations accumulate during the transformation process and may deregulate Bcl-6 mRNA, but an increase in Bcl-6 mRNA expression is not uniformly required for transformation from FL to DLBCL[878]. A subset of patients with histologic transformation from low-grade FL to intermediate- or high-grade lymphoma have relatively long-term survival; patients with limited disease and no previous exposure to chemotherapy have a favorable prognosis[839]. Progression of FL to a higher-grade malignancy is often associated with treatment failure and frequently heralds a poor prognosis[839,863,879,880]. Growth fraction, as assessed by Ki-67 staining, and Trump expression (transferrin-receptor-related protein) correlates with histologic grade but not with recurrence or progression of FL[881]. Abnormalities of chromosome 8q24 are associated with a blastic variant of FL[882,883].

MANTLE CELL LYMPHOMA

MCL (Figures 4.29 and 4.30) is an aggressive lymphoma characterized by monomorphic-appearing cells with irregular, indented nuclei, distinct immunophenotypic profile (CD5[+]/CD20[+]/CD23[-]/CD43[+]) and overexpression of cyclin D1 (Bcl-1) due to juxtaposition of the *BCL1* locus (the *CCND1* gene coding for cyclin D1) to *IgH* gene [t(11;14)(q13;q32)]. Patients usually present with generalized lymphadenopathy. Bone marrow involvement is observed in 50–80%, hepatosplenomegaly in 30–60%, B symptoms in 50% and extranodal involvement in 20% of patients[201,249,884,885]. Genome-wide array-based comparative genomic hybridization revealed additional chromosomal imbalances in MCL (−1p, −6q, −11q, −13q, −20p12.1–12.3, −22q12.1–12.3, +3q, +4p12–13, +8q)[886].

MCL exhibits the worst prognosis among B-cell lymphomas of small lymphocytes (including B-SLL/CLL, FL, MZL and lymphoplasmacytic lymphoma). Most patients are diagnosed with advanced stage III/IV disease. The median survival is 32–48 months[249,884] and 5-year survival is less than 10%[885]. In patients younger than 65 years, a dose-intensive consolidation comprising high-dose radiochemotherapy, immunochemotherapy and autologous stem cell transplantation after a CHOP-like induction results in an improved progression-free survival[887,888]. However, relapses are still observed at a high frequency. The addition of rituximab to transplantation protocols appears to be a very promising strategy for patients with relapsed MCL after autologous stem cell transplantation[889,890].

Parameters associated with poor prognosis or shorter survival include poor performance status, splenomegaly, B symptoms, leukocyte count $> 10 \times 10^9$/l, high LDH level, blastic variant and high/intermediate- or high-risk IPI[249]. Stage IV, high/intermediate- or high-risk IPI and increased LDH level are associated with a lower response rate to chemotherapy[249]. However, the value of the IPI in MCL is not well established, partly because most of the patients are within high-risk categories. In a series by Raty *et al.*, high Ki-67 expression, Ann Arbor stage III–IV and age over 60 years had an independent influence on survival in a multivariate analysis, whereas serum LDH, the number of extranodal sites and performance status did not[15].

The most common chromosomal aberration in MCL is 13q14 deletion followed by 17p deletion and +12. Trisomy 12 is the only single cytogenetic parameter predictive of a poor outcome[456]. A complex karyotype (Figure 4.31) is associated with a poor prognosis in MCL[456]. Although both leukemic and nodal MCL show similar genomic patterns of losses (involving 6q, 11q22–q23, 13q14 and 17p13) and gains (affecting 3q and 8q), genomic loss of chromosome 8p occurs more frequently in patients with leukemic disease[891]. This indicates the presence of a novel tumor suppressor gene locus on 8p, whose deletion may be associated with leukemic dissemination.

Morphologic progression of MCL is associated with an increase in large blastoid cells, resulting in the so-called blastoid variant[892,893]. The blastoid variant of MCL is a very aggressive subtype of lymphoma with median overall survival of 14.5 months as compared with 53 months for patients with a common form of MCL[892,894]. A subset of blastoid variants of MCL may have *p53* gene mutations[211]. Additionally, blastoid MCL subtypes are characterized by distinctly elevated mitotic counts (51/10 vs. 21/10 high-power fields in common MCL), proliferation indices (53% vs. 27% in common MCL), frequent *BCL1* rearrangements at the major translocation cluster locus (59% vs. 40%), and overexpression of p53 (21% vs. 6%)[379]. Blastoid MCL subtypes display a tendency to have a tetraploid number of chromosomes (36% of lymphoblastoid and 80% of pleomorphic types vs. 8% of common variants), a feature clearly separating these neoplasms from other types of B-cell NHL and possibly being related to cyclin D1 (Bcl-1) overexpression[379]. Comparative genomic hybridization (CGH) analysis showed an increased number of chromosome imbalances, being associated with blastoid variants of MCL (e.g. gains of 3q, 7p and 12q, and losses of 17p), which may have prognostic significance[895]. CGH losses of 17p correlated with *p53* gene deletions and mutations. Leukocytosis, an elevated LDH level and a high

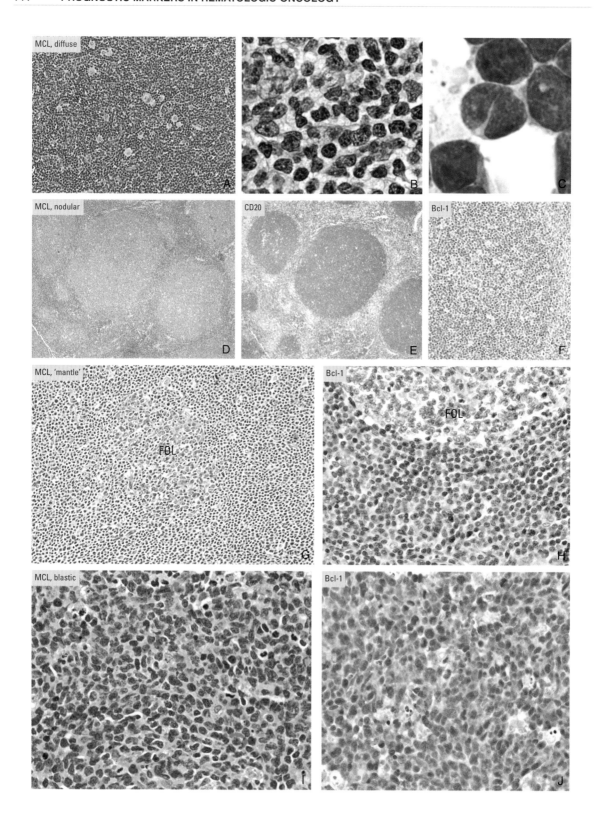

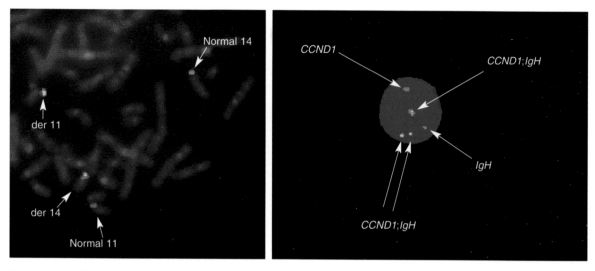

Figure 4.30 Translocation t(11;14)/*CCND1-IgH* (FISH analysis)

proliferative activity at diagnosis as assessed by the mitotic count and Ki-67 index are associated with an increased risk of blastoid transformation, and elevated serum LDH and blood leukocytosis with a short time interval to transformation[896]. Loss of expression and/or deletions of the *p21*[WAF1] and *p16*[INK4a] genes (cyclin-dependent kinase inhibitors suggested as candidates for tumor suppressor genes) are detected in aggressive MCL but not in the typical variants. The *p21*[WAF1] and *p16*[INK4a] alterations occur in a subset of tumors with a wild-type *p53* gene[897]. Deletions of the *INK4a/ARF* gene locus are found in up to 30% of MCL and are associated with poor prognosis[897,898]. Figure 4.32 shows the use of the proliferation gene-expression signature to predict the length of survival in patients with MCL.

LYMPHOPLASMACYTIC LYMPHOMA/WALDENSTRÖM'S MACROGLOBULINEMIA

Lymphoplasmacytic lymphoma is a low-grade lymphoma characterized by a mixture of small lymphocytes, lymphocytes with plasmacytoid features and plasma cells (Figure 4.33). Occasional cells display intranuclear inclusions (Dutcher bodies). In most patients, adenopathy develops slowly over many years. Extranodal sites may be involved as well, although most of these cases represent marginal zone B-cell lymphoma with plasmacytic differentiation. The overall survival is lower than in other low-grade B-cell lymphoproliferations (excluding MCL)[899,900]. Lymphoplasmacytic lymphoma is characterized

Figure 4.29 Mantle cell lymphoma (MCL), morphologic variants. A–C, MCL, diffuse pattern. Note typical presence of scattered histiocytes (A). Lymphoma cells are irregular (B, histology) with cleaved nuclei (C, touch smear). D–F, MCL, nodular pattern (D, histology; B–C, immunohistochemistry). Lymphomatous cells express CD20 (E) and cyclin D1/Bcl-1 (F). G–H, MCL, mantle zone pattern (G, histology; H, Bcl-1 staining by immunohistochemistry). Lymphomatous cells surround residual follicle (FOL), better visualized by immunohistochemical staining for cyclin D1/Bcl-1 (H). I–J, MCL, blastic variant. Highly atypical tumor cells (I) express cyclin D1/Bcl-1 (J)

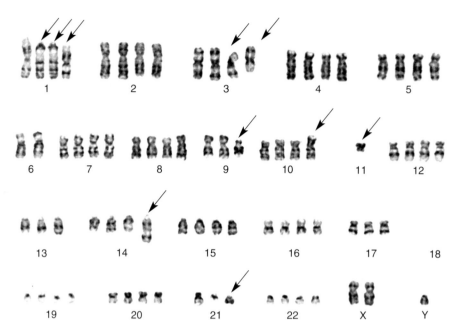

Figure 4.31   Mantle cell lymphoma with complex chromosomal abnormalities (near-tetraploid cells with t(11;14), +21, XXY); cytogenetic analysis

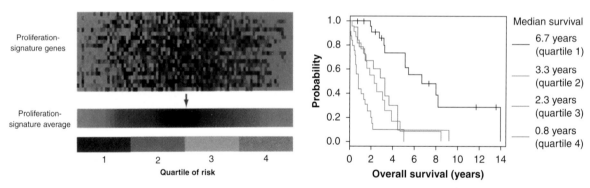

Figure 4.32   Mantle cell lymphoma (MCL). The panel shows the use of the proliferation gene-expression signature to predict the length of survival in patients with MCL. Elevated levels of expression of genes in the proliferation gene-expression signature in a biopsy specimen of MCL was associated with short survival. The relative level of expression of the proliferation-signature genes is represented by the color bars; the biopsy samples are ordered from left to right according to the increasing relative expression of the proliferation-signature genes. The levels of expression of 20 signature genes were averaged, and the resulting average was used to subdivide patients with MCL into four quartiles. The Kaplan–Meier plot illustrates the striking differences in the length of survival among these four risk groups

From: Staudt LM. Molecular diagnosis of the hematologic cancers. N Engl J Med 2003;348:1777–84. © 2003 Massachusetts Medical Society, used with permission

by t(9;14)(p13;q32) in 50% of patients. This translocation involves the *PAX5* gene on chromosome 9, which encodes a B-cell-specific transcription factor involved in the control of B-cell proliferation and differentiation. Figure 4.34 shows lymphoplasmacytic lymphoma with complex chromosomal aberrations including t(9;14). The presence of abnormal cytogenetic findings [e.g. −8; del(6q)] correlate with poor

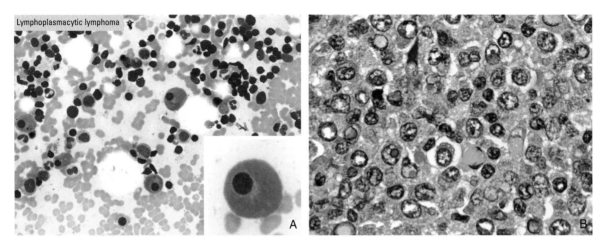

Figure 4.33 Lymphoplasmacytic lymphoma, bone marrow. A, aspirate smear with mixed population of lymphocytes and plasma cells (inset: 'flame cell'); B, histology with atypical lymphoplasmacytic infiltrate. Dutcher bodies (intranuclear inclusions) are present

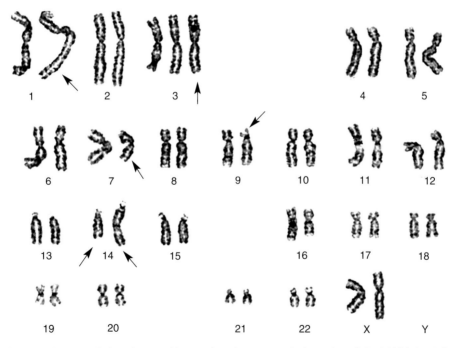

Figure 4.34 Lymphoplasmacytic lymphoma with complex chromosomal aberrations [+3, del(7)(q22q34), del(14)(q32), t(9;14)]

prognosis in lymphoplasmacytic lymphoma[901]. Lack of IgH translocations differentiates Waldenström's macroglobulinemia from multiple myeloma and many lymphomas including FL, MCL and DLBCL.

About 4–15% of lymphoplasmacytic lymphomas show transformation into a DLBCL[900].

Waldenström's macroglobulinemia is a B-cell lymphoproliferative disorder characterized by high

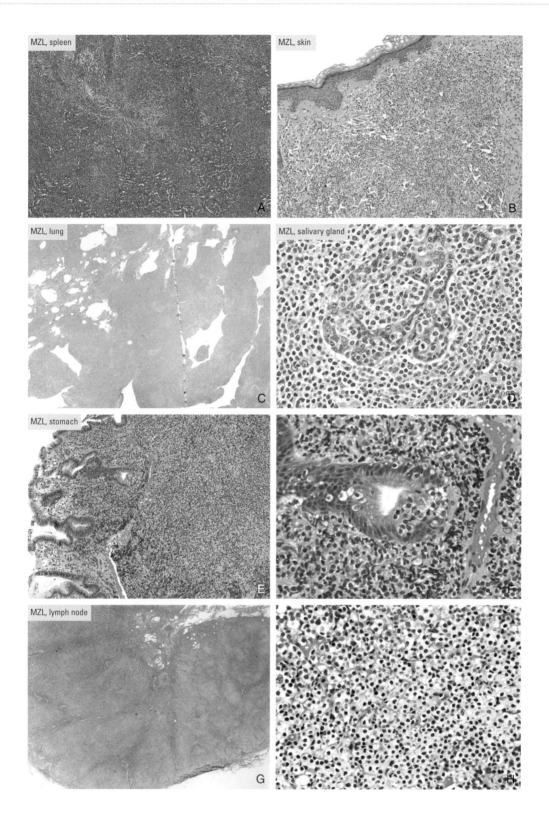

serum immunoglobulin M paraprotein and the accumulation of clonal lymphoplasmacytic cells in the bone marrow. With advancing disease, patients may acquire organomegaly, anemia and hyperviscosity. Waldenström's macroglobulinemia does not have the t(9;14)(p13;q32) translocation but often has deletions of 6q21[902]. Waldenström's macroglobulinemia has a chronic, indolent course with a highly variable prognosis. The median survival ranges from 5 to 6 years[16,130,131,903,904]. The median age is 66 years, and the 5-year overall survival is 72%[905]. Some of the pretreatment parameters, including older age, male sex, general symptoms and cytopenias, carry a poor prognosis in Waldenström's macroglobulinemia[903]. By contrast, high initial tumor burden (indicated by organomegaly, high IgM level and high percentage of marrow lymphoid cells) does not seem to be significantly associated with short survival[903]. In the multivariate analysis, age, hemoglobin level, serum β_2-microglobulin level, performance status, multiple cytopenias and serum albumin predict survival and are capable of stratifying patients with different therapeutic needs[16,130]. Advanced age, serum β_2-microglobulin level of ≥ 3 mg/l and hemoglobin level of < 120 g/l are adverse prognostic factors[131,906]. The prognostic value of a high level of a monoclonal component remains controversial[906]. Stratification of patients according to the IPI has limited value[16]. The second malignancy in patients with Waldenström's macroglobulinemia is observed in 10%, histological transformation in 3% and rapid rise of the M component in 6% of patients[905].

MARGINAL ZONE B-CELL LYMPHOMA

MZL is a low-grade B-cell lymphoma that can involve the spleen (SMZL), lymph nodes (nodal MZL) and extranodal sites (MALT lymphoma). Histomorphologic features of MZL are presented in Figure 4.35.

Splenic marginal zone lymphoma

SMZL is a disease of the elderly, with median age at presentation of 65 years[907]. SMZL is considered to be an indolent extranodal B-cell lymphoma, with reported survival of 78% at 5 years[213,908]. Prognostic factors are poorly defined and only loss or mutation of the p53 (TP53) gene is consistently associated with a poor outcome[214]. Other prognostic factors include lack of response to therapy, involvement of non-hematopoietic sites and bone marrow[909], age >70 years, hemoglobin level < 11 g/dl, lymphocytes $> 16 \times 10^9$/l and platelets $< 100 \times 10^9$/l[910], lymphocytosis $> 9 \times 10^9$/l, raised β_2-microglobulin and presence of autoimmune problems[911].

A subset of SMZL may carry 7q31 deletions. Loss of 7q may play an alternative role in the inactivation of the p53 pathway, thereby favoring tumor progression[912]. Loss of an extra copy of 3q and the acquisition of genetic aberrations involving 19p13 and 7p–q22 may play a role in the blastic transformation of SMZL[913]. A more aggressive clinical course has been related to a high proliferation fraction[914], increased number of large lymphocytes and p53 mutations[662].

The incidence of large cell transformation in SMZL seems to be lower than in FL (25–60%) and MCL (11–39%)[663,862,865,892,893,912]. Approximately 10% of patients with SMZL undergo transformation to a high-grade lymphoma, with median times from diagnosis to transformation of 2–4 years[907]. Onset of B symptoms, lymphadenopathy, involvement of the central nervous system (CNS) and the presence of large cells in blood suggest disease transformation[907]. There are no statistically significant differences in proliferation fraction (Ki-67 staining) in initial SMZL tumors of cases with large cell transformation from overall SMZL cases[912]. SMZL may display del(10)(q22q24), del(7q) or trisomy 3[915]. The

Figure 4.35 Marginal zone B-cell lymphoma: spleen (A), skin (B; SALT-lymphoma), lung (C; BALT-lymphoma), salivary gland (D), stomach (E–F; mucosa-associated lymphoid tissue (MALT)-lymphoma; high magnification shows lymphoepithelial lesions) and lymph node (G–H; high magnification shows cytologic features of monocytoid B-cells)

reported median survival of patients with SMZL ranges from 8 to 13 years[909,910,916]. Most disease-related deaths are associated with transformation to DLBCL[214].

Extranodal marginal zone B-cell lymphoma of MALT type

Extranodal marginal zone B-cell lymphoma of mucosa-associated lymphoid tissue (MALT) is a distinct low-grade lymphoma, which can occur in the stomach, salivary gland, thyroid, skin and other organs that acquire lymphoid tissue after chronic inflammatory events, such as *Helicobacter pylori*-associated chronic gastritis (Figure 4.36), or autoimmune disorders such as Hashimoto's thyroiditis and myoepithelial sialadenitis/Sjögren's syndrome[917–919].

Trisomy 3 and t(11;18)(q21;q21) are the most frequent abnormalities in low-grade MALT lymphomas[920–922]. In contrast to trisomy 3, which is nearly always accompanied by other numerical and structural chromosomal alterations, t(11;18)(q21;q21) is usually a single aberration[921,922]. The t(11;18) leads to fusion of the *API2* gene at 11q21 and the *MALT1* gene at 18q21[280–282]. The *API2–MALT1* fusion gene is characteristic for MALT lymphomas and is very rare in splenic MZL or DLBCL. *API2* is a member of the *IAP* (inhibitor of apoptosis) gene family and is essential for suppression of caspase-dependent apoptosis[284]. The t(11;18)(q21;q21)/*API2–MALT1* is present in up to 40% of cases and is strongly associated with failure to respond to eradication of *Helicobacter pylori*[511,923,924]. Based on the response to *Helicobacter pylori* eradication therapy and presence of the *API2–MALT1* fusion gene, Inagaki *et al.* divided gastric MALT lymphomas into three groups: eradication-responsive and fusion-negative (group A); eradication-non-responsive and fusion-negative (group B); and eradication-non-responsive and fusion-positive (group C)[924]. The most common group A tumors are characterized by low clinical stage and superficial gastric involvement, and group C tumors by low *Helicobacter pylori* infection rate, low-grade histology, advanced clinical stage and nuclear Bcl-10

expression. Group B tumors have frequent nodal involvement, deep gastric wall involvement, advanced clinical stage and sometimes an increased large cell component. Another recurrent translocation in MALT lymphoma, t(1;14)(p22;q32), is associated with the juxtaposition of the entire *BCL10* gene to the immunoglobulin heavy-chain gene-enhancer region leading to activation of nuclear factor kappa B (NF-κB). Both t(11;18)(q21;q21) and t(1;14)(p22;q14) are associated with nuclear expression of Bcl-10, although the value of Bcl-10 immunohisto-chemical staining as a surrogate marker for the *API2–MALT1* gene fusion is uncertain. The frequency of both t(11;18)(q21;q21) and Bcl-10 expression is significantly higher in tumors that have disseminated beyond the stomach than in those confined to the stomach[467].

Partial inactivation of the *p53* gene may play a role in the development of low-grade MALT lymphoma[925], whereas, similarly to other hematologic neoplasms, complete inactivation may be associated with high-grade transformation[208]. Homozygous deletions of *p16* also play a role in large cell transformation[208]. Transformation of MALT lymphoma to DLBCL is heralded by the emergence of increased numbers of transformed blasts that form sheets or clusters[926–928]. In a series reported by Thieblemont *et al.*, progression to high-grade lymphoma (>50% large cells) occurred in 8% of MALT lymphomas[929], and most series reported that morphologic transformation of MZL to DLBCL occurs much more frequently in extranodal lymphomas of MALT type than in nodal and splenic MZL[930–935].

Gastric MALT lymphoma usually remains localized for long periods within the tissue of origin. Bone marrow involvement at presentation is uncommon[936,937]. Disseminated disease appears to be more common in non-gastrointestinal MALT lymphomas[929,938]. MALT lymphomas harboring t(11;18) are unlikely to transform to a higher-grade lymphoma[921,939,940], but exceptions may occur[941]. Of t(11;18)-negative MALT lymphomas, 60% harbor numerical chromosomal abnormalities, including trisomy 3, 7 and/or 18. Patients with t(11;18)+ or aneuploidy+ MALT

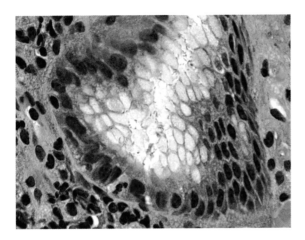

Figure 4.36 *Helicobacter pylori*, gastric mucosa

lymphomas have similar clinical behavior, with approximately half of the tumors recurring and one-fourth of the tumors involving the bone marrow[941]. In contrast, MALT lymphomas that lack chromosomal abnormalities recur in only 20% of cases and usually do not involve the bone marrow[941].

Elevated LDH, advanced stage, and high-risk IPI score are associated with poorer outcome[928]. The patients without lymph node involvement at presentation have a 5-year survival of 97%, and those with nodal involvement have 75% 5-year survival. The involvement of multiple mucosal sites at diagnosis did not appear to change the outcome[929]. The presence of monoclonal gammopathy in extranodal MZL correlates with advanced disease and bone marrow involvement[942].

Nodal marginal zone B-cell lymphoma

Nodal MZL occurs most commonly in the cervical lymph nodes, is more aggressive than MALT lymphoma, and presents with an advanced stage III/IV disease[933,943]. Patients with nodal MZL have lower 5-year overall survival and failure-free survival than patients with MALT lymphoma. The overall 5-year survival is 56% and 5-year failure-free survival is 28%[933]. When analysis is restricted to those patients with zero to three adverse risk factors in the IPI,

patients with nodal MZL still have a significantly lower overall and failure-free survival at 5 years than patients with extranodal MZL[933]. Transformation to large cell lymphoma at the time of diagnosis is seen in 20% cases of nodal MZL[933].

DIFFUSE LARGE B-CELL LYMPHOMA

DLBCL is an aggressive lymphoma of mature B cells characterized by a marked degree of morphologic and clinical heterogeneity occurring in nodal and extranodal sites. The World Health Organization (WHO) classification divides DLBCL into several morphologic and clinical variants (Figure 1.8; Chapter 1): centroblastic, immunoblastic, anaplastic, T-cell-rich/histiocyte-rich, thymic (primary mediastinal), intravascular, ALK+ and plasmablastic[225,486], with the centroblastic variant being the most frequent type (>80%). The majority of DLBCL are positive for CD45 and B-cell markers (CD19, CD20, CD22, CD79a and PAX5). A subset of tumors may express CD10 and/or Bcl-6. Patients with DLBCL have highly variable clinical courses and the prognosis depends on many clinical, morphological, phenotypic and genetic parameters (Table 4.2). A significant proportion of DLBCL seem to occur from a transformation of an unknown indolent lymphoma[944,945]. Current treatment of DLBCL is based on the combination of chemotherapy including cyclophosphamide, doxorubicin, vincristine, prednisone (CHOP) or a dose-intense CHOP-like regimen, and rituximab (R-CHOP). Approximately 60% of patients with DLBCL relapse after conventional anthracycline-based combination therapy[944,945].

Clinical and laboratory parameters

The IPI is widely used as a predictive model in DLBCL patients of all ages and stages (*see also* IPI, Chapter 1). The IPI combines patient age with easily measured clinical parameters, which can serve as surrogate markers of tumor burden: performance status, stage, extranodal involvement and serum LDH levels. Stage of disease and the B-symptom

Table 4.2   Prognostic factors in diffuse large B-cell lymphoma

Factor	Prognosis
Age >60 years	Unfavorable
Increased β_2-microglobulin	Unfavorable
Morphology: centroblastic	Favorable (?)
immunoblastic	Unfavorable (?)
CD10/Bcl-6 expression (germinal center B-like phenotype)	Favorable
MUM1/CD138 expression (activated B-like phenotype)	Unfavorable
Bcl-2 expression	Unfavorable
p53 expression/*p53 (TP53)* mutations	Unfavorable
High Ki-67 index	Unfavorable
18q amplification	Unfavorable
17p loss	Unfavorable

status are significantly associated with survival[946]. Low stage (I and II) and lack of B symptoms are favorable indicators of overall survival and failure-free survival[946]. Apart from advanced stage, age >60 years, poor performance status and elevated serum LDH levels are independent predictors of poor survival. Serum β_2-microglobulin and LDH levels are significant and independent variables for predicting time to treatment failure and survival[124,947–949]. The serum levels of β_2-microglobulin correlate with tumor burden. Conconi *et al.* showed that the β_2-microglobulin/IPI may be more useful than IPI alone for identifying the subset of patients with very poor prognosis and may help in selection of the patients with DLBCL at higher risk for treatment failure[947]. Serum soluble interleukin-2 receptor (sIL-2R) and β_2-microglobulin are able to predict time to progression in patients with DLBCL[950]. Other laboratory parameters of prognostic significance include cytokines and selenium[189]. Serum selenium concentration at presentation was reported to predict positively for dose delivery, treatment response and long-term survival in aggressive NHL[189].

Patients with bone marrow involvement (Figure 4.37) that consists of ≥50% large cells or bone marrow involvement of ≥70% have a poorer overall survival[951,952]. Those who presented with an infiltrate of less than 50% large cells and an IPI of ≤3 have a significantly longer post-relapse survival time. A diffuse or interstitial pattern of bone marrow involvement is predictive of both poor overall survival and failure-free survival[952]. Two parameters – IPI ≤3 and bone marrow large cells less than 50% – identify a group of patients with long-term survival after relapse[952]. The presence of rearranged immunoglobulin (IgR) heavy chain and immunoglobulin light chain in peripheral blood and/or bone marrow correlates with clinical stage, histopathological detection of bone marrow involvement and the IPI. IgR+ cases have a significantly lower complete remission rate (51%) than IgR− patients (71%), and a significantly poorer overall survival at 5 years (25% vs. 66%). There is a significant difference in the estimated overall survival at 5 years between patients with negative bone marrow histology and negative PCR (IgR−) results (66%), patients with negative bone marrow histology but positive IgR (37%), and patients with positive bone marrow histology (12%)[953].

Morphologic and phenotypic parameters

The cytology of neoplastic cells has long been debated as a prognostic factor, with controversial results. In some studies, patients with centroblastic lymphoma had a better prognosis (and overall survival), when compared with immunoblastic lymphoma or anaplastic variant of DLBCL[106]. Baars *et al.* showed that patients with immunoblastic lymphoma had a significantly worse prognosis than

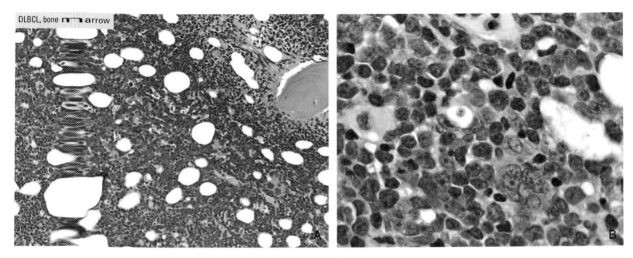

DLBCL, bone marrow

Figure 4.37 Diffuse large B-cell lymphoma (DLBCL), extensive bone marrow involvement (A, low magnification; B, high magnification)

patients with centroblastic lymphoma, with a 5-year overall survival for patients with centroblastic morphology of 56.3% and for patients with immunoblastic morphology 39.1%[954]. The 5-year disease-free survival was 53.2% for the patients with centroblastic and 26.9% for the patients with immunoblastic NHL[954]. Diametrically different conclusions were drawn from another study[107] in which there were no significant differences in survival between the three major groups of DLBCL: the 5-year survival was 51% for patients with centroblastic lymphoma, 45% for immunoblastic lymphoma and 33% for anaplastic variant. However, even this study showed that the 5-year overall survival and failure-free survival of patients with DLBCL not containing immunoblasts was significantly better than the survival of those containing immunoblasts[107]. DLBCL with plasmablastic/plasmacytoid morphology is characterized by the frequent presence of B symptoms, extranodal disease, higher IPI, poor response to chemotherapy and shorter disease-free survival (6 months) and overall survival (14 months) when compared with centroblastic DLBCL[200]. FISH studies showed frequent monoallelic $p53$ deletions (85%). Tumor cells are often CD20[+], cIgM[+], MUM1[+],

CD138[+/−] and Bcl-6[−], corresponding to an activated B-cell phenotype. T-cell/histiocyte-rich large B-cell lymphoma is an aggressive disease that often presents with adverse prognostic factors and appears to have lower survival than typical DLBCL[955]. However, when treatment is adapted to the disease risk, the outcome is equivalent to that observed in patients with DLBCL[956]. In the series reported by Bouabdallah *et al.*, clinical characteristics of patients with T-cell/histiocyte-rich large B-cell lymphoma included male predominance, median age of 47 years, normal performance status in 89% of patients and increased LDH level in 60% of patients. The disease was disseminated in 81% of patients (48% had two or more involved extranodal sites). The complete response rate to chemotherapy was 63%, and 5-year overall survival and event-free survival rates were 58% and 53%, respectively[956].

Expression of Bcl-2, Bcl-6, caspase 8, CD5, CD10, CD44, Ki-67 (MIB1) and p53 appears to have prognostic implications in DLBCL. DLBCL display Bcl-2 expression in 30–60% of cases, more frequently in nodal than in extranodal tumors[532,534–536]. The prognostic importance of Bcl-2 protein expression in patients with DLBCL is well established[257,272,453,531,538].

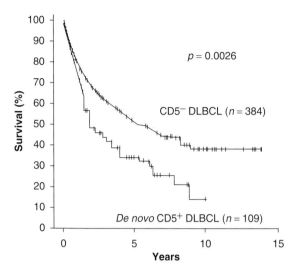

Figure 4.46 Overall survival for patients with *de novo* CD5⁺ diffuse large B-cell lymphoma (DLBCL) and with CD5 DLBCL. *De novo* CD5⁺ DLBCL showed significantly worse survival than CD5⁻ DLBCL

From: Yamaguchi M, *et al. De novo* CD5⁺ diffuse large B-cell lymphoma: a clinicopathologic study of 109 patients. Blood 2002;99:815–21. © 2002 by The American Society of Hematology, used with permission

commonly observed in children aged 4–7 years with frequent involvement of the mandible and maxilla and abdominal organs, especially the kidneys. The sporadic forms occur mainly in young adults and presents as abdominal disease. A significant subset of BL is associated with EBV infection. Morphologically, BL comprises a monotonous infiltrate of medium-sized cells with numerous mitoses, apoptotic cells and scattered macrophages with engulfed apoptotic bodies, creating a 'starry-sky' appearance (Figures 4.48 and 4.49). The majority of BL cases have t(8;14) (q24;q32), resulting in the juxtaposition of the c-*MYC* gene on chromosome 8 with the *IgH* heavy chain locus on chromosome 14. The remaining cases have either t(2;8)(p12;q24) or t(8;22)(q24;q11).

All three variants of BL have a rapid, aggressive clinical course with frequent relapses. While debate is ongoing over the most relevant prognostic factors in BL, several studies have identified advanced age, advanced stage, poor performance status, CNS or bone marrow involvement, anemia, the presence of circulating blasts and an elevated LDH level as

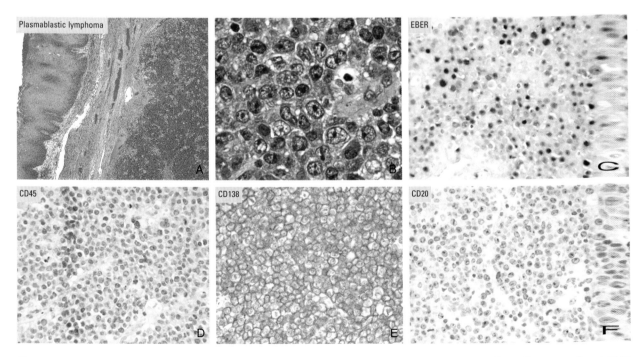

Figure 4.47 Plasmablastic lymphoma, oral mucosa. A–B, histology; C–F, immunohistochemistry. Tumor cells are positive for EBER (C) and CD138 (E). CD45 (D) and CD20 (F) are not expressed in this case

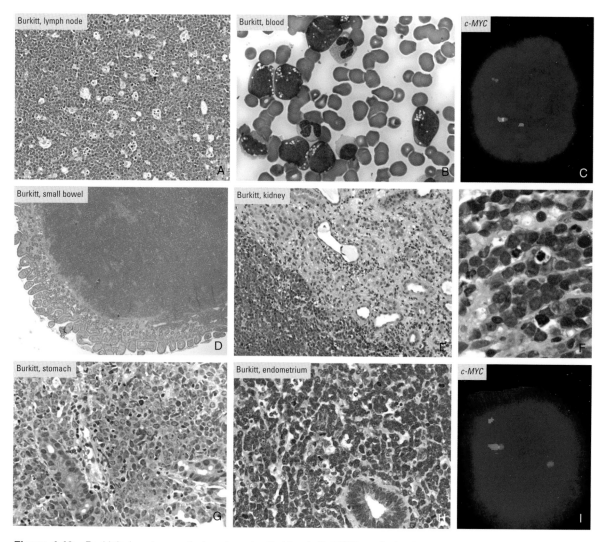

Figure 4.48 Burkitt's lymphoma. A, lymph node; B, blood; C, FISH analysis showing t(8;14); D, small bowel; E–F, kidney; G, stomach; H–I, endometrium (I, FISH probe)

indicative of a poor outcome in adult BL[1003–1006]. Valnet-Rabier *et al.* reported that the expression of c-FLIP was found to be strongly related to a poor prognosis in BL, mostly characterized by adults with a chemoresistant disease, resulting in a high death rate within the first year of diagnosis[743]. The 2-year overall survival with c-FLIP expression was 24% compared with 93% in the absence of this marker. Most patients attain a complete response within 4–6 weeks of therapy: approximately 80% of patients achieve a complete response to treatment with disease

free-survival at 4 years of 50%[1005,1007]. Failure to achieve a complete response is a poor prognostic factor[1003]. Without intensive chemotherapy (salvage therapy) or stem cell transplant those patients relapse and die of progressive disease[1003,1006,1008]. The overall survival for adult patients undergoing high-dose therapy and autologous stem cell transplantation is 53% at 3 years. The major factor predicting outcome after transplantation was disease status: the 3-year overall survival was 72% for patients transplanted in first complete remission, compared with 37% for

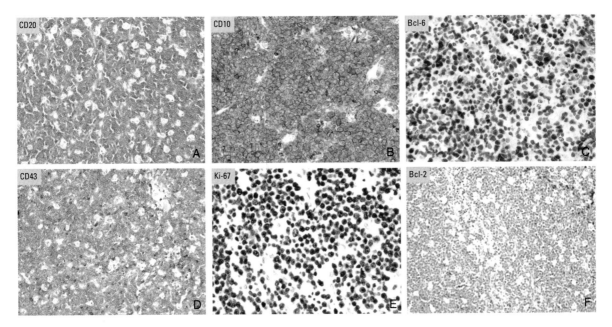

Figure 4.49   Burkitt's lymphoma, immunophenotype: tumor cells are positive for CD20 (A), CD10 (B), Bcl-6 (C), CD43 (D) and Ki-67 (E). Bcl-2 is not expressed (F)

patients in chemosensitive relapse, and 7% for chemoresistant patients[1009]. For patients transplanted in first complete remission, disease bulk at the time of autologous stem cell transplantation was the only factor predictive of progression-free survival and overall survival[1009]. During the early treatment period, rapid tumor cell death is responsible for a tumor lysis syndrome, leading to severe hyperkalemia, hyperphosphatemia and severe renal failure. The response to treatment and prognosis is improved with intensive chemotherapy and CNS protection[108,111]. Recently, rituximab has emerged as an important treatment choice in management of BL, especially in patients with poor prognostic features at diagnosis or with chemoresistant disease[1010].

BL in children with localized disease and current treatment has a good prognosis, with 5-year event-free survival exceeding 90%[1011]. Recent treatment improved the outcome for disseminated lymphoma, as well[1011]. Children and adolescents with disseminated disease had a 4-year event-free survival of 57% and

4-year overall survival of 64%[108]. The prognostic indicators in children with BL include treatment protocol, age, LDH levels and bone marrow involvement. The lower failure rate is observed among patients treated with shorter but more intensive therapy[108]. Initial serum LDH level of >500 IU/l, bone marrow involvement and age of ≥15 years are associated with inferior prognosis[108,180]. Increasing the intensity of chemotherapy negated LDH levels as a significant prognostic factor in recent studies[1012]. Recent treatment strategies improve the outcome for patients with advanced disease. Recent studies demonstrated an 84% 5-year event-free survival in patients with bone marrow involvement with or without CNS involvement[1013]. Although previously regarded as a poor prognostic indicator[1014], recent studies do not consider CNS involvement as an independent poor prognostic factor[108,180]. The presence of abnormalities on 1q and imbalances on 7q were associated with a short survival[1015]. Figure 4.50 presents unusual BL with phenotypic expression of cyclin D1 (Bcl-1) without t(11;14).

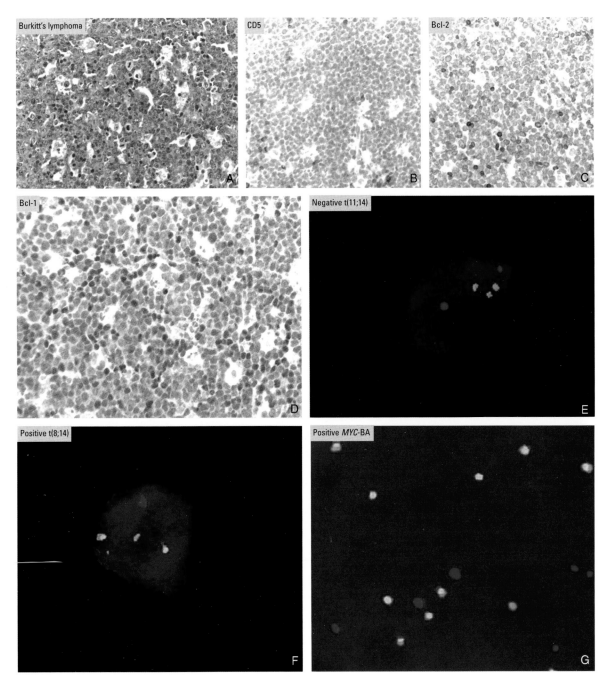

Figure 4.50   Burkitt's lymphoma with unusual cyclin D1 (Bcl-1) expression. A, histology with typical starry-sky pattern. Tumor cells are negative for CD5 (B) and Bcl-2 (C), but express cyclin D1/Bcl-1 by immunohistochemistry (D) without translocation t(11;14) (E). F, positive t(8;14); G, positive FISH analysis for *MYC* break-apart probe

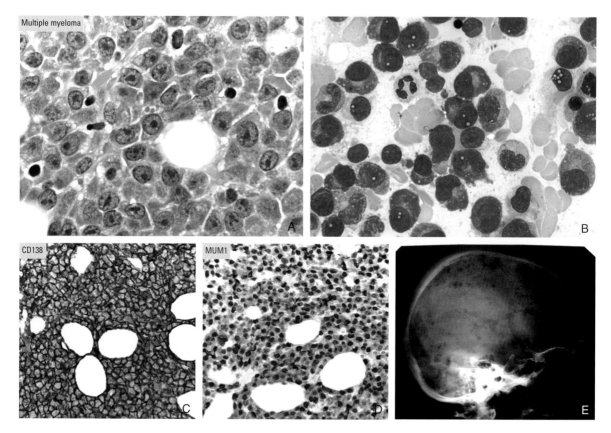

Figure 4.51   Multiple myeloma. Bone marrow is replaced by atypical plasma cells with nucleoli (A, histology; B, aspirate smear). Neoplastic plasma cells are positive for CD138 (C) and MUM1 (D). Radiologic imaging shows typical bone lesions (E)

MULTIPLE MYELOMA (PLASMA CELL MYELOMA)

Multiple myeloma (MM), also termed plasma cell myeloma (Figure 4.51), is a clonal disorder of B cells at a last stage of differentiation characterized by bone marrow infiltration by plasma cells and production of a monoclonal immunoglobulin. MM can emerge from a pre-existing benign disorder (monoclonal gammopathy of undetermined significance; MGUS) or *de novo*, bypassing the MGUS stage. The prognosis is highly variable, with survival ranging from a few days to more than 10 years[1016,1017]. Some patients present with a very aggressive form of plasma cell myeloma, i.e. primary plasma cell leukemia. The overall survival at 1, 2 and 5 years for MM patients is 72%, 55% and 22%, respectively[1018]. Numerous prognostic factors are associated with poor prognosis in MM, e.g. advanced clinical stage, extensive bone marrow involvement, features of bone marrow failure (anemia, thrombocytopenia), high level of β_2-microglobulin, deletion of chromosome 13, hypodiploid karyotype, increased plasma cell labeling index/high S-phase, monosomy of chromosome 17/deletion of *p53*, and lack of cyclin D1 expression[127,128,382,523,1019–1022].

Clinical and laboratory features

Before the introduction of the alkylating agents in the early 1980s, MM usually slowly progressed until death after about 2 years[1023]. Treatment with high-dose chemotherapy followed by bone marrow transplantation has improved disease-free survival and overall survival. Although not curative, autologous stem cell transplantation is a major advance in MM therapy; it improves the likelihood of a complete response and prolongs disease-free survival and overall survival. However, even with autologous hematopoietic progenitor cell transplant, most patients with MM will relapse and ultimately die as a result of their disease. Patients treated with intensified chemotherapy followed by myeloablative therapy and autologous stem cell rescue as first-line treatment for MM showed a higher complete remission and a longer time to progression when compared with patients treated with intensified chemotherapy alone; however, they did not have better event-free survival and overall survival[1024]. With modern treatments, the complete remission rate is 20–60%, with a median overall survival of 4.4–7 years and a median event-free survival of 24–43 months[1024–1026]. In patients with advanced MM treated with thalidomide, age greater than 60 years, short interval between diagnosis and onset of thalidomide, requirement for red blood cell transfusion, IgA isotype, platelet count of $< 80 \times 10^9/l$ and serum albumin level of $< 30\,g/l$ at the start of thalidomide were associated with a poor outcome[1027]. Among patients without any of these unfavorable risk features, 1-year overall survival and event-free survival were 87% and 78%, respectively. By contrast, patients with at least one unfavorable feature had 1-year overall survival and event-free survival of 40% and 32%, respectively. The median overall survival of patients with relapse after initial treatment was 17 months, and 84% of patients died within 5 years[1018]. Patients with a significant decrease in serum monoclonal protein after the first cycle of chemotherapy (at least 30% decrement in M-protein) have a better prognosis than patients with minimal early response to chemotherapy[1028]. Circulating MM cells may be the best indication of the patient's response to treatment[1029].

Secondary features that represent a host response to MM – anemia, bone disease, immunodeficiency, low platelet count ($< 150 \times 10^9/l$), high creatinine levels ($\geq 2\,mg/dl$), low albumin levels ($< 3\,g/dl$), and increased level of β_2-microglobulin ($> 2.5\,mg/l$) and increased levels of calcium usually correlate with

advanced clinical stage – are important negative prognostic factors for MM patients and correlate with event-free survival and overall survival[127,338,381,382,1018,1030,1031]. Multivariate analysis indicates that serum creatinine and calcium levels are significant indicators of 2-year survival in MM patients[1032]. High serum levels of interleukin (IL)-6 (and IL-6Rα) are associated with a poor prognosis. IL-6 increases the proliferation of myeloma cells, prevents apoptosis by blocking caspase 9 activation and facilitates resistance to antitumor agents. The incidence of adverse prognostic factors (e.g. β_2-microglobulin levels, S-phase fraction, LDH levels, renal function) is higher in primary plasma cell leukemia than in MM[384]. In contrast to MM, the majority of leukemic plasma cells are diploid. Factors predicting event-free survival in MM include chromosome 13 deletion, β_2-microglobulin levels of $> 3\,mg/l$, and $> 90\%$ response to treatment.

Marked dysplasia (Figure 4.52), frequent mitoses (Figure 4.53) and a high plasma cell labeling index ($\geq 1\%$) are associated with poor prognosis. The proliferative activity of plasma cells is an independent prognostic factor in MM patients. The patients with S-phase value of $\leq 1\%$, 1–3% and $> 3\%$ had median survival of 34, 22 and 12 months, respectively[1033]. High S-phase is a poor prognostic indicator. CD45 expression by MM cells is associated with a better prognosis and is higher in patients with early disease (MGUS and smoldering MM).

Chromosomal aberrations

Approximately 70% of patients with MM have numerical chromosomal abnormalities[1034]. Monosomy 13 is one of the most frequent aberrations in MM[436]. The complete or partial deletion of chromosome 13 or translocations involving 13q (−13) by conventional cytogenetics are associated with a poor outcome, a higher relapse rate (77% vs. 44%) and a shorter event-free and overall survival even with high-dose treatment and autologous stem cell transplantation[338,381,440,1031,1034]. Kroger *et al.* showed in a multivariate analysis that 13q− remained a significant

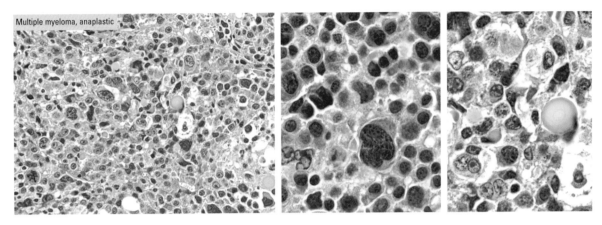

Figure 4.52   Multiple myeloma with anaplastic features

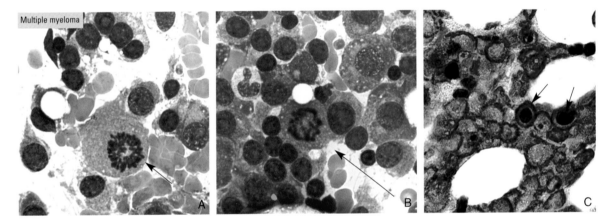

Figure 4.53   Multiple myeloma with mitoses. A–B, aspirate smear showing plasma cells with atypical mitoses (arrows); C, histologic section with dual staining for CD138 (red) and Ki-67 (brown). Proliferating cells have dark brown nuclei (arrows)

risk factor for a higher relapse rate and a shorter event-free survival after dose-reduced allogeneic stem cell transplantation; 2 or more cycles of prior high-dose chemotherapy were associated with a significantly higher probability of death while patients with deletion 13q had a nearly 2 times higher risk of death[1035]. Monosomy 13 correlates with the risk of transformation of MGUS to overt MM[1036]. In the series of Shaughnessy *et al.*, among all MM patients with cytogenetic abnormalities and standard prognostic factors examined prior to therapy, only hypodiploidy and chromosome 13 aberrations (–13), alone or in combination, were associated with the shortest event-free survival and overall survival[1022].

The shortest post-relapse overall survival was observed with hypodiploidy and monosomy 13[1022]. Superior prognosis was associated with the absence of any chromosomal abnormalities at both diagnosis and relapse (10-year overall survival, 40%)[1022].

Trisomies of chromosomes 6, 9 and 17 are associated with prolonged survival in MM. Deletion of chromosome 11q have been reported to predict poor outcome in MM patients. Some of the 14q32 abnormalities may influence the natural history of MM; t(4;14)(p16;q32) is rarely observed in MGUS, whereas t(14;16)(q32;q24) is often associated with plasma cell leukemia[1037]. The t(11;14)(q13;q32) (Figure 4.54) results in upregulation of cyclin D1

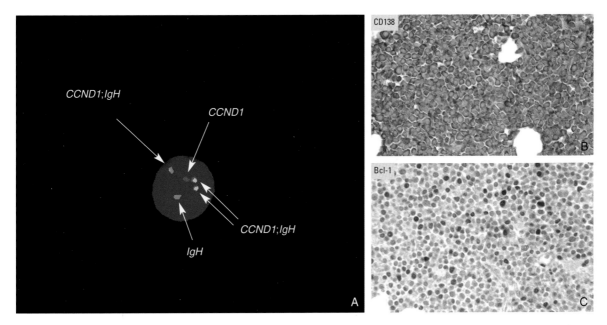

Figure 4.54 Multiple myeloma with t(11;14). A, FISH studies; B–C, immunohistochemical staining for CD138 (B) and cyclin D1 (Bcl-1) (C)

(Bcl-1) and is the most common translocation detected in MM[1038]. The presence of this translocation correlates with lymphoplasmacytic morphology and/or small mature plasma cell morphology, CD20 expression, lower levels of serum monoclonal protein, lower plasma cell labeling index and, less often, appearance of hyperdiploid DNA content[704,1038]. No correlation was found between del(13) and β_2-microglobulin serum levels, but strong associations were found between β_2-microglobulin and 14q32 abnormalities[1037]. Patients lacking any 14q32 abnormality were essentially in the good prognostic group, whereas patients with t(4;14) or t(14;16) were mostly in the poor prognostic group[1037,1039]. The t(4;14) occurs in 12% of MM patients[481]. Patients with t(4;14) have significantly shorter progression-free survival and overall survival[481]. The t(4;14) is associated with a poor prognosis in MM patients receiving intensive chemotherapy and autologous stem cell transplant. In the series reported by Moreau *et al.*, patients with t(4;14) displayed a poor outcome (short event-free survival and short overall survival), those with t(11;14) displayed long survival and patients with neither t(4;14) nor t(11;14) presented an intermediate outcome[1040]. The t(9;14) and t(6;14) involve *PAX5* and *IRF4*, respectively. Complex chromosomal abnormalities (Figure 4.55) are associated with a poorer prognosis. There are possible differences in chromosomal aberrations between younger and older patients. Breaks in chromosomes 1p13, 6q21 and 11q13 are more common in the younger age group, whereas older patients more often show loss of chromosome Y as a sole abnormality or +5.

Molecular markers

Comparative genomic hybridization showed the existence of marked differences in chromosomal imbalances between MM and plasma cell leukemia, which may help to explain the different clinical course of these disorders.[1041,1042] Losses of chromosomal material are significantly more frequent in plasma cell leukemia than in MM[1042]. MM patients often show gains at chromosome 15q, 11q, 3q, 9q

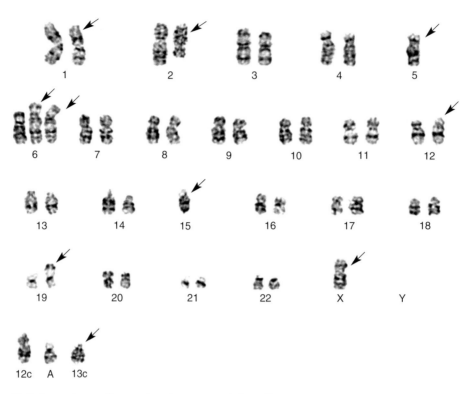

Figure 4.55   Multiple myeloma with complex chromosomal aberrations

and 1q, whereas all patients with plasma cell leukemia show gains in 1q[1042]. It has also been reported that activating mutations of Ki-*RAS* (but not N-*RAS*) represent an adverse prognostic factor in MM. Patients with *RAS* mutations had a median survival of 2.1 years; patients with wild-type *RAS* had a median survival of 4.0 years[1043]. Hideshima *et al.* divided MM patients into five categories based on five recurrent Ig translocations and cyclin D expression: TC1 tumors (high levels of cyclin D1 or cyclin D3 as a result of an Ig translocation); TC2 tumors (low to moderate levels of cyclin D1 despite the absence of a t(11;14) translocation); TC3 tumors (a mixture of tumors that do not fall into one of the other groups, with most expressing cyclin D2); TC4 tumors (high levels of cyclin D2, and also MMSET); and TC5 tumors (highest levels of cyclin D2, and also high levels of either c-Maf or Maf B)[341]. Patients with a t(4;14) translocation (TC4) have a shorter survival with either standard or high-dose therapy,

patients with a t(14;16) (TC5) have a poor prognosis and patients with tumors that have a t(11;14) translocation (TC1) have better survival following aggressive therapy[382,523,1019,1021,1022,1040].

MGUS

Patients with MGUS have a median survival rate only slightly shorter than that of a comparable US population but are at increased risk for progression to MM, lymphoma, Waldenström's macroglobuline-mia and primary amyloidosis. The risk of progression of MGUS to plasma cell malignancy is indefinite and persists even after more than 30 years of follow-up, with no reliable predictors of malignant evolution[1044]. Patients with MGUS of the IgM class progress to lymphoplasmacytic lymphoma/ Waldenström's macroglobulinemia, B-CLL, and other lymphomas, whereas patients with IgG or IgA MGUS progress to MM, plasmacytoma or primary amyloidosis. Long-term follow-up of 241 patients with MGUS revealed progression to MM or related disorders in 27% of patients; 6% of patients were alive without evidence of the disease, and the remaining patients died without evidence of MM or a related disorder[1044]. The average risk of progression of patients with an IgM MGUS is 1.5% per year[1045]. One of the few differential genetic lesions between MM and MGUS is the presence of *RAS* mutations in MM[338]. Rasmussen *et al.* suggested that *RAS* mutations provided a genetic marker if not a causal event in the evolution of MGUS to MM[633]. Perez-Andres *et al.* observed a progressive increase in the soluble levels of β_2-microglobulin from MGUS to MM and plasma cell leukemia patients[1046].

The POEMS syndrome (coined to refer to polyneuropathy, organomegaly, endocrinopathy, M protein, and skin changes) has a median survival of 165 months, independent of the number of syndrome features, bone lesions, or plasma cells at diagnosis[1047]. Additional features of the syndrome often develop, but the complications of classic MM are rare.

CHAPTER 5

Peripheral (mature/post-thymic) T-cell lymphoproliferative disorders

T-cell lymphomas are a diverse group of lymphoid neoplasms manifesting heterogeneous clinical, histologic, immunophenotypic and cytogenetic features[18,20,183,1048–1052]. T-cell lymphomas represent approximately 10% of all non-Hodgkin's lymphomas (NHL) in Western countries. The classification of T-cell lymphoma is based largely on the histomorphologic features and clinical parameters. Predominantly nodal distribution is characteristic for angioimmunoblastic T-cell lymphoma (AILT), peripheral T-cell lymphoma, unspecified (PTCL), and anaplastic large cell lymphoma (ALCL). Extranodal location is seen in mycosis fungoides (MF), cutaneous ALCL, extranodal NK/T-cell lymphoma (nasal type), enteropathy-type T-cell lymphoma, hepatosplenic T-cell lymphoma and subcutaneous panniculitis-like T-cell lymphoma. The presence of human T-cell leukemia/lymphoma virus type I (HTLV-I) defines adult T-cell leukemia/lymphoma (ATCL), whereas expression of ALK1 associated with t(2;5) is observed in ALCL. The majority of T-cell lymphoproliferative disorders are aggressive, with only MF and cutaneous ALCL frequently following an indolent course (Figures 5.1 and 5.2). Response to conventional therapy generally is poor. New treatment modalities, including purine analogs, monoclonal antibodies (alemtuzumab) and stem cell transplantation offers improved response rates and better remissions[729].

Three distinct prognostic subgroups can be distinguished on survival analysis: favorable (cutaneous ALCL), 5-year overall survival 78%; intermediate (PTCL, ALCL, AILT), 5-year overall survival 35–43%; unfavorable (NK/T-cell lymphoma, nasal type and enteropathy-type T-cell lymphoma), 5-year overall survival 22–24%[20]. Most of the pretreatment characteristics, including International Prognostic Index (IPI) risk groups, are not significantly different between B-cell and T-cell lymphomas. The rates of complete remission (71% vs. 54%) and progressive disease (39% vs. 63%) significantly favored patients with B-cell lymphoma. Also, the 5-year overall survival (49% vs. 27%), 5-year disease-free survival (48% vs. 21%) and event-free survival (35% vs. 10%) are significantly better in B-cell lymphoma[21]. Patients with T-cell lymphoma have inferior survival in all IPI risk groups. Multivariate analysis revealed T-cell phenotype as the most significant factor associated with short overall survival and event-free survival in patients with lymphoma. T-cell phenotype is an independent prognostic factor, the significance of which is at least comparable to the IPI for patients with aggressive NHL[21]. The results of treatment of patients with aggressive T-cell lymphomas are generally worse than those for patients with diffuse large B-cell lymphoma (DLBCL). Patients with T-cell lymphomas have a poorer response to therapy and shorter

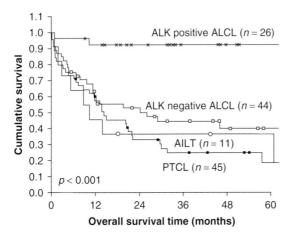

Figure 5.1 Comparison of overall survival time, according to lymphoma subtype: anaplastic large cell lymphoma (ALCL) vs. peripheral T-cell lymphoma, unspecified (PTCL) vs. angioimmunoblastic T-cell lymphoma (AILT) and anaplastic lymphoma kinase (ALK) expression

From: ten Berge *et al.* ALK-negative anaplastic large cell lymphoma demonstrates similar poor prognosis to peripheral T-cell lymphoma, unspecified. Histopathology 2003;43:463–9. © 2003 by Blackwell Publishing Limited, used with permission

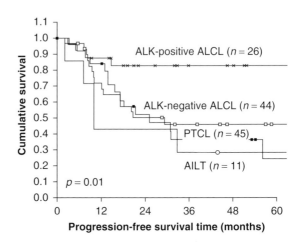

Figure 5.2 Comparison of progression-free survival, according to lymphoma subtype: ALCL vs. peripheral T-cell lymphoma, unspecified (PTCL) vs. angioimmunoblastic T-cell lymphoma (AILT) and anaplastic lymphoma kinase (ALK) expression

From: ten Berge *et al.* ALK-negative anaplastic large cell lymphoma demonstrates similar poor prognosis to peripheral T-cell lymphoma, unspecified. Histopathology 2003;43:463–9. © 2003 by Blackwell Publishing Limited, used with permission

survival than comparable patients with aggressive B-cell lymphomas[2,1053–1056].

T-CELL PROLYMPHOCYTIC LEUKEMIA

T-cell prolymphocytic leukemia (T-PLL) is a rare mature (post-thymic) T-cell lymphoproliferative disorder that affects adults, occurs more frequently in men and is characterized by an aggressive clinical course and poor outcome[1057–1060]. T-PLL is composed of small to medium-sized lymphocytes with prominent nucleoli (Figure 5.3). The principal disease characteristics are organomegaly (especially splenomegaly and lymphadenopathy; Figure 5.4), anemia, thrombocytopenia, skin lesions and prominent (often rapidly increasing) lymphocytosis in the blood (most often $> 100 \times 10^9/l$). A subset of patients experiences an initial (median 33 months, range: 6–103 months) indolent clinical course with

stable moderate leukocytosis, with subsequent progression to an aggressive stage[1061]. The majority of cases are associated with abnormalities of chromosome 14 (Figure 5.5); inv(14)(q11;q32), t(14;14)(q11;q32) and i(8)(q10)[1057]. The translocations involving chromosome 14 juxtapose the locus of the *TCRαβ* gene with the *TCL1* and *TCL1b* genes at 14q32. Chromosome 14 abnormalities are often accompanied by a complex karyotype (Figure 5.5). Prior to the appearance of pentostatin and alemtuzumab in clinical protocols, the outcome for T-PLL patients was exceedingly poor (median survival < 1 year). Alemtuzumab (Campath; a humanized monoclonal antibody directed against the CD52 antigen) is an effective agent in T-PLL and represents a significant improvement over other types of therapy[1062]. While the use of alemtuzumab in particular has improved remissions, the disease remains incurable[727]. Best results are achieved if

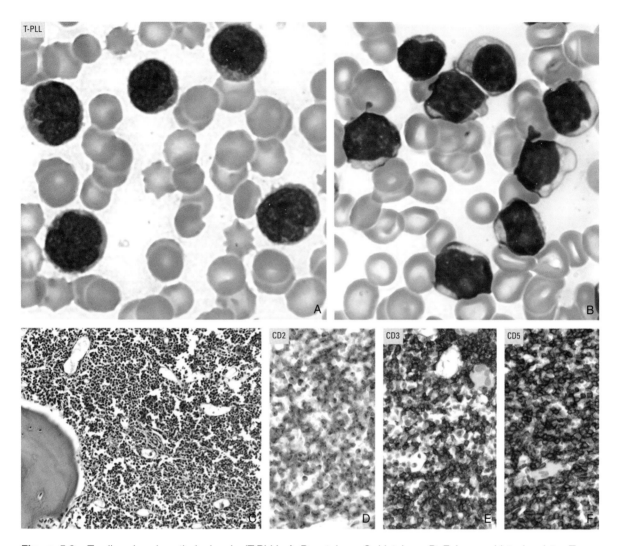

Figure 5.3 T-cell prolymphocytic leukemia (T-PLL). A–B, cytology; C, histology; D–F, immunohistochemistry. Tumor cells have irregular nuclear outlines and nucleoli (A–B). Bone marrow is diffusely infiltrated by leukemic cells (C), which express CD2 (D), CD3 (E) and CD5 (F)

treatment with alemtuzumab is followed by allogeneic transplant[726,1062].

T-LARGE GRANULAR LYMPHOCYTE LEUKEMIA

T-large granular lymphocyte leukemia (T-LGL) is a clonal disorder of large granular lymphocytes (Figure 5.6) characterized by an indolent course, lymphocytosis and cytopenia(s). Patients are asymptomatic (28%) or experience fatigue (60%), B symptoms (12%) and recurrent infections (15%)[1063,1064]. The median age is about 60 years (range: 4–88)[1064]. Morbidity is associated with cytopenia (neutropenia and/or anemia)[225,1065,1066]. Associated co-morbid conditions include rheumatoid arthritis (26%), and the presence of autoantibodies or hypergammaglobulinemia[1063,1064]. Rare cases progress to a more aggressive disorder[1067]. Treatment with cyclosporine improves clinical parameters (e.g. neutrophil counts

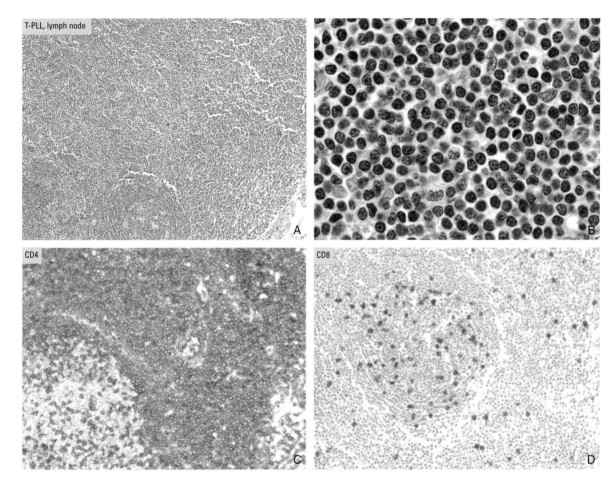

Figure 5.4   T-prolymphocytic leukemia (T-PLL) with lymph node involvement. A–B, histology; C–D, immunohistochemistry. Lymph nodes show a prominent interfollicular infiltrate by small atypical lymphoid cells with inconspicuous nucleoli (A–B). Tumor cells are positive for CD4 (C) and do not express CD8 (D)

and transfusion dependence)[1065]. HLA-DR4 predicts the hematological response to cyclosporine in T-LGL leukemia[1065]. Patients may also benefit from treatment with cyclophosphamide, methotrexate and corticosteroids[1063]. The prognosis is generally favorable, with 10-year survival greater than 80%[1057,1063]. The most deaths are related to sepsis[1057]. The risk factors associated with poor prognosis include fever at diagnosis, low percentage of CD57+ cells, severe neutropenia and B symptoms[1068,1069].

The LGL lymphoproliferations with NK-cell phenotype (Figure 5.7) have most often an aggressive clinical course, tend to occur in younger patients and

are more likely to present with B symptoms, marked hepatosplenomegaly, thrombocytopenia and a rapid increase in the number of leukemic cells[1070].

ADULT T-CELL LEUKEMIA/LYMPHOMA

ATCL is a peripheral (mature/post-thymic) T-cell lymphoproliferative disorder caused by the retrovirus human T-cell leukemia/lymphoma virus type I (human T-lymphotropic virus I, HTLV-I)[1071,1072]. Tumor cells have prominent nuclear irregularities, often referred to as 'cloverleaf' or 'flower' cells (Figure 5.8). ATCL affects adults with leukemic or

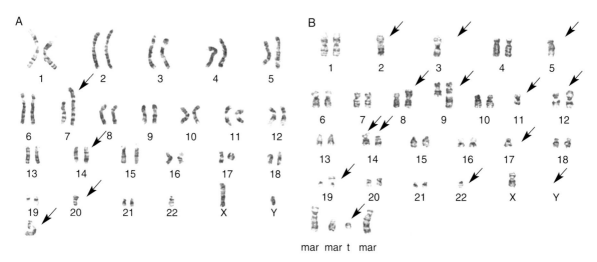

Figure 5.5 Two cases of T-prolymphocytic leukemia with complex chromosomal abnormalities. A, inv(14)(q11.2q32), add(7)(p22), r(17), −19, −20, −22, +1. B, 43–46, X–Y, −2, −3, −5, add(6)(q13), +del(6)(q15), t(8;8)(p11.2;q12), add(9)(q34), −11, add(11)(q23), −12, add(12)(p13), add(14)(p11.2), inv(14)(q11.2q32), −17, add(19p), −22

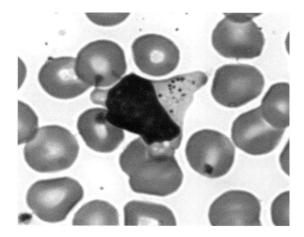

Figure 5.6 T-large granular lymphocyte leukemia, blood

subleukemic presentation, cutaneous involvement, lymphadenopathy and/or organomegaly. Hypercalcemia is present in up to 50% of patients and may result in renal failure. Patients are at increased risk for bacterial and viral infections. Several clinical variants of ATCL are recognized: chronic, smoldering, acute and lymphomatous. Chronic and smoldering variants are clinically indolent, whereas acute and lymphomatous variants show a highly aggressive

clinical behavior and a very poor outlook (median survival 9–10 months), mostly due to chemoresistance and severe immunosuppression[1073–1077]. The 4-year survival rate is 66% for the smoldering type, 27% for the chronic type, and 5–6% for the lymphoma and acute types[1078,1079]. Indolent variants of ATCL can progress to very aggressive variants, occasionally referred to as 'crisis variants'[1080]. On the other hand, spontaneous regression can also be observed in sporadic cases[1078,1079]. The prognostically relevant subclassification of ATCL is based mainly on clinical and hematologic parameters[1075]. High tumor burden reflected by increased lactate dehydrogenase (LDH) level, high leukocytosis, tumor bulk, hypercalcemia, age >40 years and poor performance status are associated with poor prognosis. Patients with increased interleukin-6 (IL-6) levels have inferior overall survival compared with patients with normal IL-6 levels[142]. Survivin is expressed in ATLC and the level of expression is higher in the acute type when compared with chronic/smoldering types[750]. Higher expression of survivin mRNA is associated with shorter survival[750]. Other poor prognostic factors include hypercalcemia, poor clinical performance and infectious complications, especially

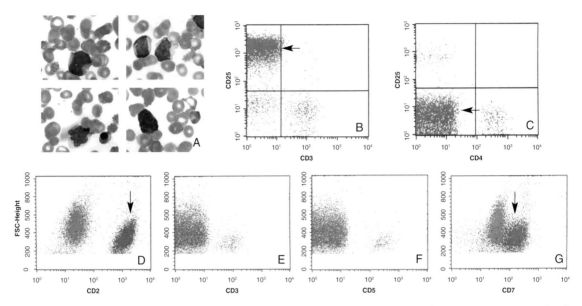

Figure 5.7 Aggressive NK-cell lymphoma/leukemia, blood. A, cytomorphology, B–G, immunophenotyping by flow cytometry. Leukemic cells express CD56 (B, arrow), CD2 (D, arrow) and CD7 (G, arrow) and are negative for CD4/CD8 (C, arrow), CD3, (E) and CD5 (F)

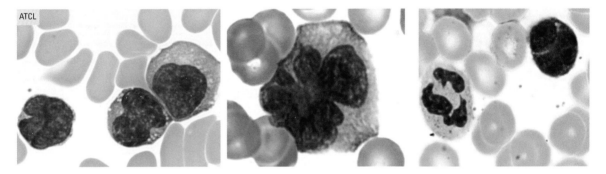

Figure 5.8 Adult T-cell leukemia/lymphoma, blood. Atypical lymphocytes with characteristic nuclear irregularities

opportunistic pulmonary infections. The prognosis in patients with adenopathy (Figure 5.9) depends on histologic features: pleomorphic infiltrate of medium to large cells and anaplastic infiltrate are associated with a highly aggressive course; Hodgkin-like infiltrate is associated with progressively decreased survival; while patients with the lymphadenitis type of lesion are considered to have a non-neoplastic status[1081]. There is also a strong correlation between the clinicopathologic features of cutaneous infiltrate and prognosis. Patients with ATCL with papules and nodules have a poorer prognosis than those with erythema[1082]. The median survival time of patients with monoclonal proviral DNA integration in cutaneous lesions was 14 months, which was shorter than that of patients with negative proviral DNA (72 months)[1082]. Nodular or diffuse cutaneous infiltrate of medium to large cells predicted poorer prognosis than perivascular infiltration of small lymphocytes[1082]. Patients with ATCL benefit from

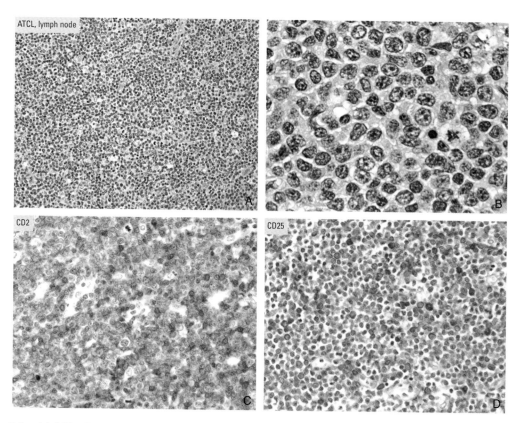

Figure 5.9 Adult T-cell leukemia/lymphoma, lymph node. A–B, histology; C–D, immunohistochemistry. Leukemic cells diffusely infiltrate the lymph node (A). They display pleomorphic nuclei and occasional mitoses (B) and are positive for CD2 (C) and CD25 (D)

aggressive chemotherapy, antiretroviral therapy, bone marrow transplantation and new drugs (proteasome inhibitors, retinoids, immunotherapy and angiogenesis inhibitors)[1076,1083]. Antiviral therapy employing zidovudine and interferon has shown promising results, as have antibody-based therapies to the IL 2 receptor (IL-2R, CD25) in combination with other agents or allogeneic transplantation.

PERIPHERAL T-CELL LYMPHOMA, UNSPECIFIED

PTCL forms a heterogeneous group of tumors with variable clinical features, histology (Figure 5.10), genetic alteration, response to treatment and prognosis. Despite aggressive therapy, the prognosis is

dismal, with more than half of the patients dying of their disease[202]. The estimated overall survival is 41–49% at 5 years[17,18,183]. The IPI is a significant prognostic factor for both progression-free and overall survival[17,19,1084,1085]. Besides IPI, systemic symptoms and bone marrow infiltration have been found to correlate with prognosis[1085]. Bone marrow is involved in 20–40% of PTCL (Figure 5.11) and appears to worsen the prognosis[183,202]. The overall 5-year survival for the low-risk group (IPI 0–1) is 64–75% and for the high-risk group (IPI ≥2) it is 30%[20,1085]. The IPI appears to be the best current prognostic model in PTCL. However, only about one-third of patients have low-risk disease. Using age, performance status, LDH level and bone marrow involvement as four factors independently

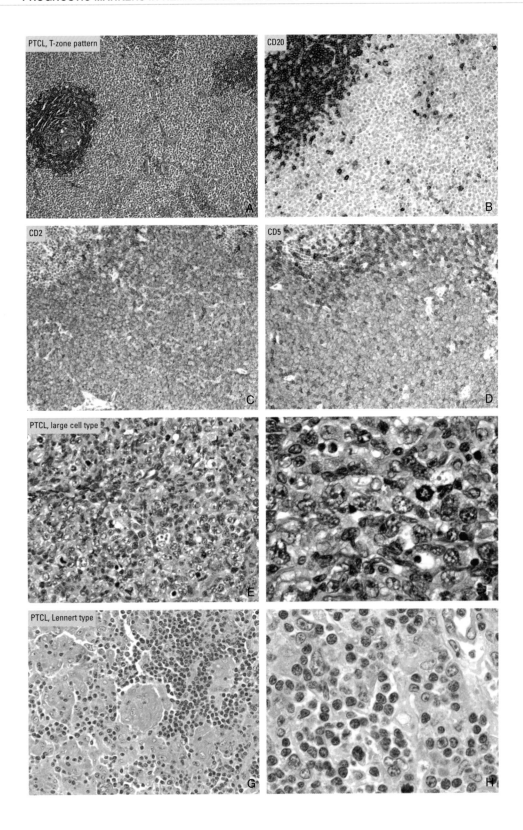

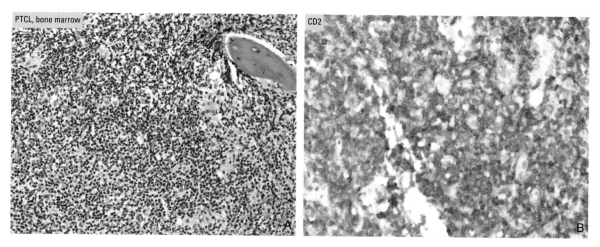

Figure 5.11 Extensive bone marrow involvement by peripheral T-cell lymphoma, unspecified (PTCL). A, histology; B, immunostaining for CD2

predictive of survival, Gallamini *et al.* proposed dividing PTCL into four prognostic groups: group 1, no adverse factors (5-year and 10-year survival of 62% and 54%, respectively); group 2, one factor (5-year and 10-year survival of 53% and 39%, respectively); group 3, two factors (5-year and 10-year survival of 33% and 18%, respectively); and group 4, three or four factors (5-year and 10-year survival of 18% and 12%, respectively)[183]. Age older than 60 years, LDH value at normal levels or above, performance status ≥2 and bone marrow involvement are factors independently predictive for shorter survival[183].

Patients with PTCL have an extremely poor prognosis when relapsed or refractory to conventional chemotherapy. Treatment by front-line autotransplantation can prevent relapse in patients with adverse IPI factors. However, patients presenting with a non-anaplastic T-cell phenotype, more than one extranodal site, or marrow involvement still have a higher risk of relapse. These factors should be taken into account when designing post-autotransplantation maintenance studies[1086].

ANGIOIMMUNOBLASTIC T-CELL LYMPHOMA

AILT is a mature T-cell lymphoma characterized by a sudden onset of constitutional symptoms and lymphadenopathy. Morphologically it is characterized by effacement of lymph node architecture by a polymorphous infiltrate that includes clusters of atypical lymphoid cells with clear cytoplasm, admixture of small lymphocytes, histiocytes, eosinophils and plasma cells, a marked increased in the number of arborizing vessels and scattered Epstein–Barr virus (EBV)+ B immunoblasts (Figure 5.12). Patients present with generalized adenopathy and B symptoms, and often have hepatosplenomegaly, skin rashes and pruritus, polyclonal hypergammaglobulinemia, autoantibodies, thrombocytopenia, or hemolytic

Figure 5.10 Peripheral T-cell lymphoma, unspecified (PTCL). A–D, PTCL with T-zone pattern. Lymphomatous cells are distributed in the interfollicular/paracortical area (A). Residual follicles are positive for CD20 (B) and tumor cells express CD2 (C) and CD5 (D). E–F, PTCL, large cell type. G–H, PTCL, Lennert type. Numerous histiocytic aggregates are present

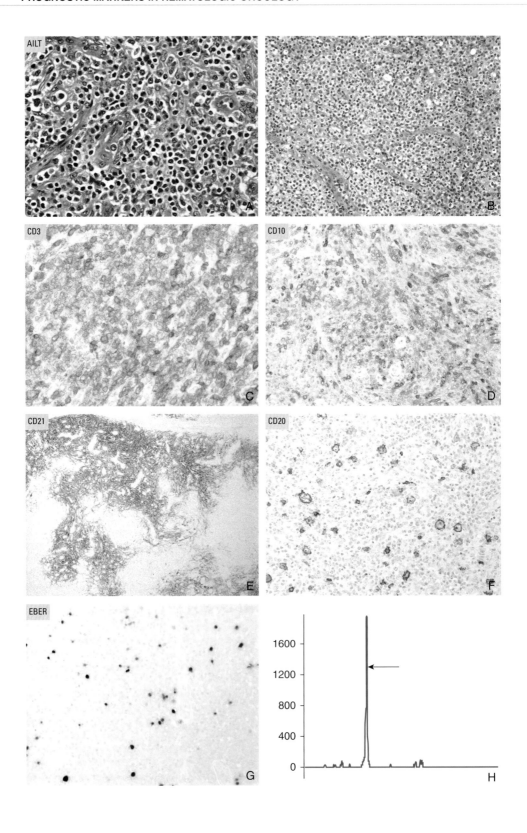

anemia. Patients with AILT have an aggressive clinical course and a poor prognosis with conventional treatment (corticosteroid and immunosuppressive agents). Overall, about 80% of patients die within 5 years, and 60–75% within 2 years[1087]. Treatment with high-dose chemotherapy with or without autologous stem cell transplantation may offer long-term disease-free survival[1088]. IPI is currently the best indicator of prognosis[17]. Complex karyotype is an independent poor prognostic factor.

HEPATOSPLENIC γδ T-CELL LYMPHOMA

Hepatosplenic γδ T-cell lymphoma is a disease with distinct clinical, morphologic and phenotypic characteristics with poor prognosis. Despite a satisfactory response to induction treatment in the majority of patients, the long-term therapeutic results are poor. A platinum–cytarabine-based induction regimen shows better results than CHOP or CHOP-like treatments. The median survival time is 16 months[447]. Many patients have isochromosome 7q. Figure 5.13 presents the morphologic features of hepatosplenic lymphoma.

NK/T-CELL LYMPHOMA, NASAL TYPE

This is an aggressive lymphoma of the upper respiratory tract, especially the nasal cavity (Figure 5.14), although it may occur at different locations, including testis, bone, skin and subcutaneous tissue. Among T-cell lymphomas, nasal-type NK/T-cell lymphoma and enteropathy-type T-cell lymphoma belong to the most aggressive tumors, with a worse prognosis than in PTCL. Extranodal NK/T-cell lymphoma, nasal type has an estimated overall survival of 0% at 5 years[1089]. Takahara *et al.* showed that high LDH level, large cells, immunoblastoid polymorphous histology, and *p53* (*TP53*) missense mutations were

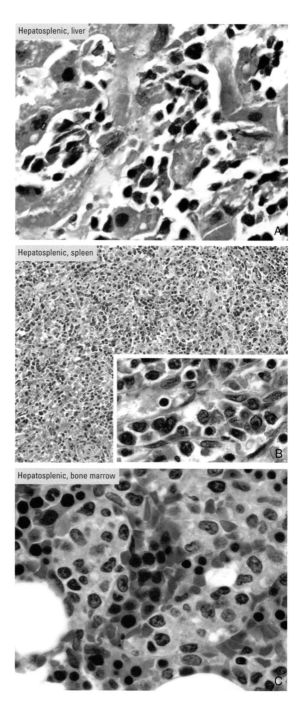

Figure 5.13   Hepatosplenic γδ T-cell lymphoma. A, liver; B, spleen; C, bone marrow

Figure 5.12   Angioimmunoblastic T-cell lymphoma (AILT). Effacement of the lymph node by atypical lymphoid infiltrate with increased vascularity (A) and clusters of large cells with clear cytoplasm (B). Tumor cells express CD3 (C) and aberrantly CD10 (D). The follicular dendritic cell meshwork is expanded (E). The neoplastic T-cell infiltrate is accompanied by large B-cell immunoblasts, reactive with CD20 (F) and EBER (G). Clonality of T cells was confirmed by PCR studies (H)

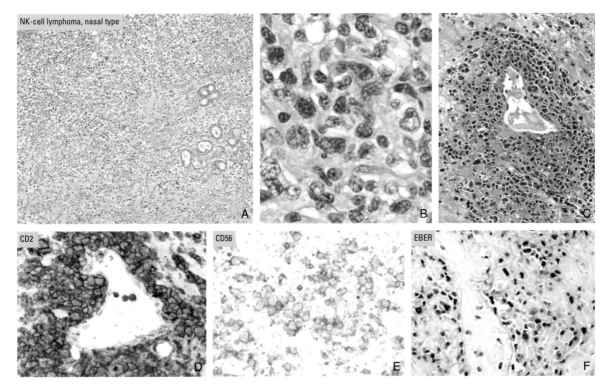

Figure 5.14   NK-cell lymphoma, nasal type. Atypical large cell infiltrate within the respiratory mucosa (A–B) with prominent perivascular distribution (C). Tumor cells are positive for CD2 (D), CD56 (E) and EBER (F)

significantly related to worse cause-specific survival in nasal NK/T-cell lymphoma[1090]. Nasal type NK/T-cell lymphoma occurring outside the nasal cavity is more aggressive, has shorter survival times and poorer response to treatment than that located within the nasal cavity. Multivariate analysis showed that *p53* missense mutation was the most independent among these three factors. Other prognostic factors for aggressive NK/T-cell neoplasm include age (≤ 40 vs. >40 years old) and the source of stem cells for transplantation (bone marrow vs. blood).

CUTANEOUS T-CELL LYMPHOMAS

Primary cutaneous T-cell lymphomas represent a heterogeneous group of neoplasms derived from skin-homing T-cells. The majority of cutaneous T-cell lymphomas represent mycosis fungoides (MF) and CD30+ T-cell lymphoproliferative disorders, such as cutaneous anaplastic large cell lymphoma (ALCL) and

lymphomatoid papulosis (LyP). Other less common neoplasms include blastic NK-cell lymphoma/leukemia, extranodal NK/T-cell lymphoma (nasal type), secondary peripheral T-cell lymphomas and subcutaneous panniculitis-like T-cell lymphoma.

Prognostic factors in primary cutaneous T-cell lymphomas include type of skin involvement, increased blood eosinophil count and increased serum level of LDH[1091]. Blood eosinophilia is strongly associated with disease progression and disease-specific death in primary cutaneous T-cell lymphoma[1091]. Prognostic studies of primary cutaneous lymphomas other than MF and Sézary's syndrome showed that serum LDH level, B symptoms and parameters related to tumor extension (i.e. distribution, maximum diameter and number of skin lesions) were significantly associated with survival. When these variables were considered together in a multivariate analysis, the European Organization for Research and Treatment of Cancer (EORTC) prognostic group and distribution of

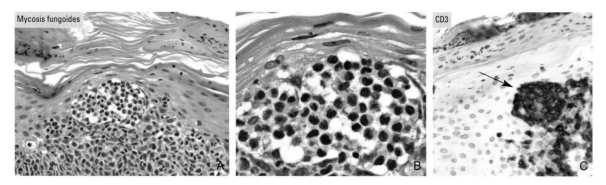

Figure 5.15 Mycosis fungoides. Atypical dense lymphoid infiltrate in the upper dermis (A) with prominent epidermotropism (B). The immunostaining with CD3 (C) highlights malignant cells within the epidermis

skin lesions remained statistically significant and independent prognostic factors. This study confirmed the good predictive value of the EORTC classification for primary cutaneous lymphoma and showed that the distribution of skin lesions at initial evaluation is an important prognostic indicator[1092]. A high number of chromosomal imbalances (≥5) in cutaneous T-cell lymphomas is associated with a shorter survival[411]. Gain in 8q and loss of 6q and 13q correlates with a significantly shorter survival, whereas the most frequent aberrations (loss in 17p and gain in 7) do not influence the prognosis[411]. Dual CD4−/CD8− cutaneous T-cell lymphomas (representing predominantly γδ T-cell lymphoma) remain largely restricted to the skin but often show rapid and multifocal cutaneous spread and uniformly aggressive behavior[1093]. Cutaneous γδ T-cell lymphomas, which are not defined as a specific entity in the WHO classification, are associated with significantly decreased survival[1094]. The median survival for individuals with γδ T-cell lymphoma is 15 months, whereas the median survival of individuals with αβ cutaneous T-cell lymphoma is 166 months[1094].

Mycosis fungoides and Sézary's syndrome

MF (Figure 5.15) is a cutaneous CD4+ T-cell lymphoma characterized by multifocal disease and protracted clinical course except for cases with large cell transformation. MF represents the most indolent of the cutaneous T-cell lymphomas, with 10-year relative survival ranging from 100% to 40% depending on the degree of skin involvement[1095].

MF may progress to aggressive cutaneous or extracutaneous large T-cell lymphoma[1096–1099]. Figures 5.16 and 5.17 present large cell transformation of cutaneous lymphoma. The probability of progression to extracutaneous disease within 20 years of diagnosis is approximately 40%[1095]. Clinicopathologic or biologic criteria predictive of transformation are unknown except for the expression of CD25 antigen (IL-2R), which may identify a subset of MF patients at risk[707]. Independent of clinical stage, patients who had the same T-cell receptor (*TCR*) gene rearrangement detected in multiple biopsy specimens at the time of diagnosis are more likely to have progressive disease than those who have different gene rearrangement[1100]. The transformation of MF is associated with rapid deterioration of clinical status. The change in histologic appearance and clinical behavior of MF is similar to transformations of other hematopoietic and lymphoid neoplasms. Disease is usually classified as transformed if biopsy showed large cells (≥4 times the size of a small lymphocyte) in more than 25% of the infiltrate or if they formed microscopic nodules[1096,1098,1099]. The transformation is more common in patients with tumors and with more advanced clinical stage of the disease. Survival in patients with transformed cutaneous lymphoma is significantly shorter than in patients without transformation; survival after diagnosis of transformation is short[1096–1098]. Patients with transformation have a

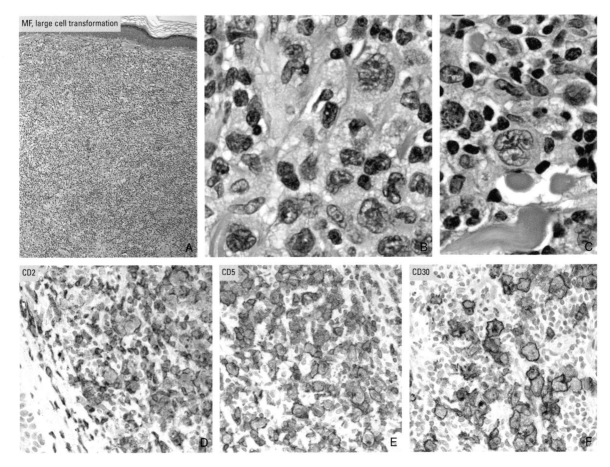

Figure 5.16   Large cell transformation of mycosis fungoides (MF). Dense lymphoid infiltrate involving the dermis (A), composed of pleomorphic cells with numerous large anaplastic lymphocytes (B–C). Neoplastic cells are positive for CD2 (D), CD5 (E) and CD30 (F)

relatively poor survival, especially if transformation occurs early (within 2 years) in the course of disease or if they are at a higher stage. Patients with extracutaneous transformation had a shorter median survival after transformation than those with transformation limited to skin; extracutaneous transformation apparently indicates a poorer prognosis than cutaneous transformation[1096]. In a univariate analysis by Vergier *et al.*, only extracutaneous progression was associated with a worse prognosis (5-year actuarial survival: 7.8% vs. 32%). Sex, age, clinical or skin disease, stage at transformation, transformation speed, percentage of large cells or CD30 expression did not have a prognostic value. When

performing multivariate analysis, age (at least 60 years) and extracutaneous spreading were found to be associated with a poor prognosis[1099].

Sézary's syndrome is an aggressive erythrodermic cutaneous T-cell lymphoma with a poor prognosis. It remains practically incurable, with a median survival of 2–3 years[1101]. The prognostic factors in multivariate analysis are age at diagnosis, interval before diagnosis and the presence of the EBV genome in keratinocytes[1101]. Univariate analysis revealed the LDH level as a prognostic indicator. Fast evolution of the disease, increased level of LDH and increased level of serum β_2-microglobulin are associated with poor prognosis in MF/Sézary's syndrome[126]. Chromosomal

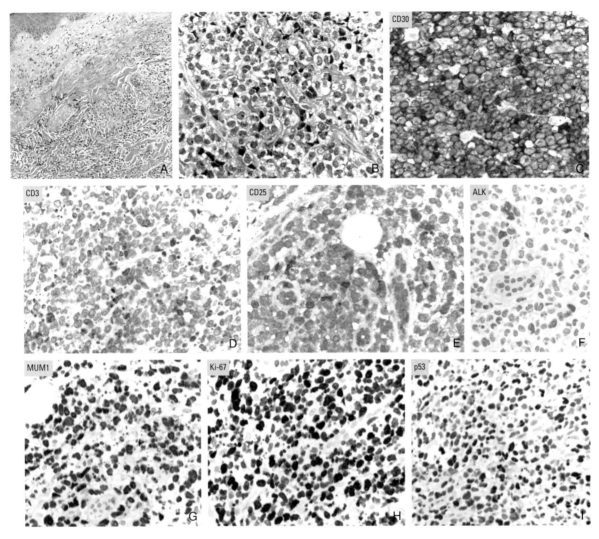

Figure 5.17 Large cell transformation of cutaneous T-cell lymphoma. A–B, histology; C–I, immunohistochemistry. Tumor cells involve the dermis (A). They are predominantly large and pleomorphic (B) and express CD30 (C), CD3 (D), CD25 (E), MUM1 (G), Ki-67 (H) and p53 (I). ALK is not expressed (F)

abnormalities occur in 43% of patients[1102], usually involving chromosomes 1, 6, 10, 14, and 17.

Primary cutaneous anaplastic large cell lymphoma

Cutaneous ALCL arises *de novo* in the skin, affects older patients, and does not express ALK (Figure 5.18). Cutaneous ALCL is generally accepted to be at the malignant end of the spectrum of CD30+

cutaneous lymphoproliferative disorders that include LyP[217,1103]. Primary cutaneous ALCL has a more favorable prognosis than systemic ALCL. Although primary cutaneous ALCL and LyP are usually ALK−, survival is generally better than for ALK+ systemic ALCL. A subset of patients with cutaneous ALCL shows partial or complete spontaneous regression, showing overlapping features with lymphomatoid papulosis. Spontaneous regression occurs in approximately 25–42% of primary cutaneous ALCL and in

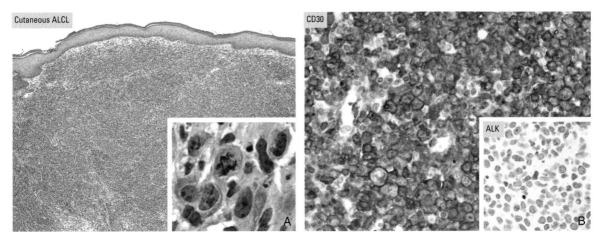

Figure 5.18 Cutaneous anaplastic large cell lymphoma (ALCL). A, histology showing extensive lymphoid infiltrate of large cells (*inset; high magnification*); B, tumor cells are strongly positive for CD30 (*inset: negative expression of ALK*)

virtually all cases of LyP[1104,1105]. Only patients with disseminated skin involvement are at greater risk of developing extracutaneous disease[1106]. Patients with multifocal skin lesions more often acquired extracutaneous disease (17% vs. 8%) and more often died of lymphoma (12% vs. 3%) than patients with solitary or localized skin lesions[1105]. However, univariate analysis demonstrated that none of extent of skin lesions, age at diagnosis, presence of spontaneous remission or histologic subtype were significantly related to disease progression or survival[1105]. Regional lymph node involvement usually does not predict a poor prognosis in patients who present with primary cutaneous ALCL[1104,1105]. CD30 expression is an important prognostic parameter for this group of primary cutaneous large cell lymphomas. CD30[+] cutaneous lymphomas generally presented with localized skin disease, and had a favorable prognosis when compared to CD30[−] lymphomas[1105,1107]. The latter often presented with or rapidly developed generalized disease. Five-year survival for primary cutaneous ALCL is greater than 90% and is nearly 100% for lymphomatoid papulosis[1105,1106]. Patients with CD30[−] primary cutaneous T-cell lymphomas have an unfavorable prognosis, irrespective of the presence or absence of extracutaneous disease at the time of diagnosis, cell size and expression of a CD4[+] or CD8[+]

phenotype[1108]. Patients with systemic CD30[+] ALCL with concurrent or secondary skin lesions have a poor response to treatment and poor prognosis, with 5-year survival rates of 44% after diagnosis and 23% after development of skin lesions – suggesting that appearance of skin lesions in CD30[+] ALCL is a poor prognostic sign[1106].

Lymphomatoid papulosis

LyP belongs to the spectrum of CD30[+] lymphoproliferative disorders involving the skin. It was first described by Macaulay as a continuous self-healing eruption that is clinically benign but with histologic features that resemble malignant lymphoma[1109]. Patients present with popular, papulonecrotic or nodular skin lesions, often in different stages of evolution next to each other. LyP patients have an increased risk of developing lymphoma, compared with the normal population[1110]. The most common types of lymphoma in LyP patients are mycosis fungoides, Hodgkin's lymphoma and cutaneous (or rarely extracutaneous) CD30[+] large T-cell lymphoma[1105,1111–1113]. The risk for systemic disease within 10 years of diagnosis is 4%[1105]. Overall 5-year survival is 98% (disease-related 5-year and 10-year survivals are 100%)[1105].

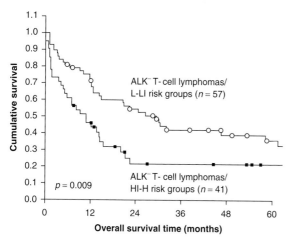

Figure 5.19 Comparison of overall survival time in ALK⁻ T-cell lymphomas (comprising ALK⁻ anaplastic large cell lymphoma (ALCL), peripheral T-cell lymphoma, unspecified (PTCL) and angioimmunoblastic lymphoma (AILT)), according to the International Prognostic Index (IPI): low–low-intermediate (L-LI) vs. high-intermediate– high (HI-H) risk groups

From: ten Berge *et al*. ALK-negative anaplastic large-cell lymphoma demonstrates similar prognosis to peripheral T-cell lymphoma, unspecified. Histopathology 2003; 43:462–9. © 2003 by Blackwell Publishing Limited, used with permission

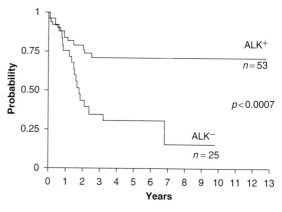

Figure 5.20 Overall survival of ALK⁺ versus ALK⁻ lymphoma

From: Falini B, *et al*. ALK+ lymphoma: clinicopathological findings and outcome. Blood 1999;93:2697–706. © 1999 by The American Society of Hematology, used with permission

Subcutaneous panniculitis-like T-cell lymphoma

Subcutaneous panniculitis-like T-cell lymphoma is a cytotoxic T-cell lymphoma characterized by primary involvement of the subcutaneous fat in a manner mimicking panniculitis with a progressive clinical course[1114,1115]. Dissemination to lymph nodes and other organs is rare and occurs late in the clinical course[225]. Histologically, the lesions are reminiscent of panniculitis and are composed of a mixture of small and large atypical lymphoid cells. Patients with subcutaneous panniculitis-like T-cell lymphoma frequently show clinical features of hemophagocytic syndrome. Estimated 5-year survival is 80%[1089]. However, patients with CD56⁺ tumors and TCRγδ phenotype have an aggressive clinical course[735,736,1116]. The median survival rate for patients with CD56⁺

tumors is 12 months[736]. CD56 expression, therefore, appears to be an important factor in determining the clinical course of subcutaneous lymphomas. CD56⁺ subcutaneous panniculitis-like T-cell lymphomas show overlap of some clinical, histologic and prognostic features with extranodal NK/T-cell lymphoma, nasal type. The latter is positive for EBV/EBER, usually shows germline configuration of TCR genes and occurs mostly in Asia. Subcutaneous panniculitis-like T-cell lymphomas are EBV⁻[735].

Cutaneous NK/T-cell lymphoma, nasal type

Cutaneous NK/T-cell lymphoma, nasal type is an aggressive tumor associated with rapid clinical progression, treatment failure, multiple relapses, and an average survival of 15 months[1117].

ANAPLASTIC LARGE CELL LYMPHOMA

ALCL is an aggressive lymphoma characterized by large pleomorphic cells with irregular nuclei ('hallmark' cells), preferential paracortical and intrasinusoidal lymph node involvement and expression of

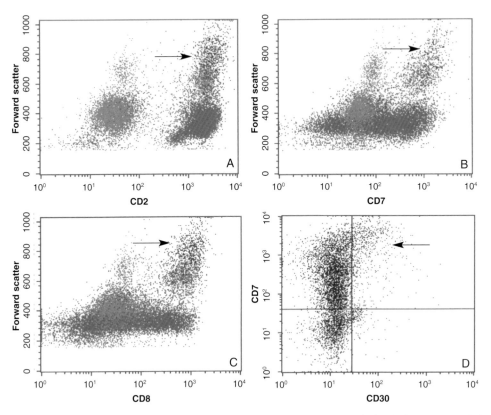

Figure 5.21   Anaplastic large cell lymphoma, leukemic phase. Flow cytometry of blood shows a population of large cells (increased forward scatter; arrows) expressing CD2 (A), CD7 (B), CD8 (C) and CD30 (D)

CD30[1118]. ALCL includes a subset of tumors that carry t(2;5)(p23;q35)[1118]. The t(2;5) disrupts the nucleophosmin (*NPM*) gene at 5q35 and the anaplastic lymphoma kinase (*ALK*) gene at 2p23, generating a novel *NPM–ALK* gene. *NPM–ALK* fusion leads to a chimeric mRNA molecule and a unique 80-kDa NPM–ALK fusion protein referred to as p80[620]. Several cytogenetic and molecular studies have demonstrated that chromosomal aberrations other than t(2;5)(p23;q35) may give rise to *ALK* fusion genes in ALCL. These alternative partners to the *NPM* gene include *TPM3* (non-muscle tropomyosin) associated with t(1;2)(q21;p23), *TFG* (*TRK*-fused gene) associated with t(2;3)(p23;q21), *CLTC* (clathrin heavy-chain gene) associated with t(2;22)(p23;q11) and *MSN* (moesin)[1119–1121]. In contrast to the nuclear and cytoplasmic distribution

of the NPM–ALK protein, variant ALK fusion proteins show a variable subcellular localization. The t(2;5)(p23;q35) and variant translocation involving 2p23 result in overexpression of the ALK protein by ALCL, which can be detected by routine immunohistochemistry[22,1119,1120,1122,1123]. ALK+ ALCL occurs most commonly in the first 3 decades of life, is more common in men, presents as aggressive stage III–IV disease with systemic symptoms, frequently has extranodal involvement and is characterized by a good response to chemotherapy[22,182,1124–1126]. ALK+ ALCL shows a wide range of morphological characteristics, including common, lymphohistiocytic, small cell, giant cell and Hodgkin-like types[1126]. ALCL without ALK expression occurs in older patients, with similar distribution in male and female patients, and is associated with a lower incidence of

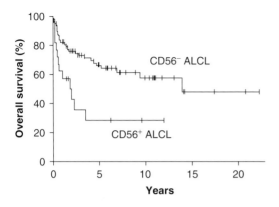

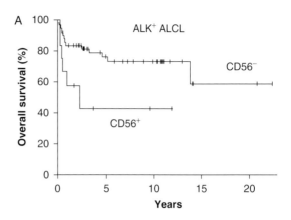

Figure 5.22 Overall survival of CD56⁺ and CD56⁻ cases of anaplastic large cell lymphoma (ALCL). The CD56⁺ group has a significantly worse prognosis ($p = 0.002$)

From: Suzuki R, *et al*. Prognostic significance of CD56 expression for ALK-positive and ALK-negative anaplastic large cell lymphoma. Blood 2000;96:2993–3000. © 2000 by The American Society of Hematology, used with permission

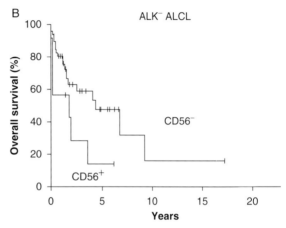

Figure 5.23 Prognostic difference between CD56⁺ and CD56⁻ anaplastic large cell lymphoma (ALCL) according to ALK expression. The CD56⁺ group shows a significantly lower survival for both ALK⁺ (A, $p = 0.02$) and ALK⁻ (B, $p = 0.04$) subtypes

From: Suzuki R, *et al*. Prognostic significance of CD56 expression for ALK-positive and ALK-negative anaplastic large cell lymphoma. Blood 2000;96:2993–3000. © 2000 by The American Society of Hematology, used with permission

stage III–IV disease and extranodal involvement. Figures 5.19 and 5.20 compare the survival of patients with ALK⁺ lymphoma versus other type of T-cell lymphoma.

Unfavorable factors affecting overall survival of patients with ALCL include age >60, CD56⁺, stage III/IV, lack of ALK expression, B symptoms, extranodal disease in ≥2 sites and increased LDH[734]. ALK⁻ ALCL demonstrates similar poor prognosis to PTCL[1127]. In the group of ALK⁻ ALCL and PTCL, only age and the IPI are of significant prognostic value[1127]. Patients with ALK⁺ ALCL have better overall survival than patients with ALK⁻ ALCL[22,182]. The 5-year overall survival of ALK⁺ versus ALK⁻ ALCL is 71–79% versus 15–46%, respectively. Other studies, which did not investigated ALK expression, have reported excellent outcome for (systemic) ALCL occurring in children and young adult patients[1128–1131]. This may be associated with a large proportion of chimeric ALK⁺ ALCL in younger patients. ALCL carrying variants of the NPM–ALK fusion protein can be grouped with classic t(2;5)⁺ tumors with a better prognosis than ALK⁻ ALCL[1132].

Within the good prognostic group of ALK⁺ cases, 5-year survival in patients in the low/intermediate-risk group (IPI 0–1) is 94%, and in patients in the high/intermediate-risk group (IPI ≥2) it is 41%[22]. Therefore, IPI in conjunction with ALK expression and patient age can serve to design optimal therapeutic strategies for individual patients (e.g. less aggressive therapy for children with ALK⁺ ALCL with IPI ≤2 and aggressive chemotherapy followed by stem cell support for patients with IPI ≥2 or ALK⁻ tumors). Leukemic blood involvement in ALCL is uncommon, but may occur at the time of initial presentation or during the course of disease (Figure 5.21). It is most often associated with small cell histologic features and the t(2;5)(p23;q35)[1133]. Most of the cases with leukemic blood involvement have a poor response to therapy or early relapse[1133] and require more aggressive therapy (including hematopoietic stem cell transplantation). In children with ALCL, the strongest adverse prognostic factors are lung or mediastinum involvement in conjunction with skin involvement. Children with completely excised stage I tumor (low risk) or no skin, lung,

mediastinum, spleen or liver involvement (standard risk) have a 3-year event-free survival of ~90%, and children with biopsy-proven involvement of skin, lung, mediastinum, liver or spleen (high risk) have a 3-year event-free survival of ~60%. CD56, a neural cell-adhesion molecule, can be expressed by a subset of ALCL, with the CD56⁺ cases showing a much poorer prognosis than CD56⁻ cases in both the ALK⁺ and ALK⁻ subgroups[734]. Figures 5.22 and 5.23 illustrate the prognostic significance of CD56 expression in ALCL. Bcl-2, a major negative regulator of apoptosis, was detected in 60% of ALK⁻ ALCL but Bcl-2 was not expressed in ALK⁺ ALCL[1134]. Patients with Bcl-2⁺ ALCL showed a trend toward an unfavorable prognosis, but this did not reach statistical significance[1134].

CHAPTER 6

Hodgkin's lymphoma

CLASSICAL HODGKIN'S LYMPHOMA

Hodgkin's lymphoma (HL, Figure 6.1) is a malignant lymphoma of B cells characterized by Reed–Sternberg and Hodgkin cells accompanied by reactive lymphocytes, granulocytes, eosinophils, histiocytes and plasma cells, and often a variable amount of fibrosis. Tumor cells are positive for CD30 and often CD15 and PAX5. A subset of cases expresses CD20, Epstein–Barr virus (EBV)/EBV-encoded RNA (EBER) and Bcl-2. CD45, T-cell antigens and ALK1 are not expressed. Neoplastic cells in classical HL originate from germinal center B-lymphoid cells with defective immunoglobulin transcription, which escape from apoptosis. Based on the number of neoplastic cells, the amount of fibrosis and composition of background cells, HL is divided into nodular sclerosis (NS), mixed cellularity, lymphocyte-rich and lymphocyte-depleted subtypes. With the modern therapeutic approach, HL is now considered to have a favorable prognosis. The long-term effect in successfully treated patients is a second malignancy, which occurs at rates exceeding those in the general population[1135]. These cancers may occur years to decades after remission and arise in the breast, thyroid, gastrointestinal tract, lung, skin, urogenital tract and brain. There is also an increased risk of acute leukemia and non-Hodgkin's lymphoma (NHL). A second malignancy is the leading cause of death in long-term survivors of HL.

Clinical parameters

The clinical stage of HL (Ann Arbor classification updated at Cotswold; Table 1.3) determines the treatment regimen and the prognosis. Tumor burden is the most important prognostic factor in HL[1136,1137]. In a series reported by Specht and Nissen, both lymphocytopenia and bone marrow involvement had independent prognostic significance, and these two factors emerged as the most important prognostic factors in disseminated HL, and both appeared to be related to the patient's total tumor burden[1136,1137]. Advanced stage of the disease (III–IV), age over 60 years, extranodal disease, mediastinal mass (widening of the mediastinum by more than one-third), bulky disease (>10 cm maximum dimension of nodal mass) and B symptoms (fever, drenching sweats, weight loss) are associated with worse prognosis[254,1138,1139]. Based on stage and risk factors (large mediastinal mass, B symptoms, bulky disease, extranodal disease, high erythrocyte sedimentation rate and three or more lymph node areas involved) the German Hodgkin Lymphoma Study Group (GHSG) defined three risk groups in classical HL: (1) early stages (patients in stage I–II without risk factors), (2) intermediate stages (I–IIA with one or more risk factors) and (3) advanced stages (all patients in stages III–IV and selected patients in stage IIB with large mediastinal mass and/or extranodal disease). Hasenclever and Diehl constructed

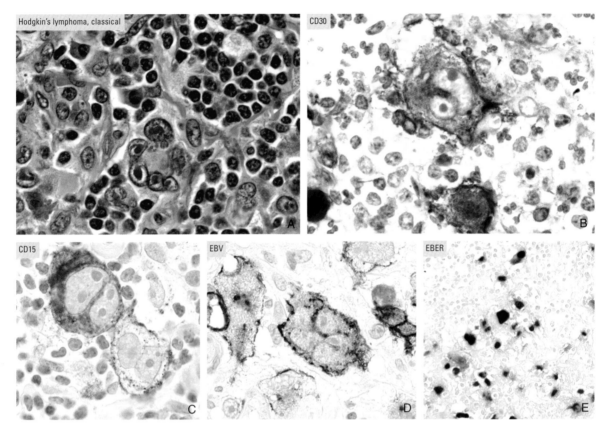

Figure 6.1 Classical Hodgkin's lymphoma. Reed–Sternberg cells (A) are positive for CD30 (B), CD15 (C), Epstein–Barr virus (EBV) (D) and EBER (E)

a prognostic index (International Prognostic Score) based on seven factors that had similar independent prognostic effects: a serum albumin level of < 4 g/dl, a hemoglobin level of < 10.5 g/dl, male sex, age ≥ 45 years, stage IV disease (Ann Arbor classification), leukocytosis (≥ 15 × 10⁹/l) and lymphocytopenia (< 0.6 × 10⁹/l or less than 8% of white blood cell count)[27]. The score predicted the rate of freedom from progression of disease as follows: 0 (no factors), 84%; 1, 77%; 2, 67%; 3, 60%; 4, 51%; and 5 or higher, 42%[27]. In patients with HL undergoing an autologous stem cell transplantation after a first relapse, advanced stage at diagnosis, complementary radiotherapy before transplantation, a short first complete response and detectable disease at transplantation adversely influenced time to treatment failure, while bulky disease at diagnosis, a short first complete response, detectable disease at transplantation and ≥ 1 extranodal areas involved at transplantation are adverse factors for overall survival[1140].

Morphologic and phenotypic features

A British National Lymphoma Investigation study proposed to divide NS HL into low grade (NS1) and high grade (NS2)[1141]. It was suggested that HL with extensive areas of lymphocyte depletion or with numerous anaplastic Hodgkin cells (NS2) is associated with a poor response to initial therapy, an increased relapse rate and decreased survival when

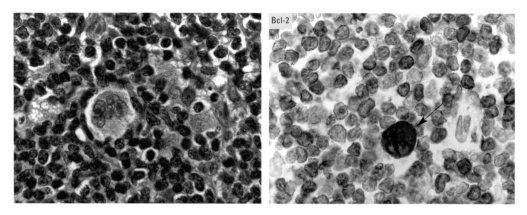

Figure 6.2 Classical Hodgkin's lymphoma. Reed–Sternberg cells express Bcl-2 (arrow)

compared with other NS variants (NS1)[1141]. Grading of NS has been widely debated in the literature, with some reports supporting and other not confirming British findings[1142–1145]. In a recent grading system proposed by von Wasilewski *et al.*, NS cases were divided into low risk and high risk, based on eosinophilia, lymphocyte depletion and atypia of Hodgkin/Reed–Sternberg cells. The presence of eosinophilia, lymphocyte depletion and atypia of the Hodgkin/Reed–Sternberg cells was a significant indicator of prognosis in intermediate and advanced stages[1146].

The better overall survival in HL is associated with the expression of CD15[547,1147,1148], MCL1[547] and EBV latent membrane protein 1 (LMP1)[254,547]. Multivariate Cox regression using expression of three markers (CD15, CD30, CD20), age, sex, histology, stage, B symptoms (fever, sweats, weight loss >10% of body weight), hemoglobin and erythrocyte sedimentation rate as factors showed that lack of CD15 expression in classical HL was an independent negative prognostic factor for relapses and survival[1148]. Neoplastic cells in a subset of HL patients express Bcl-2 (Figure 6.2). Rassidakis *et al.* reported that Bcl-2 expression was independently associated with inferior failure-free survival along with age 45 or older, Ann Arbor stage IV, low serum albumin and high serum lactate dehydrogenase (LDH) levels in patients treated with doxorubicin, bleomycin,

vinblastine and dacarbazine[546]. In a study by Morente *et al.*, a high proliferation index (Ki-67) and loss of retinoblastoma protein (pRb) expression were found to be adverse prognostic factors influencing, respectively, lower overall survival and failure to achieve complete remission, but histopathological type, p53, Bcl-2 and CD15 expression lacked significant influence on the outcome[254]. Both time to treatment failure and overall survival are decreased in CD20+ HL as compared with CD20− HL[703]. Reed–Sternberg cells expressing CD20 are shown in Figure 6.3. Although mast cells can be detected in virtually every case of HL, with increasing numbers being seen in the nodular sclerosis type, patients with high mast cell infiltration were reported to have worse relapse-free survival[1149]. Similarly, tissue eosinophilia appears to be a strong negative prognostic indicator in NS HL[1150].

There is a relationship between the expression of cell cycle proteins and patients' outcome. A high proliferation index (Ki-67) and loss of pRb expression were also found to be adverse prognostic factors influencing, respectively, lower overall survival and failure to achieve complete remission. Multivariate analysis confirmed the independent significance of these two parameters and additionally identifies EBV LMP1 expression as a favorable prognostic marker, in relation to overall survival.

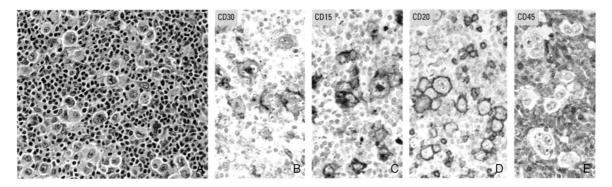

Figure 6.3 Classical Hodgkin's lymphoma. A, histology; B–E, immunohistochemistry. Reed–Sternberg cells are positive for CD30 (B), CD15 (C) and CD20 (D) and do not express CD45 (E)

Molecular markers

Tissue microarray analysis revealed deregulation of the genes involved in the G_1/S and G_2/M transitions and inactivation of the tumor suppressor pathways including p14^{ARF}–p53–p21^{WAF1}, p16^{INK4a}–pRb and p27^{KIP1} [255]. The abnormalities of p14^{ARF} are associated with Hdm2 overexpression and subsequently *p53* (*TP53*) inactivation, whereas the p16^{INK4a}–pRb pathway is inactivated by loss of p16^{INK4a} and/or cyclin D overexpression. Additionally, neoplastic cells in HL show high expression of cyclins and cdk involved in the G_1/S and G_2/M transitions and have defective regulation of apoptosis due to overexpression of Bcl-2 (23%), Bcl-X$_L$ (19%) and survivin (89%), loss of BAX expression (3%) and increased nuclear expression of p65/RelA[255]. Bcl-2, Bcl-X$_L$ and nuclear factor κB (NF-κB) activation are involved in the resistance to apoptosis by Hodgkin and Reed–Sternberg cells. The presence of NF-κB and its activation are related to changes in the expression of a set of proteins that play a role in the control of cell cycle progression, apoptosis and gene transcription, such as p21, p16, p27, pRb, cyclins E and D3, cdk1, cdk2, and survivin[255]. Shorter survival of patients with HL is related to overexpression of Bcl-2, p53, Bcl-X$_L$, BAX, and high proliferative (Ki-67/MIB1) and apoptotic indexes[255].

NODULAR LYMPHOCYTE-PREDOMINANT HODGKIN'S LYMPHOMA

Nodular lymphocyte-predominant HL (NLPHL) is a distinct type of HL representing approximately 5% of all HL cases[1151]. It is characterized by nodular architecture on low magnification and the presence of large neoplastic cells with irregular multilobed nuclei, often referred to as 'popcorn' cells or *L&H* cells (Figure 6.4). Overall survival rates are similar in patients with NLPHL (86%) and classical HL (82%) at clinical stages IA and IIA treated with anthracycline-based chemotherapy plus high-dose extended irradiation; they share the same excellent prognosis[1152]. A small subset of patients with NLPHL in whom lymph node biopsy shows NLPHL with a typical purely nodular pattern also may have lymphoma in the bone marrow. Bone marrow involvement is associated with laboratory, radiologic, or morphologic evidence of aggressive disease and poor prognosis[1153].

NLPHL and T-cell/histiocyte-rich large B-cell lymphoma may occur concurrently or subsequently in the same patient[225,1154–1156]. The presence of a diffuse T-cell/histiocyte-rich-like pattern is more common in patients with recurrent disease than in those without recurrence[223]. The presence of a diffuse

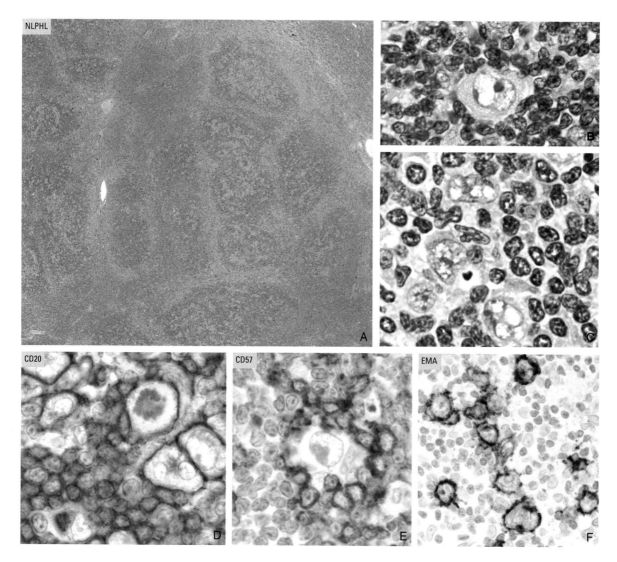

Figure 6.4 Nodular lymphocyte-predominant Hodgkin's lymphoma (NLPHL). A, low magnification of the lymph-node histologic section shows the characteristic nodular pattern. B–C, high magnification shows large cells with irregular nuclei and prominent nucleoli ('popcorn' cells or L&H cells). Neoplastic cells are positive for CD20 (D) and epithelial membrane antigen (EMA) (F). CD57+ small T cells form rosettes around tumor cells (E)

pattern (T-cell-rich B-cell lymphoma-like) is an independent predictor of recurrent disease[223]. Analysis of sequential biopsies from patients with recurrent disease suggests that the presence of prominent extranodal L&H cells might represent early evolution to a diffuse pattern[223].

Patients with NLPHL may develop more aggressive lymphomas, most often diffuse large B-cell lymphoma (DLBCL) (Figure 6.5). The median time to the development of DLBCL in those with prior NLPHL was only 1 year (range, 0.5–24 years). The median age of the patients at the

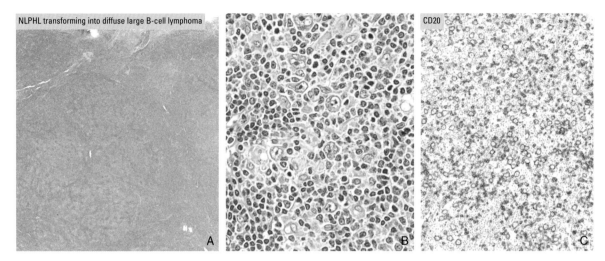

Figure 6.5 Nodular lymphocyte-predominant Hodgkin's lymphoma (NLPHL) transforming into diffuse large B-cell lymphoma. A, Low power shows typical features of NLPHL; B–C, high magnification and CD20 staining shows numerous large B cells with relatively few small B lymphocytes

time of diagnosis of DLBCL was 46 years (range, 18–72 years) and the male/female ratio were 17:4. The median overall survival and failure-free survival of the entire group were 35 months and 11 months, respectively, and the predicted 5-year overall survival and failure-free survival were 31 and 18%, respectively. There are no significant differences in the survival outcomes between patients with DLBCL arising in NLPHL and age- and sex-matched patients with *de novo* DLBCL[221].

CHAPTER 7

Precursor B- and T-lymphoblastic leukemia/lymphoma (acute lymphoblastic leukemia)

PRECURSOR B-LYMPHOBLASTIC LEUKEMIA/LYMPHOMA

Precursor B-lymphoblastic leukemia/lymphoma (acute lymphoblastic leukemia; B-ALL) is a lymphoproliferative disorder of immature B-cells with blastic morphology (Figure 7.1), which often express CD10, CD34 and terminal deoxynucleotidyl transferase (TdT). A number of clinical, phenotypic and genetic features are prognostically significant in B-ALL. The total white blood cell (WBC) count at the time of diagnosis is the single most powerful clinical predictor of remission induction and duration, and long-term survival for all age groups[1157–1159]. Patients with high WBC counts often have extramedullary disease at diagnosis and are at high risk for relapse in the central nervous system (CNS) and testes. Age at diagnosis, certain chromosomal changes, immunophenotype and persistence of leukemia after induction therapy comprise other important prognostic parameters[1160–1162]. Table 7.1 presents prognostic factors in ALL.

Clinical features

Age is an important prognostic factor in ALL. Advanced age, high WBC count and Philadelphia chromosome-positive (Ph$^+$) ALL are the major risk factors for attaining complete remission. In adults with ALL, increasing age is associated with shorter remission duration and survival. Children younger than 1 year or older than 10 years have a worse prognosis when compared with children in the age group of 2–6 years[1162]. Among patients with Ph$^+$ ALL, children between 1 and 9 years old have a better prognosis than patients in other age groups. Improvements in the treatment of childhood ALL result in a long-term disease-free survival of about 80%[1160,1163]. Children with drug-resistant ALL have a worse prognosis than children with drug-sensitive leukemia[1164–1166].

Boys with ALL have a higher incidence of relapse and a shorter survival when compared with girls[1161,1167–1169]. These results are independent of other prognostic parameters, including age and presenting leukocyte count[1161,1167]. The difference in outcome can partially be explained by differences between boys and girls in the distributions of the ALL immunophenotype and DNA index[1170]. Pieters *et al.* showed that leukemic cells from boys were more resistant to thioguanine than were those from girls[1164]. Multivariate analysis indicates a poorer

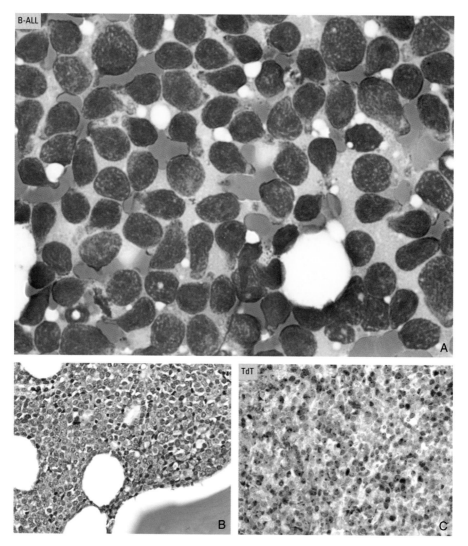

Figure 7.1 Precursor B-lymphoblastic leukemia (B-ALL). A, cytomorphology (aspirate smear) shows blasts with occasional 'hand-mirror' cells; B, histology section from bone marrow core biopsy shows total replacement of the bone marrow by immature mononuclear cells, which are positive for terminal deoxynucleotidyl transferase (TdT) (C)

outcome for Blacks when compared with Whites, in part related to different biologic characteristics of ALL[1169,1171–1173]. The use of intensified chemotherapy for ALL has diminished the prognostic significance of race in some[1174,1175] but not other studies[1173,1176].

Hyperleukocytosis is a poor prognostic indicator in B-ALL. By univariate analysis, massive lymphadenopathy, splenomegaly, hepatomegaly and/or presence of a mediastinal mass at diagnosis, reflecting high tumor burden, is a prominent poor prognostic feature[1162,1177]. However, in multivariate analysis, the prognostic significance of these parameters is diminished by other factors, such as WBC count, early response to therapy and age[1177,1178].

Morphologic and phenotypic features

In childhood ALL, the relationship between lymphoblast L1 and L2 morphology and prognosis is controversial. According to some studies L2

Table 7.1 Prognostic factors in acute lymphoblastic leukemia

Factor	Prognosis
WBC count	
$<10 \times 10^9/l$	Favorable
$>200 \times 10^9/l$	Unfavorable
Age	
3–7 years	Favorable
$<1, >10$ years	Unfavorable
Gender	
Female	Favorable
Male	Unfavorable
Lymph node enlargement, splenomegaly and/or hepatomegaly	Unfavorable
Testicular or CNS involvement	Unfavorable
FAB	
L1	Favorable
L2	Unfavorable
Ploidy	
Hyperdiploidy	Favorable
Hypodiploidy <45	Unfavorable
Trisomy 4, 10 and/or 17	Favorable
t(9;22)	Unfavorable
Remission	
<14 days	Favorable
>28 days	Unfavorable
MRD	
$<10^{-3}$	Favorable
$\geq 10^{-3}$	Unfavorable

WBC, white blood cell; CNS, central nervous system; MRD, minimal residual disease

morphology is associated with a poor prognosis[1179–1181], whereas in others the association disappears after adjustment for other known risk factors[1182–1184]. In a more recent study, French–American–British (FAB) L2 morphology was found to be an adverse risk factor, independent of other risk factors, in the setting of contemporary intensified chemotherapy, influencing both the early response to treatment and, in the low-WBC group, the ultimate outcome[1185].

The phenotype of blasts (Figure 7.2) is an independent prognostic parameter in B-ALL. B-ALL are divided into early pre-B-ALL (pro-B-ALL; TdT+/CD19+/CD10−), common ALL (CD10+/ CALLA+), pre-B-ALL (CD10+/−; cytoplasmic IgM+) and mature B-ALL (surface IgM+). Early pre-B-ALL is associated

with a favorable prognosis[1186]. In a series by Cimino et al., adult patients with early-pre-B-ALL had the ALL1–AF4 fusion transcript, originating from the t(4;11) translocation in 36.4%, and the BCR–ABL chimeric product of t(9;22) in 9%[480]. B-ALL with t(9;22) often displays aberrant expression of pan-myeloid antigens (CD33 or less often CD13). Pediatric patients with ALL blasts possessing myeloid antigens may represent a high-risk group for length of remission and survival[685]. Adult patients with early-pre-B-ALL and t(4;11) or t(9;22) have a poor prognosis, and the absence of both of these translocations correlates with a significantly better clinical outcome after intensive polychemotherapy[480]. CD10/CALLA expression does not appear to have

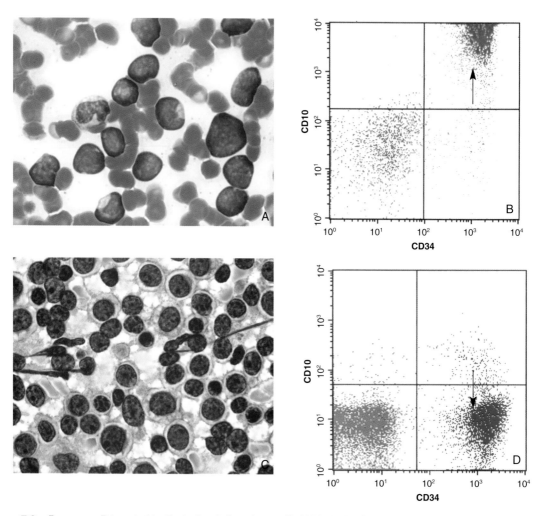

Figure 7.2 Precursor B-lymphoblastic leukemia/lymphoma (B-ALL). A–B, CD10+ (CALLA+) B-ALL (A, cytology; B, flow cytometry display of CD34 vs. CD10 expression); C–D, CD10– B-ALL. Green dots represent leukemic cells; red dots represent residual benign lymphocytes

independent prognostic significance[391,679,1187]. The outcome of patients with pre-B-ALL and common ALL is similar. Pre-B-ALL is associated with a poorer outcome compared with early pre-B-ALL[1188]. A subset of patients with pre-B-ALL and common ALL is Ph+, and their prognosis remains poor. Mature B-ALL occurs in older children and is characterized by L3 morphology and a higher incidence of CNS involvement. In univariate analysis, fluorescence intensity of CD45 and CD20 is significantly associated with event-free survival, whereas other

phenotypic markers showed no significant correlation with outcome. Patients whose blasts were greater than the 75th centile of intensity for CD45 fared significantly worse than those with lower-density CD45, and those whose blasts were greater than the 25th centile of intensity for CD20 had a poorer event-free survival[1189]. The intensity of both CD45 and CD20 is independently correlated with outcome. There was no significant correlation between intensity of expression of either antigen and traditional clinical risk factors, ploidy, or t(9;22) or t(1;19). In multivariate analysis, both CD45 intensity greater than the 75th centile and CD20 intensity greater than the 25th centile were significantly correlated with poor outcome, independently of previously reported poor prognostic factors including National Cancer Institute (NCI) risk group, ploidy, trisomies of 4 and 10, and adverse translocations including t(1;19), t(9;22) and t(4;11)[1189]. The overall survival of patients with B-ALL expressing CD1d is shorter than in CD1d⁻ ALL.

Cytogenetic and molecular features

B-ALL with hyperdiploidy (> 50 chromosomes) is associated with a favorable prognosis[387,388,390–392]. Hyperdiploidy in association with trisomies of chromosomes 4, 10 and/or 17 is associated with a particularly favorable prognosis[1190–1192]. Near-tetraploid tumors (92–94 chromosomes) are associated with a high frequency of treatment failure and therefore differ in prognosis from other hyperdiploid ALL[395]. Hypodiploid tumors with less than 45 chromosomes, especially those with 24–28 chromosomes, have a significantly worse prognosis despite intensive treatment[394,397,398,1193,1194].

Chromosomal translocations are strong predictors of adverse treatment outcome in ALL. The t(9;22) (q32;q11) leading to the BCR–ABL fusion, the molecular equivalent of the Philadelphia chromosome, is present in approximately 20% of adults and 5% of children with ALL[1195–1198]. Features associated with t(9;22)⁺ ALL include high WBC count, older age, male predominance and FAB L2 blast morphology[1196]. There is a strong adverse prognostic significance of t(9;22) in ALL, even after adjustment for other prognostic features[388,499,1199]. Irrespective of the breakpoint site, the presence of any BCR–ABL transcript predicted a lower chance of initial treatment response and a lower probability of disease-free survival at 3 years. This bad outcome was not influenced by post-induction high-dose treatment stratifications[499]. In some t(9;22)⁺ ALL patients with favorable prognostic features (age between 1 and 9 years, low WBC count) the outcome is better because the disease

can be controlled by transplantation and intensive chemotherapy[1198]. The t(1;19)(q23;q13) translocation, associated with fusion of the E2A and PBX1 genes on chromosomes 1 and 19, respectively, is present in 20–30% of pre-B-ALL[1200] and is associated with a poor prognosis[186,469]. Rearrangements of the mixed-lineage leukemia gene MLL (also known as ALL1, Htrx and HRX) are associated with aggressive acute leukemias and poor prognosis in both children and adults. The t(4;11)(q21;q23), similarly to the Philadelphia chromosome, is associated with high-risk features (high WBC count, age < 1 year) and poor prognosis[1201,1202], although recent treatment protocols improved the outcome. The MLL–AF4 rearrangements are the molecular hallmark of ALL with t(4;11). The t(4;11)/MLL–AF4 is identified in approximately 50% of B-ALL in infants below 6 months of age[1203] and is associated with a poor prognosis[400,478,479]. Figure 7.3 presents B-ALL with deletion of the MLL gene. The cryptic translocation t(12;21) is common in childhood ALL. The presence of a reciprocal translocation of the chromosome 12p13 and the 21q22 results in a fusion of the TEL gene on chromosome 12 and the RUNX1 (AML1) gene on chromosome 21. TEL–RUNX1 transcripts, detectable by polymerase chain reaction (PCR) and/or fluorescence in situ hybridization (FISH), are associated with an early pre-B immunophenotype, younger children and non-hyperdiploidy, and have a favorable prognosis, although relapse may occur in a subset of patients[1204–1206]. It is suggested that the favorable prognosis of t(12;21) may be associated with the intensity of therapy[1207,1208]. TEL–RUNX1-positive patients are relatively more sensitive to L-asparaginase[651]. Intensive chemotherapy with regimens appropriate for Burkitt's lymphoma reversed the poor prognosis previously associated with ALL with the translocations involving the c-MYC locus at 8q24 [t(8;14), t(2;8) and t(8;22)][1011,1209,1210]. Genes involved in multidrug resistance, cell cycle control, DNA repair, drug metabolism and apoptosis have been associated with prognosis in ALL (see Chapters 1 and 2 for details)[307,308,602,648,651,1164,1166,1211]. The gene expression profile can differentiate lineage and molecular

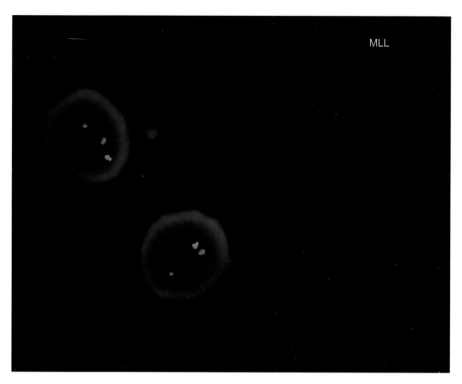

Figure 7.3   B-lymphoblastic leukemia/lymphoma (B-ALL) (patient 2 years old) with deletion of the *MLL* gene

subtypes of ALL[353,355,1212], but can also identify genes associated with drug resistance and treatment outcome[307].

In childhood ALL, minimal residual disease (MRD) is an independent prognostic factor allowing for risk stratification[44,1213]. The most widely applied MRD assays in ALL are flow cytometric identification of leukemia immunophenotypes and PCR amplification of antigen-receptor genes, both yielding concordant results in the vast majority of cases[84,1214]. Early clearance of leukemic cells is a favorable prognostic indicator in childhood ALL. Approximately half of the children with ALL achieve significant clearance of leukemic cells after 2–3 weeks of remission-induction chemotherapy, and these patients have an excellent treatment outcome[1215]. The level and kinetics of MRD by real-time quantitative PCR (RQ-PCR) correlates better with the risk of relapse than qualitative results (MRD+ vs. MRD−); patients with low levels of MRD and those with

decreasing levels after treatment have a lower risk of relapse[89–93]. Bone marrow and peripheral blood MRD in patients with ALL is associated with a very high risk for disease recurrence[1216]. In a series by Coustan-Smith *et al.*, the 4-year cumulative incidence of relapse in patients with B-ALL was 80% for those who had peripheral blood MRD at the end of remission induction therapy, but only 13% for those with MRD confined to the marrow[1216].

Adult ALL

ALL is uncommon in adults. The major prognostic factors include age, WBC count, time to response, chromosomal aberrations, MRD and drug resistance. Factors associated with a better prognosis include age < 30 years, WBC count $< 30 \times 10^9/l$, t(10;14) and complete remission within 4 weeks. Factors associated with a poor prognosis include elevated total WBC count ($> 50 \times 10^9/l$), t(9;22), t(4;11), t(1;19), hypodiploid ploidy, −7, +8, expression of myeloid antigens (CD13, CD33), and persistent MRD[1213,1217–1220]. The 5-year survival rate is 24% and it decreases markedly with age (37% for patients 15–45 years old and 3% for patients ≥75 years old)[123]. Most current prognostic systems use a cut-off of either 35 years (German), 50 years (New German) or 60 years (Sloan–Kettering, Cancer and Leukemia Group B (CALGB)) for favorable (below) and unfavorable (above) prognosis[1217–1220]. The difference in prognosis for elderly patients is most likely to be associated with reduced tolerance to intensive therapy, co-morbidity and higher incidence of unfavorable genetic changes (e.g. Philadelphia chromosome)[1221–1223]. Similarly to pediatric patients, adults with leukemia harboring aberrations of 19p13 usually do not respond to intensive therapy and have a short survival[1224]. Based on the cytogenetic–molecular aberrations and disease-free survival (DFS), Mancini *et al.* divided adult ALL into three prognostic categories: (1) no genetic abnormalities or isolated del(9p) (p15–p16), predicting relatively favorable outcome (median DFS >3 years); (2) t(9;22)/*BCR–ABL*, t(4;11)/*MLL–AF4*, t(1;19)/ *E2A–PBX1*, predicting highly adverse prognosis (median DFS 7 months); and (3) 6q deletions, other miscellaneous structural aberrations and hyperdiploidy predicting an intermediate prognosis (median DFS 19 months)[1225]. In adult patients, analysis of DFS rates for MRD[+] and MRD[−] patients established that MRD positivity was associated with increased relapse rates at all times, being most significant at 3–5 months post-induction and beyond[99]. For autologous stem cell transplantation, MRD tests before the procedure are predictive of outcome, which differs from allogeneic stem cell transplantation, in which outcome is related to results of the tests after the procedure rather than before[99]. Status of MRD can be used in risk stratification of patients with ALL in conjunction with conventional prognostic factors such as WBC count, age, immunophenotype, cytogenetics and molecular genetics[1226]. MRD-based risk stratification allows a highly significant prediction of relapse in adult ALL[1226,1227].

PRECURSOR T-LYMPHOBLASTIC LEUKEMIA/LYMPHOMA

Several of the clinical and laboratory prognostic factors that are used reliably for B-precursor ALL are much less predictive in T-acute lymphoblastic leukemia (T-ALL) – e.g. improved treatment protocols and diminished prognostic significance of hyperleukocytosis in T-ALL – but remain predictors of a worse outcome in B-ALL[1228]. The poor prognostic features of T-ALL are associated with high initial WBC count, age older than 15 years, massive splenomegaly and hepatomegaly, FAB L2 blast morphology and an abnormal karyotype[1229,1230]. Tumor cells have blastic morphology, are often either dual CD4/CD8-positive or dual CD4/CD8-negative and may express CD1a and TdT (Figure 7.4). Patients with a WBC count less than $50 \times 10^9/l$ who lack massive splenomegaly and have blasts expressing CD5 have a good prognosis[1230]. Among T-ALL patients, those with the least mature phenotype have a significantly worse outcome, those with a thymic phenotype have a favorable outcome and those with the most mature phenotype have a poor prognosis.

Better survival in T-ALL is associated with a normal karyotype and with t(10;14), whereas the presence of any derivative chromosome is associated with worse survival[1231]. Five different T-cell oncogenes (*HOX11*, *TAL1*, *LYL1*, *LMO1* and *LMO2*) are often aberrantly expressed in the absence of chromosomal abnormalities. Using oligonucleotide microarrays, Ferrando *et al.* identified several gene expression signatures that were indicative of leukemic arrest at specific stages of normal thymocyte development: *LYL1*[+] signature (pro-T), *HOX11*[+] (early cortical thymocyte) and *TAL1*[+] (late cortical thymocyte)[356]. Hierarchical clustering analysis of gene expression signatures grouped samples according to their shared oncogenic pathways and identified *HOX11L2* activation as a novel event in T-cell leukemogenesis. These findings have clinical importance, since *HOX11* activation is significantly associated with a favorable prognosis, while expression of *TAL1*, *LYL1*

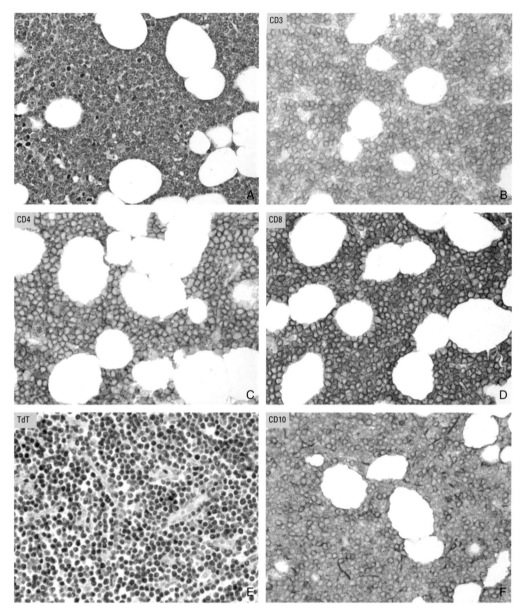

Figure 7.4   Precursor T-lymphoblastic leukemia/lymphoma (T-ALL). A, histology; B–F, immunohistochemistry. Tumor cells are positive for CD3 (B), CD4 (C), CD8 (D), terminal deoxynucleotidyl transferase (TdT) (E) and CD10 (F)

or *HOX11L2* confers a much worse response to treatment[356]. T-ALL with expression of *HOX11* as a result of *MLL–ENL* fusion has a favorable prognosis[356]. *NUP214–ABL1* expression defines a new subgroup of individuals with T-ALL who could benefit from treatment with imatinib (Gleevec)[1232].

BLASTIC NK-CELL LEUKEMIA/ LYMPHOMA

Blastic NK-cell leukemia/lymphoma (DC2 acute leukemia) is a highly aggressive neoplasm that involves the skin and often disseminates into other

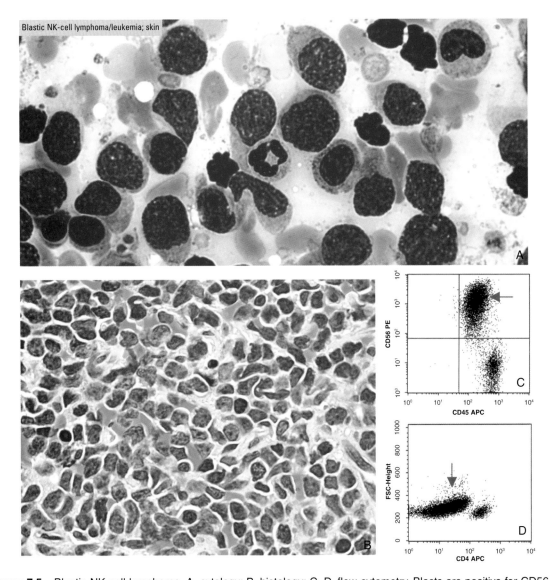

Blastic NK-cell lymphoma/leukemia; skin

Figure 7.5   Blastic NK-cell lymphoma. A, cytology; B, histology; C–D, flow cytometry. Blasts are positive for CD56 (C) and CD4 (D)

organs, with leukemic blood and bone marrow involvement. It is suggested that it arises from transformed CD56⁺ 'plasmacytoid' monocyte-like dendritic cells (DC2). Tumor cells express CD56 CD43, HLA-DR and CD4 (Figure 7.5). The 5-year survival is 0%[1089].

CHAPTER 8

Acute myeloid leukemia

Acute myeloid leukemia (AML) represents a heterogeneous disorder with variability in clinical presentation, cellular morphology, therapeutic response and overall prognosis. Generally, AML can be defined as a clonal malignancy of transformed multipotent hematopoietic progenitor cells leading to accumulation of immature cells in the bone marrow that replace normal elements, causing cytopenias and their complications (fatigue, infections and bleeding). The diagnosis and prognosis is most accurately provided by pretreatment assessment of the morphology, immunophenotype and underlying chromosomal/molecular aberrations responsible for the disease, e.g. patients with acute promyelocytic leukemia (APL) are treated with an all-*trans*-retinoic acid (ATRA) and anthracycline-based treatment program, and patients with other types of AML are typically given conventional chemotherapy (e.g. cytarabine- and anthracycline-containing induction regimens). Post-induction treatments include stem cell transplantation and experimental approaches. Over the past decades, improvement in the diagnosis (especially identification of prognostically relevant cytogenetic groups), new treatment strategies and advances in supportive care have increased the survival rate in patients with AML[1233,1234]. Despite this, however, nearly two-thirds of patients diagnosed with AML will die of the disease or of complications of treatment. Minimal residual disease (MRD) level, cytogenetics and number of cycles to achieve complete remission are the most important prognostic factors in patients with AML.

Clinical features

Clinical features (e.g. age, albumin level, prior chemotherapy, performance status and antecedent myelodysplasia (MDS)), leukocyte count, treatment protocol and number of induction courses, morphologic/phenotypic features and chromosomal abnormalities/genotype (e.g. presence of *FLT3* mutations) are associated with the outcome of AML[1235]. Hyperleukocytosis correlates with a poor prognosis in some series, but the correlation is not as strong as it is in precursor B-lymphoblastic leukemia/lymphoma (B-ALL)[450,1236]. Early response to therapy is one of the most important prognostic factors in AML. The speed of cytoreduction correlates with survival (*see below*, MRD). The sooner the aplasia is achieved the better the prognosis[1237,1238]. Adverse factors for patients with relapsed diesease include first complete remission (CR) <6 months, second CR <6 months, salvage therapy not including allogeneic stem cell transplantation, non-inversion 16 AML, platelets $<50 \times 10^9$/l and white blood cells (WBC) $>50 \times 10^9$/l. Patients with preceding bone marrow disorder, including MDS or myeloproliferative disease, or with a history of chemotherapy, have an inferior response and survival compared with those with *de novo* AML[1239,1240]. Therapy-related AML (t-AML) is an unfavorable factor independent of cytogenetics with respect to survival[1241].

Both age and cytogenetics (Figure 8.1) are independent prognostic parameters in AML. Very young

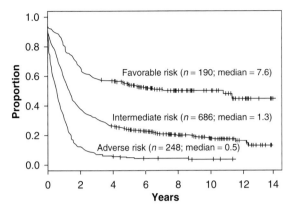

Figure 8.1   Overall survival in AML patients categorized into favorable, intermediate and adverse cytogenetic risk groups using the Cancer and Leukemia Group B (CALGB) criteria

From: Byrd JC, *et al.* Pretreatment cytogenetic abnormalities are predictive of induction success, cumulative incidence of relapse, and overall survival in adult patients with *de novo* acute myeloid leukemia. Blood 2002;100: 4325–36. © 2002 by The American Society of Hematology, used with permission

patients (< 2 years of age) and elderly patients have the worst prognoses[1235,1242]. The karyotype is an important prognostic factor in all age groups, while the age up to 49 years has no major impact on prognosis[117]. In pediatric patients with AML, patient age is inversely related to treatment outcome[1243,1244]. Children with Down's syndrome and AML are younger, have lower WBC count, display more French–American–British (FAB) M7 morphology (megakaryoblastic leukemia) and experience a better outcome than other children. Megakaryoblastic leukemia is unfavorable in others but prognostically neutral in Down's syndrome. Patients with trisomy 21 have higher survival rates[1245]. Similarly to age, initial WBC count is inversely related to outcome. Hyperleukocytosis is an independent prognostic factor, indicating a high risk, especially for early failure[1246]. Bone marrow blasts on day 15 are of prognostic value: event-free survival at 5 years estimated for patients with ≤5% and >5% blasts on day 15 is 56% versus 27%, respectively[1246].

African-Americans and Whites with AML differ with respect to important prognostic factors.

African-Americans with *de novo* AML are younger at the time of diagnosis (48 years vs. 54 years), are more commonly classified in the favorable (23% vs. 14%) and unfavorable (31% vs. 23%) cytogenetic groups and less commonly in the intermediate group (47% vs. 63%)[1247]. African-American men had a lower complete remission rate (54% vs. 64% for White men, 65% for White women, and 70% for African-American women) and a worse overall survival compared with all other patients[1247].

Morphologic and phenotypic features

Favorable morphologic features include Auer rods (M1–M4) and eosinophils (M2 and M4Eo), whereas megaloblastic features that may be seen in erythroleukemia (AML-M6), acute megakaryoblastic leukemia (AML-M7), or AML evolving from MDS are unfavorable[1239,1248,1249]. The finding of Auer rods was a positive prognostic factor with respect to complete remission rate and survival time[1249]. The detection of trilineage dysplasia correlates with unfavorable cytogenetics[188,1248]. Dysplastic features in *de novo* AML correlated with short overall survival[1248] and with decreased probability of achieving complete remission[113,114,1250]. However, in a series reported by Haferlach *et al.*, dysplasia was not found to be an independent prognostic parameter in AML[188]. With regard to FAB, the prognostic impact in not consistent in published data, but, generally, patients with AML-M0, M6 and M7 have lower survival rates. AML minimally differentiated (M0) and AML without maturation (M1) had a poor prognosis, with aggressive clinical course, early relapses and lower remission rate. AML with maturation (M2) and acute myelomonocytic leukemia (M4) respond frequently to aggressive therapy. The clinical course of acute monoblastic leukemia (AML-M5; Figures 8.2 and 8.3), acute erythroid leukemia (AML-M6; Figure 8.4) and acute megakaryoblastic leukemia (AML-M7; Figure 8.5) is usually aggressive. Infants with AML-M7 and t(1;22) have a particularly poor prognosis. Extramedullary myeloid tumor (granulocytic sarcoma; Figure 8.6) is a leukemic infiltration outside bone marrow. It may precede AML or it can occur concurrently with AML.

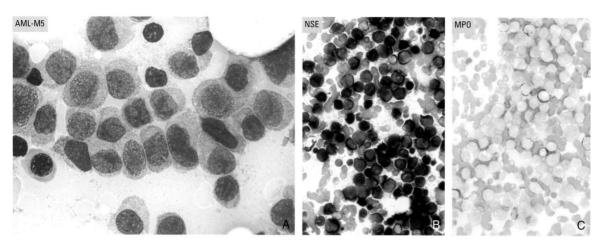

Figure 8.2   Acute monoblastic leukemia (AML-M5). A, cytology; B–C, cytochemical staining showing expression of non-specific esterase (NSE) (B) and lack of myeloperoxidase (MFO) (C)

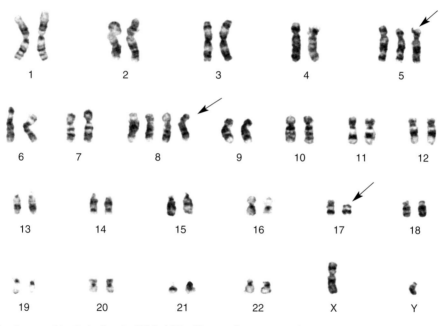

Figure 8.3   Acute monoblastic leukemia (AML-M5) with complex cytogenetics: +5, +8, +8, del(17)(p11.1), trisomy 5 and trisomy or tetrasomy 8 is often associated with monocytic leukemia; deletion of the short arm of chromosome 17 in AML usually confers a poor clinical outcome

Extramedullary disease, especially common in AML with monocytic differentiation (AML-M5), is associated with a poor prognosis. In a series reported by de Greef *et al.*, the presence of granulocytic sarcoma and platelets $<100 \times 10^9$/l or neutrophils $<1 \times 10^9$/l were associated with a reduced overall survival and increased remission rate[1251]. Acute panmyelosis with myelofibrosis has an unfavorable prognosis with a median survival of less than a year[1252,1253]. Acute panmyelosis shows considerable overlap with hyperfibrotic MDS, AML and toxic myelopathy[1252,1253].

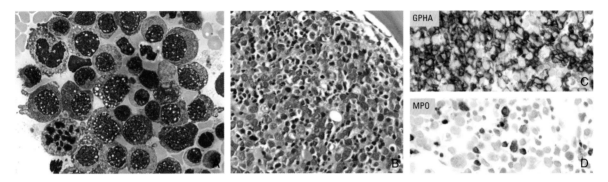

Figure 8.4   Acute erythroleukemia (AML-M6). A, cytology (aspirate smear) shows highly atypical erythroid precursors with megaloblastoid changes, mitoses and cytoplasmic irregularities; B, histology sections show almost total bone marrow replacement by atypical erythroid cells. They express glycophorin A (GPHA) (C) and lack myeloperoxidase (MPO) staining (D)

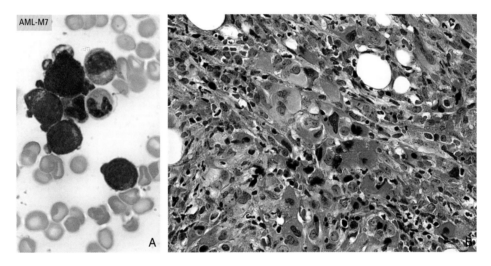

Figure 8.5   Acute megakaryocytic leukemia (AML-M7). A, cytology; B, histology. Atypical megakaryocytes and immature forms (megakaryoblasts) are present

The effect of phenotype on prognosis is variable and is interdependent with other factors (especially FAB classification). CD34 expression (Figure 8.7) has been reported as an adverse factor in some studies, but it has little impact on survival[718]. CD34 expression is a poor prognostic factor when co-expressed with CD7, but this is most likely to be due to accompanying chromosomal abnormalities or CD7 expression[677,678]. CD34 is expressed in favorable subtypes of AML, including patients with t(8;21) and inv(16)/t(16;16). CD56, a cell adhesion molecule, has been associated with the development of extramedullary disease. CD56 expression has been found to be a risk factor for AML with t(8;21) and t(15;17)[732,733]. CD56 expression in AML with t(8;21) is associated with significantly shorter complete remission duration and survival[732]. The presence of lymphoid markers, particularly when they are multiple, is often associated with a poor prognosis. However, they have not predicted a poor prognosis in children and in patients within a good cytogenetic group. There appears to be a strong association

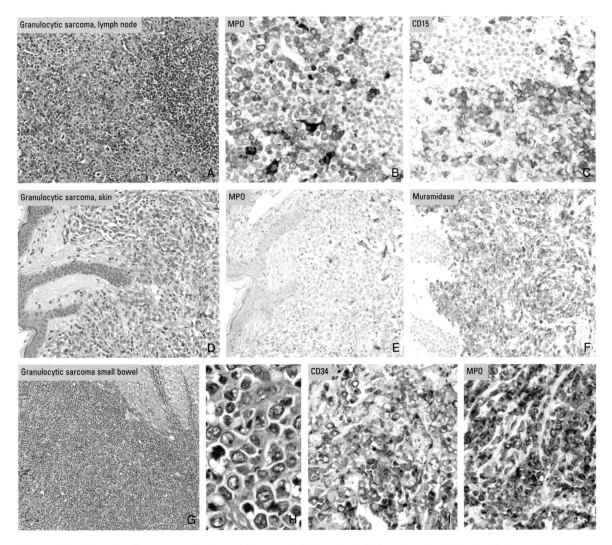

Figure 8.6   Granulocytic sarcoma (extramedullary myeloid tumor), A–C, lymph node; D–F, skin; G–J, small bowel

between early death (at less than 2 months) and the co-expression of leukocyte function-associated (LFA) antigens CD11b and CD11c[1254]; the relationship was independent of clinical features and persisted even if AML-M5 cases were excluded. The significance of this latter finding is unclear, but may be related to the known role of CD11b and CD11c LFA antigens in the cellular response to infection. Acute leukemia of ambiguous lineage (mixed lineage leukemia, AML/ALL) has an unfavorable prognosis, mostly due to a higher frequency of unfavorable prognostic factors

including older age, unfavorable karyotype including t(4;11) or the Philadelphia chromosome, and P-glycoprotein overexpression by reverse transcriptase polymerase chain reaction (RT-PCR)[1255,1256].

Cytogenetic and molecular features

Table 8.1 presents the most common chromosomal abnormalities in AML. Cytogenetic abnormalities in AML at presentation have been identified as one of the most important prognostic factors and have been

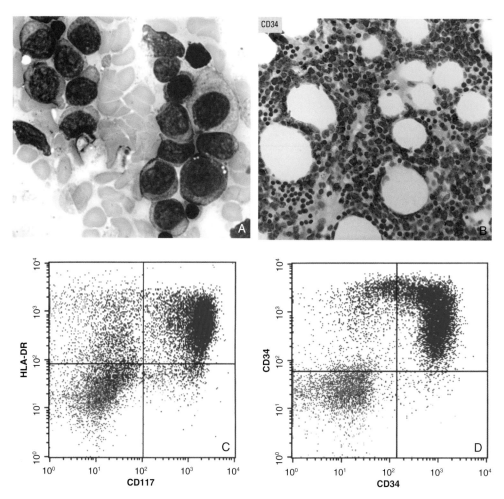

Figure 8.7   AML with CD34 expression. Cytology smear (A) shows large blasts with prominent nucleoli; blasts are positive for CD34 (B; immunohistochemistry). Flow cytometry (C–D) shows expression of CD117 and CD34

shown to be independent of age, WBC count and type of leukemia[115,1257–1259]. Cytogenetic risk status is a significant factor in predicting response of AML to therapy[1260]; for example, the outcome of patients with t(15;17) APL has substantially improved with the use of ATRA in combination with chemotherapy[1261–1264]. Figure 8.1 presents overall survival in AML patients categorized into favorable, intermediate and adverse cytogenetic risk groups.

Three abnormalities – t(8;21), t(15;17) and inv(16) – are regarded as favorable. Patients with inv(16)/t(16;16) or t(15;17) have a favorable prognosis,

most often regardless of additional abnormalities[115,119,1260]. Figure 8.8 presents t(8;21) detection by standard cytogenetic and PCR analysis, and Figure 8.9 shows inversion of chromosome 16 by fluorescence *in situ* hybridization (FISH) analysis. Neither complex karyotype nor secondary aberrations affected the outcome of patients with t(8;21) and inv(16)/t(16;16)[119]. However, the prognosis of patients with t(8;21) worsens when there is extramedullary disease, CD56 expression or del(9q)[492]. Fenaux *et al.* showed that the t(8;21) might be associated with a high incidence of early relapses[1265].

Table 8.1 Primary chromosomal abnormalities in acute myeloid leukemia

Cytogenetic abnormality	Genes	Prognosis
t(1;3)(p36;q21)	MEL1; ribophorin	Poor
t(1;7)(q10;q10)		Poor
t(1;11)(p32;q23)	AF1p, MLL	Poor
t(1;11)(p21;q23)	AF1q, MLL	Poor
t(1;22)(p13;q13)	OTT; MAL	Poor
inv(3)(q21;q26), t(3;3)(q21;q26)	EVI1; ribophorin	Poor
t(3;5)(q25.1; q35)	MLF1; NPM	Intermediate to poor
t(3;21)(q26;q22)	EVI1 or MDS1; RUNX1 (AML1)	Poor
+4		Poor
del(5q)		Very poor
t(5;17)(q35;q12)	NPM; RARα	Intermediate
t(6;9)(p23;q34)	DEK; CAN	Poor
t(6;11)(q27;q230	AF6; MLL	Poor
t(7;11)(p15;p15)	HOXA9; NuP98	Intermediate
−7/del(7q)		Very poor
+8		Intermediate to poor
t(8;16)(q11;q13)	MOZ; CBP	Poor
t(8;21)(q22;q22)	ETO; RUNX1 (AML1)	Good
t(9;11)(p21–22;q23)	AF9; MLL	Intermediate
t(9;22)(q34;q11)	ABL; BCR	Poor
t(10;11)(p12;q23)	AF10; MLL	Poor
+11	MLL	Poor
t(11;16)(q23;p13)	MLL; CBP	Poor
t(11;17)(q23;q25)	MLL; AF17	Poor
t(11;17)(q23;q21)	PLZF; RARα	Intermediate
t(11;17)(q13;q21)	NUMA; RARα	Good
t(11;19)(q23;p13)	MLL; ENL	Poor
i(12)(p10)		Poor
t(12;22)(p13;q11)	TEL; MN1	Poor
+13		Poor
t(15;17)(q22;q11)	PML; RARα	Good
inv(16)(p13)(q22)		Good
t(16;16)(p13;q22), del(16)(q22)	MYH11; CBFB	Good
t(16;22)(p11;q22)	FUS; ERG	Poor
iso(17)(q10)		Poor
t(17;17)(q11;q21)	STAT5b; RARα	
del(20q)		Poor
+21		Intermediate
+22		Intermediate
−Y		Intermediate
Complex (>3)		Very poor

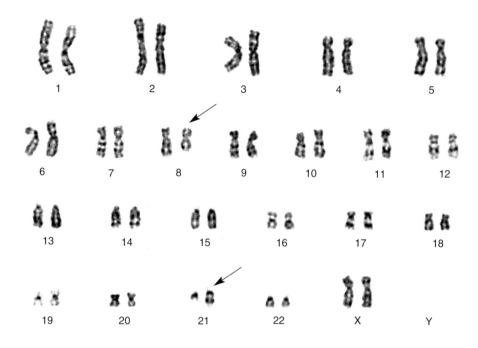

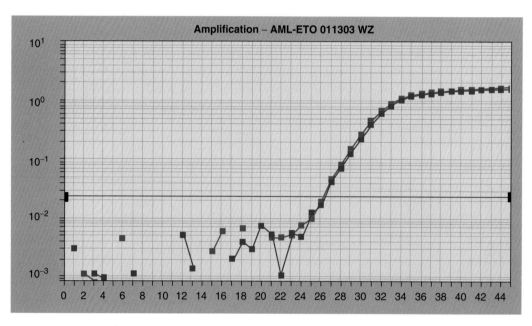

Figure 8.8 Acute myeloid leukemia with t(8;21). Cytogenetic analysis (top) shows translocation t(8;21); molecular analysis (polymerase chain reaction, bottom) shows *ETO* (eight–twenty-one fusion gene) mRNA

Trisomy 8 is the most frequently reported numerical cytogenetic abnormality in patients with AML. Patients with sole +8, and +8 with additional abnormality other than t(8;21), inv(16)/t(16;16) and t(9;11), had significantly inferior overall survival, but not complete remission, while patients with +8 and a

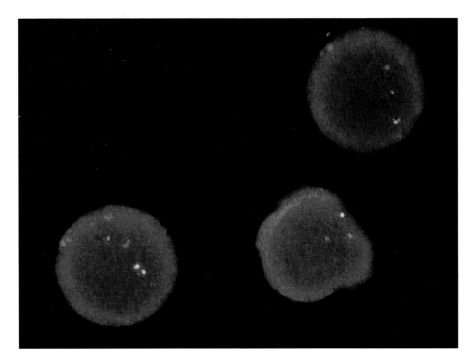

Figure 8.9   Acute myeloid leukemia with inv(16); FISH analysis

complex karyotype with three or more abnormalities had significantly inferior complete remission and overall survival[119]. The impact of trisomy 8 on AML patients is best predicted by the presence and nature of the abnormalities that accompany it[119,454].

Patients with normal karyotype, −Y, del(5q), t(9;11), del(11q), +13, del(20q) and +21 belong to the intermediate prognostic category[115,119,1260]. Patients with AML with 5q− and additional aberrations (Figure 8.10) have a worse prognosis than those with 5q− as a sole abnormality. Patients with complex karyotypes (≥3 abnormalities; Figure 8.11) had significantly worse outcomes than cytogenetically normal patients[119]. Other adverse cytogenetic changes include: inv(3) or t(3;3), t(6;9), t(6;11), −7, +8[119]. The outcome of patients with balanced 11q23 translocations depends on which partner chromosome is involved[119,1258,1266]. While the prognosis for patients with t(9;11) is not different from those with normal karyotype (intermediate prognostic category), the overall survival of patients with t(6;11) or t(11;19)

(q23;p13.1) is significantly shorter, comparable to that of the normal group[119]. Therefore, the prognosis of patients with 11q23 aberrations is coded as either unfavorable[1260,1267] or intermediate[115]. These inconsistencies in outcome may result from the multiplicity of 11q23 aberrations resulting in different fusion partners, variable molecular rearrangements, or the presence of additional chromosomal alterations imparting the prognostic impact. Young patients with a *de novo* presentation with t(9;11) belong to the intermediate category. Patients with t(6;9) have a dismal prognosis[119]. The prognosis of patients with del(9q) is intermediate/unfavorable but varies with its genotypic makeup[1260].

Internal tandem duplication of the *FLT3* gene and point mutations of the N-*RAS* gene are the most frequent somatic mutations causing aberrant signal transduction in AML. *FLT3* mutation status has a major impact on remission duration and overall survival in patients with AML and normal cytogenetics. *FLT3* mutations are present in

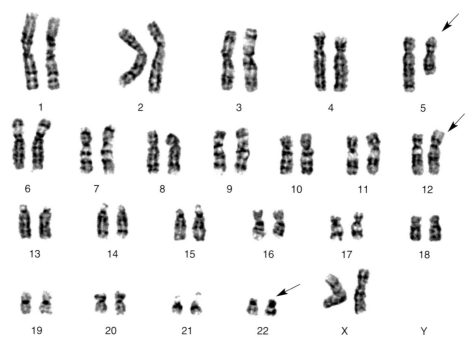

Figure 8.10   Acute myeloid leukemia with 5q− and t(12;22)

27–32% of patients and are associated with leukocytosis and a high percentage of bone marrow blast cells[120,1268]. *FLT3* mutations predominantly occur by internal tandem duplications and, less commonly, through an activation loop involving an aspartic acid residue at amino acid position 835 (Asp835 mutations). *FLT3* mutations do not correlate with complete remission rate, but they predict relapse and are associated with shorter remission duration, shorter event-free survival and shorter overall survival when compared with AML patients without *FLT3* mutations[120,122,1268,1269]. *RAS* mutations occur in 20–44% of AML patients, may be associated with lower peripheral blast and bone marrow blast percentages and have not consistently predicted prognosis[569,1270]. AML patients with *MLL* gene amplification/tandem repeats (Figure 8.12) have a poor response to treatment and dismal prognosis[1271]. Mutations in the tumor suppressor gene *p53* (*TP53*) are associated with a poor outcome[1272]. The co-expression of the apoptosis-related genes *BCL2* and *WT1* predicts poor survival in AML patients[1273]. Expression of multidrug resistance (*MDR*) genes has been identified as an adverse prognostic marker in AML[113,114,1274,1275]. Expression of MDR1/P-glycoprotein is more commonly found in older patients, often in conjunction with adverse cytogenetics, and is associated with lower complete remission rate[113,114].

Minimal residual disease

MRD can be evaluated by multiparameter flow cytometry (FC), FISH or molecular tests, such as automated real-time quantitative PCR (RQ-PCR) (Figure 8.13). Chromosomal aberrations, such as t(15;17), t(9;22), t(8;21) and t(16;16)/inv(16), are the easiest targets for MRD analysis in AML patients. In the fusion transcript-negative AML patients, *WT1*[1276] or *FLT3* expression by RQ-PCR may be employed as a tool to detect MRD. The CR

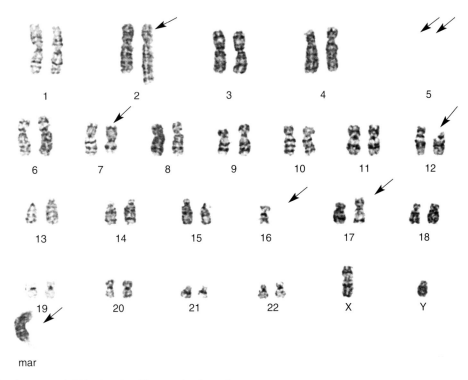

1 2 3 4 5

6 7 8 9 10 11 12

13 14 15 16 17 18

19 20 21 22 X Y

mar

Figure 8.11 Acute myeloid leukemia with complex karyotype

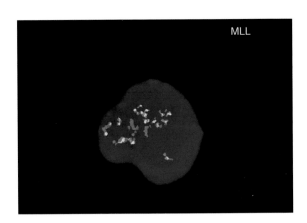

Figure 8.12 Mixed lineage leukemia (myeloid lymphoid leukemia; MLL) gene amplification in acute myeloid leukemia; FISH analysis

evaluation after induction therapy plays a crucial role in prognosis and determination of treatment strategies in AML patients. Patients with no more that 5% of

blasts show the best overall survival and the lowest relapse rate, independently of circulating blasts in blood or bone marrow cellularity[1251]. San Miguel *et al.*, using multiparameter FC, identified four different risk categories of AML: very low risk ($< 10^{-4}$ cells) with no relapse, low risk (10^{-4}–10^{-3} cells) with 3-year relapse rate of 14%, intermediate risk (10^{-3}–10^{-2} cells) with relapse rate of 50% and high risk ($> 10^{-2}$ cells) with 3-year relapse rate of 84%[72]. In APL patients, RT-PCR/MRD positivity for *PML–RARα* was predictive of clinical relapse, whereas PCR⁻ tests were associated with prolonged disease-free survival of patients with APL[77–79]. Qualitative tests (RQ-PCR) may further improve MDR detection in APL[29]. In AML with t(8;21), *RUNX1(AML1)–ETO* fusion transcript can be identified in patients in long-term remission (e.g. due to *RUNX1(AML1)–ETO* fusion expression by non-leukemic cells), which limits the role for

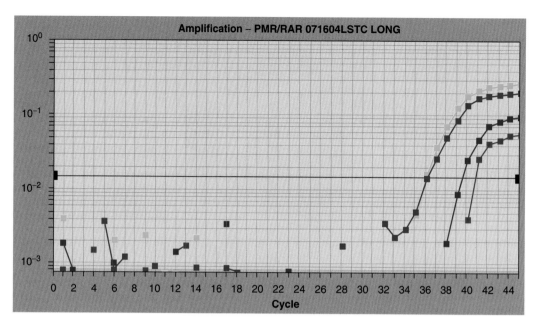

Figure 8.13   Acute promyelocytic leukemia. Minimal residual disease detected by polymerase chain reaction analysis

MRD evaluation by conventional nested RT-PCR[81]. Morschhauser *et al.* suggested that a single-step RT-PCR instead of nested PCR could be predictive of outcome in AML with t(8;21). The same group (Leroy *et al.*) recently showed that in t(8;21)[+] AML, absolute transcript levels below 10^{-3} (compared with Kasumi cell line), or a greater than 3 log decrease (compared with diagnosis levels) were significant predictors of the absence of relapse[493]. MRD levels after consolidation therapy were also significant indicators of relapse[493]. *See also Chapter 1.*

Acute promyelocytic leukemia

APL (Figure 8.14), which accounts for approximately 10% of AML cases, is a subtype of AML with a defined clinical course and a biology that differs from other forms of AML. Distinctive features of this disorder at the time of diagnosis include leukopenia coexisting with a marrow replaced with atypical promyelocytes, disseminated intravascular coagulopathy (DIC), lack of HLA-DR antigen expression and translocation between the long arms of chromosomes 15 and 17 (Figure 8.15). Before treatment with retinoids, APL was recognized for its particularly poor clinical outcome due to hemorrhagic complications related to DIC and abnormal fibrinolysis. Introduction of ATRA has transformed clinical practice for this condition, and changed APL from a fulminant disorder with devastating complications and the worst prognosis in the past, to one of the most curable forms of AML[1262,1263,1277–1279]. ATRA combined with chemotherapy for induction and also probably for maintenance provides results that are as favorable in children with APL as in adults and currently constitutes the reference first-line treatment in both age groups[1280]. APL occurring as a second tumor responds as well as *de novo* APL to upfront ATRA plus chemotherapy[1281]. The presence of adverse prognostic factors, including older age, high white blood cell count at presentation, high platelet count, expression of CD56 and presence of mutations in the *FLT3* gene (often accompanied by leukocytosis), identify patients at risk for relapse[1282].

The balanced translocation between chromosomes 15 and 17 characterizes over 95% of cases of APL[1283]. The t(15;17) was found to disrupt the *PML* gene on

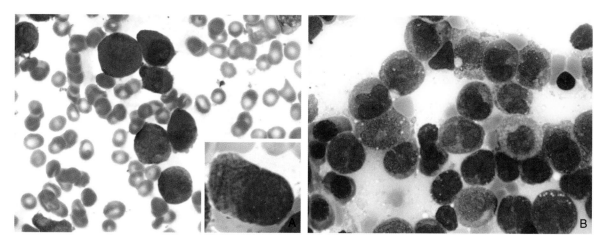

Figure 8.14   Acute promyelocytic leukemia (APL; AML-M3) – cytologic features. A, hypergranular variant; B, hypogranular variant

chromosome 15 and the gene encoding the retinoic acid receptor-α (*RARα*) on chromosome 17. The t(15;17) leads to the formation of two reciprocal fusion genes: *PML–RARα* on chromosome 15 and *RARα–PML* on chromosome 17. The resultant PML–RARα fusion protein, which retains the retinoic acid receptor-binding domain, plays a role in leukemogenesis but also mediates the response to retinoids[506]. The fusion of *PML* and *RARα* genes may result in some cases from insertion of complex rearrangements[508,1284]. Variant translocations (Figure 8.16) in which *RARα* is fused to a gene other than *PML* have also been identified in APL[506]. In these variant translocations, *RARα* is fused to the *PLZF* (promyelocytic leukemia zinc finger) [t(11;17) (q23;q21)], *NPM* (nucleophosmin) [t(5;17) (q35;q21)] and *NuMA* (nuclear mitotic apparatus) [t(11;17)(q13;q21)][507,621,1285]. The nature of the fusion partner has significant impact on the biology of the disease. The t(15;17) translocation is associated with a favorable prognosis[115,1257,1286]. APL associated with t(11;17)(q23;q21) and fusion of the *PLZF* and *RARα* genes is a discrete clinicopathologic syndrome that is resistant to the differentiation effects of ATRA and has a distinctly worse prognosis than t(15;17) APL[507]. The *PLZF–RARα* cases are often characterized by a predominance of immature precursors with regular nuclei, by an increased

number of pelgeroid features and by expression of CD56[1287]. The secondary chromosomal changes in addition to t(15;17) occur in 26–40% of APL and include most often trisomy 8 (46% of all cases with secondary abnormalities) followed by abnormalities of chromosomes 6, 7, 9, 12, 16, 17 and 21[455]. The presence of additional chromosomal changes in APL has no impact on prognosis in patients treated with ATRA and chemotherapy[455]. Mutation of the *PML* gene leading to loss of PML function is associated with ATRA resistance and poor prognosis[629].

After achievement of CR there is a definitive role of maintenance therapy with ATRA with or without low-dose chemotherapy. Treatment with extended ATRA results in a superior remission rate (87% vs. 70%), reduced relapse risk (20% vs. 36% at 4 years) and superior survival (71% vs. 52% at 4 years)[76]. Presenting WBC count was a key determinant of outcome. The 70% of patients who presented with a WBC count of $< 10 \times 10^9$/l had a better CR (85% vs. 62%) and reduced relapse risk (22% vs. 42%) and superior survival (69% vs. 43%). Within the low-count group, extended ATRA resulted in a better CR (94% vs. 76%), reduced relapse risk (13% vs. 35%) and improved survival (80% vs. 57%). There was no evidence of benefit in patients presenting with a higher WBC count ($> 10 \times 10^9$/l). Molecular monitoring after the third chemotherapy course showed a

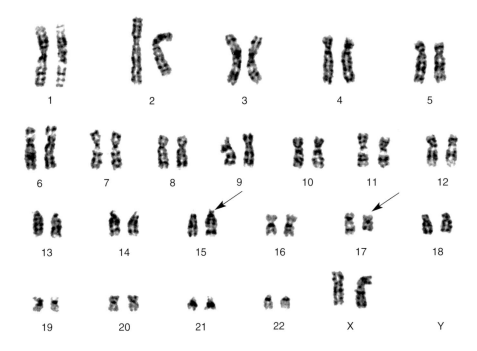

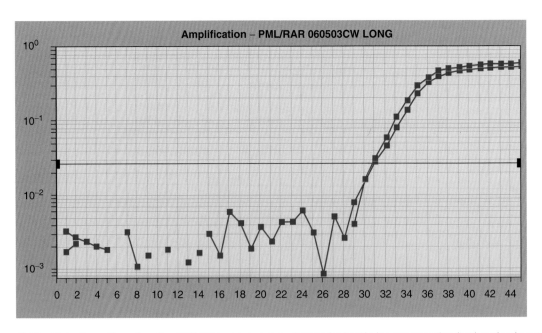

Figure 8.15 Detection of translocation t(15;17) in acute promyelocytic leukemia by cytogenetics (top) and polymerase chain reaction (bottom)

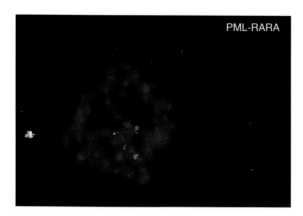
PML-RARA

Figure 8.16   Acute promyelocytic leukemia with insertion of a fragment of chromosome 17 into chromosome 15. Cytogenetic studies were negative for t(15;17)

correlation with risk of relapse. The relapse risk was 57% if the RT-PCR was positive versus 27% if the RT-PCR was negative. APL patients who present with a low WBC count benefit from combining ATRA with induction chemotherapy until remission is achieved. Molecular characterization of disease can improve diagnostic precision, and a positive RT-PCR after consolidation identifies patients at a higher risk of relapse[76]. In relapsed patients, arsenic trioxide is considered the treatment of choice. With the continued improvement in the field of stem cell transplantation, this may play an important role in the few patients with relapsed/refractory disease or those in second complete remission[1288].

CHAPTER 9

Myelodysplastic syndromes and chronic myelomonocytic leukemia

CHRONIC MYELOMONOCYTIC LEUKEMIA

Chronic myelomonocytic leukemia (CMML) is a myeloid stem cell disorder characterized by persistent monocytosis in the bone marrow (Figure 9.1) and blood ($>1 \times 10^9$/l), variable degree of marrow dyspoiesis, lack of the Philadelphia chromosome, $<20\%$ blasts in the blood or bone marrow and wide heterogeneity of clinical presentation. A large fraction of patients with CMML show unequivocal predominance of proliferative features with marked leukocytosis white blood cell (WBC) count $>13 \times 10^9$/l) and hepatosplenomegaly ('proliferative-type' CMML). Other patients show predominance of dysplastic features with only modest leukocytosis (WBC count $\leq 13 \times 10^9$/l) and often cytogenetic abnormalities ('dysplastic-type' CMML). The current World Health Organization (WHO) classification includes CMML in a new category of mixed chronic myeloproliferative/myelodysplastic disorder[225]. The natural course of the disease is variable with survival ranging from a few months to several years. The survival for patients with CMML is usually 12–40 months (median about 20 months)[1289–1295]. No treatment is effective in improving the natural course of the disease. Onida *et al.* observed no significant difference in survival time between patients who received supportive treatment, interferon-based therapy, low-dose/single-agent chemotherapy or intensive/combination chemotherapy[1289]. The rate of transformation into acute leukemia (approximately 20%) is similar in both variants of CMML: 14–32% for 'dysplastic-type' CMML and 15–19% for 'proliferative-type' CMML[1289,1295,1296]. The prognosis in the proliferative variant is generally worse than in the dysplastic variant[1289,1297]. Univariate analysis identified low hemoglobin level, low platelet count, high monocyte and lymphocyte counts, the presence of circulating immature myeloid cells, a high percentage of marrow blasts, a low percentage of marrow erythroid cells, abnormal cytogenetics, and high levels of lactate dehydrogenase (LDH) (>700 U/l) and β_2-microglobulin (>4 mg/l) as parameters associated with shorter survival[1289,1298]. Hemoglobin level below 120 g/l, presence of circulating immature myeloid cells, absolute lymphocyte count above 2.5×10^9/l and marrow blasts $\geq 10\%$ are the most significant predictors of poor prognosis in CMML and are independently associated with shorter survival by multivariate analysis[1289,1290,1292–1294,1296,1298,1299]. Karyotype analysis does not appear to yield additional prognostic information in CMML. Germing *et al.* found that the International Prognostic Scoring System (IPSS) was not useful for defining risk groups in CMML, while the Spanish Score, the modified Bournemouth Score, the Dusseldrof Score and the MD Anderson Prognostic Score identified patient groups differing significantly in survival[1289,1295].

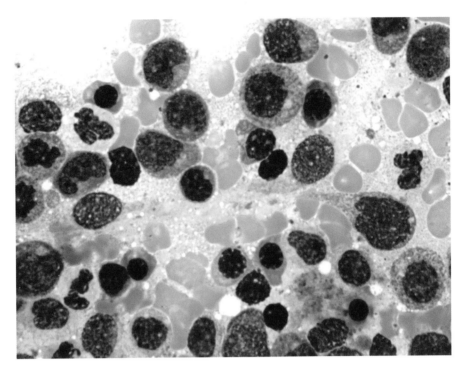

Figure 9.1   Chronic myelomonocytic leukemia (CMML); bone marrow aspirate smear

MYELODYSPLASTIC SYNDROMES

Myelodysplastic syndromes (MDS) are clonal hematopoietic stem cell disorders characterized clinically and morphologically by ineffective hematopoiesis and dyspoiesis (Figure 9.2) leading to bone marrow failure, cytopenia and high risk of progression to acute leukemia[225,1300]. MDS disorders may arise *de novo* or following chemotherapy or irradiation. Ineffective hematopoiesis in MDS has been attributed in part to a complex interaction between progenitor cells and the microenvironment that results in the premature apoptotic death of blood cell precursors. An increased frequency of apoptosis in the bone marrow cells of patients with MDS has been confirmed by many studies[1301–1303]. MDS displays clinical, pathologic and cytogenetic heterogeneity, and the natural history of the disease ranges from a chronic course that may span years to a rapid progression to acute leukemia. Based on clinical symptoms, morphology, number of blasts and chromosomal changes, the WHO classification recognizes several categories of MDS: refractory anemia (RA), refractory anemia with ringed sideroblasts (RARS), refractory cytopenia with multilineage dysplasia (RCMD), RCMD and ringed sideroblasts, refractory anemia with excess blasts (RAEB; Figure 9.3) and MDS associated with isolated deletion of 5q (5q⁻ syndrome; Figure 9.4). RAEB is further subdivided into type I (5–9% blasts in the bone marrow) and type II (10–19% blasts in the bone marrow). Based on duration of survival and incidence of progression into acute leukemia, MDS can be categorized into two risk groups: low risk (MDS with isolated 5q deletion, RA and RARS) and high risk (RCMD and RAEB). The median survival for RA patients is 66 months, RARS patients 6 years, RCMD patients 24–33 months, RAEB-I patients 18 months and RAEB-II patients 10 months[226,1304]. In the group of patients with less than 5% marrow blasts, there was a difference in median survival between patients with unilineage dysplasia (51% surviving at 67 months)

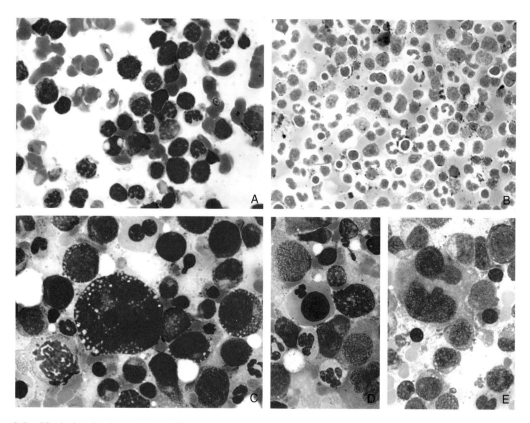

Figure 9.2   Myelodysplastic syndrome. Cytomorphologic features showing trilineage dyspoiesis. A, dysgranulopoiesis; B, ringed sideroblasts; C–D, dyserythropoiesis; E, dysmegakaryopoiesis

and those with multilineage dysplasia (median survival, 28.5 months)[1305]. Approximately 6–26%, 1–11%, 11% and 25–38% of patients with RA, RARS, RCMD and RAEB, respectively, progress into acute leukemia[226]. The projected median survival of patients with isolated del(5q) is 146 months. Patients with an increased medullary blast count and those with an additional chromosomal abnormality have a significantly shorter overall survival (24 and 45 months, respectively) than patients with isolated del(5q)[404]. MDS with erythroid hypoplasia is a rare form of MDS with clinical and morphologic features overlapping with pure red cell aplasia. This form of MDS responds to cyclosporine therapy[1306–1308].

The main prognostic factors in MDS are percentage of bone marrow blasts (< 5% vs. 5–9% vs. 10–19%), number and degree of cytopenias (less versus more

than 1 or 2 cytopenias; thrombocytopenia, anemia versus neutropenia), age and presence of chromosomal abnormalities[23,168,1300,1309–1311]. The presence of excessive fibrosis in the bone marrow (fibrotic MDS) is associated with inferior survival[1312–1314].

The presence of Auer rods does not appear to be associated with poor prognosis in MDS[1315].

Clonal cytogenetic abnormalities are present in the marrow of more than 50% of patients with MDS[1316] and are strong and independent prognostic indicators[23,1317–1319]. More common use of fluorescence *in situ* hybridization (FISH) and molecular tests in the management of patients with MDS would increase the percentage of patients with chromosomal and/or genetic aberrations. Figures 9.5 and 9.6 present survival and risk of transformation into acute leukemia in MDS based on chromosomal abnormalities. Three

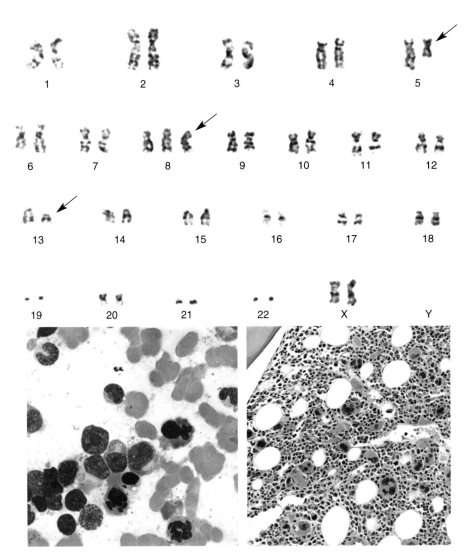

Figure 9.3   Refractory anemia with excess blasts with complex changes: 46,XX, del(5)(q13;q33), del(13)(q12q14) [1]/47, idem,+8[15]

risk-based cytogenetic groups (good, intermediate and poor) can be distinguished. The cytogenetic subgroup with good outcome includes normal karyotype, −Y alone (monosomy Y), del(5q) alone (Figure 9.3) and del(20q) alone; poor outcome includes complex karyotype (≥3 abnormalities; Figure 9.7) or chromosome 7 abnormalities (Figure 9.8); and intermediate outcome includes all other abnormalities[23]. Abnormalities of chromosomes 5 and 7 or complex aberrations are seen only in RCMD and RAEB. Patients with normal karyotype, del(5q) alone, or del(20q) alone have median survival of >24 months, whereas patients with high-risk cytogenetic changes (complex karyotype, chromosome 3 abnormalities or chromosome 7 abnormalities) have median survival of <12 months[1320]. The International Prognostic Scoring System (IPSS) for MDS has defined patients with a normal karyotype as a good risk

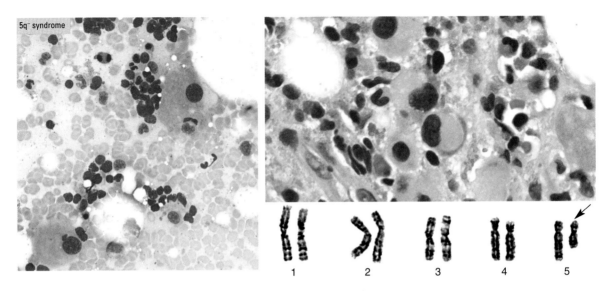

Figure 9.4 Myelodysplastic syndrome with isolated deletion of 5q (5q⁻ syndrome)

cytogenetic subgroup. It is suggested that the prognostic impact of karyotypic subgroups in MDS is modified by sex[1321]. Shorter survival was detected for men in the favorable and the intermediate subgroups, but not in the poor-prognosis subgroup, when compared with women. The better outcome for women in the favorable subgroup was mainly the result of the 5q⁻ syndrome[1321]. The cytogenetic profile of MDS, particularly of RAEB, is nearly identical to that of elderly patients with AML both in frequency and in the type of chromosomal abnormalities[118].

Patients with aplastic anemia and clonal karyotypic evolution most often show numerical and structural abnormalities of chromosome 7 (40%), followed by trisomy 8, aberrations of chromosome 13, deletion of the Y chromosome and complex cytogenetic abnormalities[1322]. Unlike in primary MDS, aberrances of chromosome 5 and 20 are infrequent. Most deaths related to leukemic transformation occurred in patients with abnormalities of chromosome 7 or complex cytogenetic alterations, or both. Evolution of chromosome 7 abnormalities was seen most often in refractory patients who had failed to respond to therapy. In contrast, trisomy

8 developed in patients with good hematologic responses who often required chronic immunosuppression with cyclosporine, and survival was excellent[1322]. Although aplastic anemia patients with monosomy 7 showed a similar prognosis to those with primary MDS, trisomy 8 in aplastic anemia appears to have a more favorable prognosis than in MDS[1322].

As mentioned above, the prognosis in MDS is extremely variable, with survival ranging from a few months to more than 20 years. Based on the multivariate analyses of a large series of patients, several different scoring systems have been proposed for MDS to predict outcome and risk of transformation to acute leukemia[168,1300,1323–1325]. Among different systems, the IPSS (Table 1.1) is most commonly applied[23]. Based on the analysis of cytogenetic, morphologic and clinical data, it has defined four prognostic subgroups: low (0), intermediate-1 (0.5–1.0), intermediate-2 (1.5–2.0) and high (≥2.5). The IPSS separated patients into distinctive subgroups of risk to undergo evolution to acute myeloid leukemia (AML), with low (31% of patients), 9.4 years; intermediate-1 (INT-1; 39%), 3.3 years; INT-2 (22%), 1.1 years; and high (8%), 0.2 years. IPSS also separated patients into similar distinctive risk groups for

A

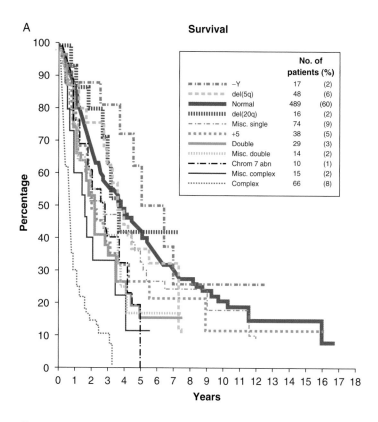

B

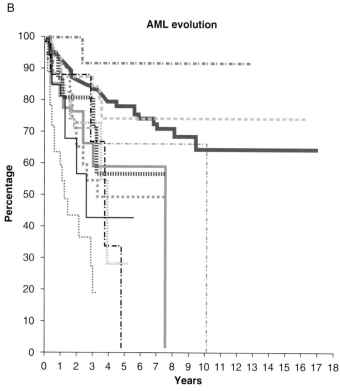

Figure 9.5 Survival (A) and freedom from acute myeloid leukemia (AML) evolution (B) of myelodysplastic syndrome patients related to their individual cytogenetic categories (Kaplan–Meier curves). The number of patients in each category and their proportional representation (in brackets) are given for the 816 patients analyzed for survival (A). Virtually identical proportions of cytogenetic abnormalities were found for the 759 patients analyzed for AML evolution (B)

From: Greenberg P, *et al.* International scoring system for evaluating prognosis in myelodysplastic syndromes. Blood 1997;89: 2079–88. © 1997 by The American Society of Hematology, used with permission

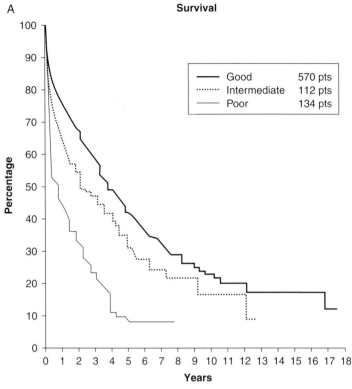

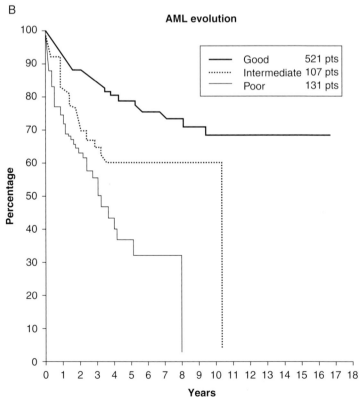

Figure 9.6 Survival (A) and freedom from acute myeloid leukemia (AML) evolution (B) of myelodysplastic syndrome patients related to their risk-based categorical cytogenetic subgroups: good, intermediate and poor. Good, normal, del(5q) only, del(20q) only, −Y only. Poor, complex (i.e. three anomalies) or chromosome 7 abnormalities. Intermediate, other abnormalities. Kaplan–Meier curves

From: Greenberg P, *et al*. International scoring system for evaluating prognosis in myelodysplastic syndromes. Blood 1997;89: 2079–88. © 1997 by The American Society of Hematology, used with permission

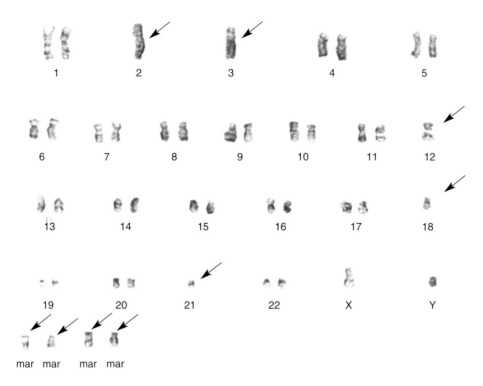

Figure 9.7   Myelodysplastic syndrome with complex chromosomal changes

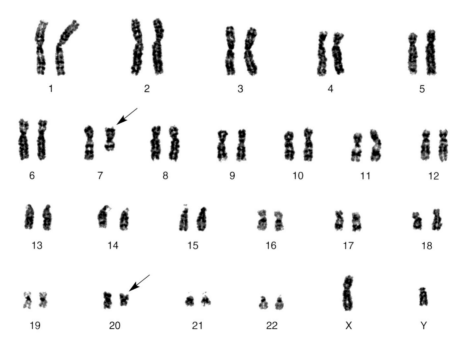

Figure 9.8   Myelodysplastic syndrome with partial deletion of chromosomes 7 and 20

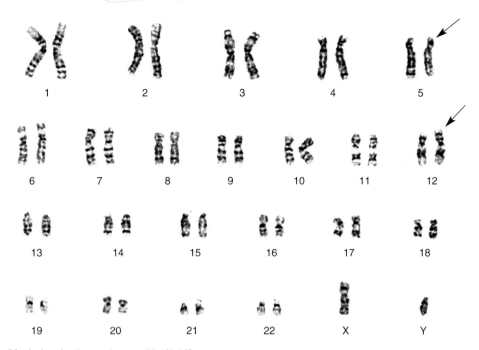

Figure 9.9   Myelodysplastic syndrome with t(5;12)

median survival: low, 5.7 years; INT-1, 3.5 years; INT-2, 1.2 years; and high, 0.4 years[23]. Stratification for age further improved analysis of survival[23]. The role of IPSS as the predominant prognostic instrument seems to be uncertain in the new WHO classification of MDS[1326]. Between 40% and 60% of *de novo* MDS patients have a normal karyotype at the time of diagnosis[1327–1330]. Normal karyotype has been considered a good-risk prognostic variable by the IPSS, although it has been shown that this group of patients has a variable clinical course and rather variable final outcome. Therefore, alternative prognostic markers other than cytogenetics may be of value for patients with a normal karyotype (or with unproductive metaphases). Evaluation of FISH may be helpful in detecting occult defects in patients with a normal karyotype on routine cytogenetic studies. Clinical variables in all MDS patients with a normal karyotype are also helpful in identifying patients with a different prognosis, suitable for risk-adapted therapeutic strategies. Multivariate analysis of patients with a normal karyotype showed that, among clinical

scoring systems, the Bournemouth score (0–1 vs. ≥2) appeared to be the best prognostic indicator for risk of leukemic transformation, and platelet count $< 10 \times 10^9$/l, presence of hemorrhagic symptoms at the time of diagnosis and morphologic classification were the main prognostic factors for prediction of survival[1330]. Also, phenotypic markers may be of value in patients lacking cytogenetic information or in whom the karyotype was normal. The presence of ≥2 phenotypic aberrations as determined by flow cytometry (e.g. mature neutrophils with HLA-DR expression or decreased side scatter) is associated with shorter survival[1331]. Flow cytometric studies have begun to characterize individual or composite immunophenotypic abnormalities as well as light scatter properties that may be helpful for diagnosis and of prognostic value for the natural course of the disease and for outcome after therapy[1332–1334].

Because of the lack of a recurrent chromosomal abnormality in MDS, few genes involved in the pathogenesis of MDS have been identified. Figure 9.9 presents MDS with the t(5;12) translocation. The t(5;12)(q33;p13), which disrupts a gene coding for a tyrosine kinase, the platelet-derived growth factor receptor-β (PDGFRB), leads to deregulation of cell growth. Patients with the PDGFRB fusion gene respond well to treatment with the tyrosine kinase inhibitor imatinib (Gleevec) and experience resolution of the cytogenetic abnormalities[1335]. Receptor tyrosine kinases include, among others, the EGF family (EGFR, ErbB2/HER2), PDGF receptor family, PDGFR receptor family (PDGFR, c-Kit, Flt3), TRK family and EPH receptor family[1336]. The mutations of c-*fms* in MDS are associated with a poor outcome[1337]. The *FLT3* mutations (internal tandem duplications, ITD) in MDS are associated with more common and rapid progression to AML and with subsequent disease progression[1338,1339]. Patients with *FLT3*/ITD-positive disease also had significantly shorter survival compared with patients without *FLT3*/ITD-negative disease. On multivariate analysis, *FLT3*/ITD was identified as an independent predictor of reduced time to development of AML and reduced overall survival[584]. The most frequent molecular abnormalities, identified in approximately 30%

of patients with advanced MDS, are point mutations in the *RAS* gene family that lead to activated RAS protein[1316]. Mutations of *p53* (*TP53*) are infrequent and are generally associated with high-risk MDS and other cytogenetic abnormalities[1316]. Therefore, they may contribute to disease progression and clonal expansion in leukemia.

Excessive apoptosis is implicated in the pathogenesis of MDS. The percentage of mononuclear cells expressing Bcl-2 and Bcl-X$_L$ was higher in RAEB and CMML than in RA and RARS. Conversely, the pro-apoptotic proteins Bad, Bak and Bcl-X$_S$ were detected in a higher percentage of cells in RA and RARS. RA and RARS were associated with an increased Bcl-X$_S$/Bcl-X$_L$ ratio. Higher expression of pro-apoptotic Bcl-2-family proteins (Bak, Bad, Bcl-X$_S$) and higher Bcl-X$_S$/Bcl-X$_L$ ratio were associated with longer survival and decreased risk of leukemic transformation in univariate analysis, whereas expression of anti-apoptotic proteins was associated with decreased survival. Consequently Bcl-2 protein expression was well correlated with the IPSS[1340].

CHAPTER 10

Chronic myeloproliferative disorders

Chronic myeloproliferative disorders represent a range of clonal hematopoietic stem cell diseases that include the four major categories chronic myeloid leukemia (CML), polycythemia vera (PV), essential thrombocythemia (ET) and chronic idiopathic myelofibrosis (CIMF). They are characterized by hyperplasia of marrow cells with increased production of granulocytes (most typical for CML), platelets (a major feature of ET) and red cells (a major feature of PV). With the exception of CML (see below), the molecular pathogenesis of chronic myeloproliferative disorders is unknown, but tyrosine kinases have been implicated. The BCR–ABL tyrosine kinase fusion causes CML, and other kinases are altered in malignant hematopoietic tumors (e.g. *FLT3* in acute myeloid leukemia (AML), *PDGFRβ* in chronic myelomonocytic leukemia (CMML), *PDGFRα* in chronic eosinophilic leukemia and *KIT* in systemic mastocytosis). Recently, mutations of *JAK2*, a cytoplasmic tyrosine kinase with a key role in signal transduction from multiple hematopoietic growth factor receptors, have been implicated in the pathogenesis of chronic myeloproliferative disorders other than CML[590].

CHRONIC MYELOID LEUKEMIA

CML is a clonal stem cell disorder characterized by a proliferation of myeloid cells at all stages of differentiation (Figure 10.1) and the t(9;22)(q34;q11),

leading to the formation of the *BCR–ABL* fusion gene[1341–1343]. The diagnosis of CML is usually based on detection of the Philadelphia chromosome (Ph), first described as a shortened chromosome 22 and then as a t(9;22) translocation (Figure 10.2). This abnormality is present in the leukemic cells of more than 95% of patients with CML[1344]. The remaining patients have complex or variant translocations involving additional chromosomes. The translocation of the *BCR* (breakpoint cluster region) gene on chromosome 22 to the *ABL* (Abelson leukemia virus) gene on chromosome 9 (Figure 10.2) leads to the formation of *BCR–ABL*. The encoded fusion protein, BCR–ABL is a constitutively active cytoplasmic tyrosine kinase. The breakpoints may occur at three different regions of the *BCR* gene: major (M-bcr), minor (m-bcr) and micro (μ-bcr). Depending on the site of the breakpoint in the *BCR* gene, the fusion protein can vary in size from 190 kDa (p190[BCR–ABL]; m-bcr), to 210 kDa (p210[BCR–ABL]; M-bcr) to 230 kDa (p210[BCR–ABL]; μ-bcr).

Clinical and laboratory features

The molecular basis of CML is well defined and highly consistent, yet prognosis varies considerably. The median survival of patients with CML after diagnosis is 4–5 years. High initial white blood cell (WBC) count, significant basophilia, the percentage of circulating blasts, massive hepatosplenomegaly,

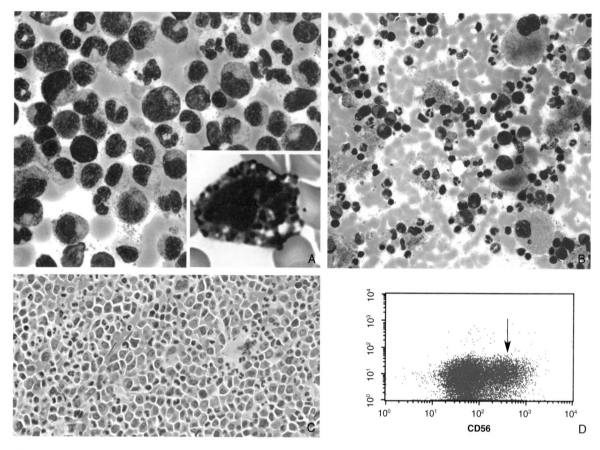

Figure 10.1 Chronic myeloid leukemia (CML). A, bone marrow aspirate showing myeloid hyperplasia with leftward shift morphology (*Inset*: basophil); B, bone marrow aspirate (low magnification) showing atypical hypolobated micromegakaryocytes; C, histologic section showing markedly hypercellular marrow with increased M:E ratio; D, flow cytometry showing upregulation of CD56 on maturing myeloid cells (arrow)

thrombocytopenia or thrombocytosis, multiple chromosomal abnormalities, marrow fibrosis, male sex, Black ethnicity, increased patient age and poor performance status are important prognostic indicators associated with poor outcome[1345]. Multivariable regression analysis indicated that spleen size and the percentage of circulating blasts are particularly important prognostic indicators[1345]. A platelet count of $>700 \times 10^9$/l is an unfavorable marker. Basophils plus eosinophils over 15%, more than 5% marrow blasts, and karyotypic abnormalities in addition to the Ph chromosome are also significant unfavorable signs. The Cox model, generated with four variables representing percentage of blasts, spleen size, platelet

count and age, provided a useful representation of risk status in CML. The Sokal and Hasford prognostic scoring systems for CML are presented in Table 10.1. Patients with high-risk prognostic scores (according to the Sokal or Hasford systems) had a significantly higher proliferation index than those with low risk scores[1346]. Bone marrow blast count demonstrated a highly significant correlation with the respective cytogenetic results of the patients and was clearly linked to the frequency and complexity of clonal evolution[1347]. The New CML score using age, spleen size, blast cell count, eosinophil count, basophil count and platelet count shows good discrimination for survival. In high-risk patients,

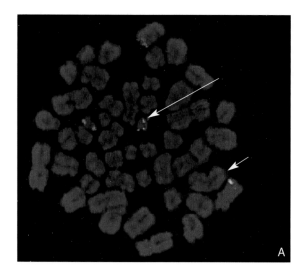

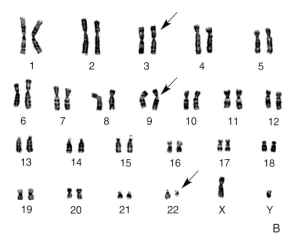

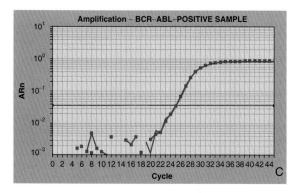

Figure 10.2 Chronic myeloid leukemia with t(9;22)/ BCR–ABL identified by fluorescence *in situ* hybridization (A), routine cytogenetics (B) and polymerase chain reaction analysis (C)

complete clinical remission had no impact on prognosis[1348]. The pretreatment characteristics that correlate with an increased risk of hematologic relapse (univariate Cox regression analysis) are hemoglobin level less than 120 g/l, an elevated platelet count, increased bands in the peripheral blood and clonal evolution[1349]. During treatment, the absence of a major cytogenetic response within the first 6 months also significantly correlated with relapse[1349]. Patients failing to achieve a major cytogenetic response by 6 months had a significantly higher rate of hematologic relapse (27%) compared with those who achieved a major cytogenetic response by 6 months (3%), and patients with clonal evolution had a significantly higher risk of hematologic relapse (50%) than those without clonal evolution (9%)[1349]. Patients carrying submicroscopic der(9) deletions were reported to have an unfavorable prognosis when treated with hydroxyurea, interferon-α, or bone marrow transplantation[497,1350], and it was suggested that the presence of der(9) deletions may be a more significant prognostic indicator than Sokal or Hasford scoring systems[1351]. Huntly *et al.* found no difference in survival between patients with and without der(9) deletions, contrasting with previous reports in cohorts with a lower proportion of patients treated with imatinib (Gleevec). However, the time to disease progression on imatinib treatment was significantly shorter for patients with deletions, both in the chronic phase and in advanced phases[1352]. In a recent series published by Quintas-Cardama *et al.*, the rates of major (82% vs. 79%) and complete cytogenetic response (76% vs. 66%) with imatinib therapy were similar in patients with and without der(9) deletions, respectively[1353]. After a median follow-up of 28 months, there was no difference in overall survival or response duration in patients with and without deletions. In a multivariate analysis, der(9) deletions had no significant impact on response, survival, or response duration, suggesting that treatment with imatinib overcomes the adverse prognostic significance of der(9) deletions in patients with CML[1353].

Table 10.1   Sokal and Hasford prognostic scoring systems for chronic myeloid leukemia

Hasford		Sokal	
Age (years)		*Age (years)*	
0 if <50;			
0.6666 if ≥50			
Spleen size		*Spleen size*	
0.042 × size (cm below costal margin)		cm below costal margin	
Peripheral blood		*Peripheral blood*	
Blasts	0.0548×% blasts	Blasts (%)	
Eosinophils	0.0413×% eosinophils	Platelets (10^9/l)	
Basophils	0.2039 when basophils >3%		
Platelets	0 if <1500×10^9/l; 1.0956 if =1500×10^9/l		
Hasford score=[0.6666 age+0.042 spleen (cm below the costal margin)+0.0584 blasts (%)+0.0413 eosinophils (%)+0.2039×basophils+1.0956 platelets]×1000		Sokal score = exp[0.011(age–43.4)+0.0345 (spleen–7.51)+0.188 [(platelet/700)^2–0.563] +0.0887 (blasts–2.1)]	
Risk categories		*Risk categories*	
Low	≤780	Low<0.8	
Intermediate	781–1480	Intermediate 0.8–1.2	
High	>1480	High>1.2	

Morphologic features

Marrow fibrosis is an independent poor prognostic indicator of CML, allowing an early prediction of therapy failure[1354–1356]. The risk of death markedly increased when marrow fibrosis occurred or progressed, independently of all other prognostic factors evaluated, including the cytogenetic response. In a study by Cervantes *et al.*, survival studies demonstrated that marked diffuse reticulin fibrosis and more than 15 megakaryocytes/mm³ of marrow tissue were associated with a poorer prognosis. However, they lost their prognostic influence when they were included in a multivariate regression model[1357]. Marrow fibrosis appears to be a significant early indicator of ineffective therapy in CML[1358]. In patients treated with interferon-α, hydroxyurea and busulfan, evolving or progressive marrow fibrosis was an independent and early predictor of therapy failure about 2 years earlier than indicated by changes in the peripheral blood, spleen size, marrow blast count and cytogenetics[1356]. Fibrosis disappeared when high-dose interferon-α was combined with low-dose cytosine arabinoside[1358]. Treatment with imatinib

appears to reduce CML-associated fibrosis in most patients[1359]. A transition of a myelofibrotic into a non-fibrotic subtype is also detectable in a subset of patients treated with hydroxyurea[1360].

CML progression

CML usually has a biphasic or triphasic course, with disease progression from the chronic phase to an accelerated phase (Figure 10.3) and/or blast phase (Figure 10.4). In most untreated patients, a progressive increase in leukocyte count is observed. Eventually the chronic phase of the disease progresses into an accelerated phase and/or blast phase (crisis) of myeloid or less often lymphoid phenotype. The progression is frequently preceded or accompanied by recurring secondary chromosomal abnormalities and oncogene alteration (most often *p53* (*Tp53*), *RB1*, *c-MYC* and *RAS* genes). The chromosomes most commonly involved include chromosomes 9 and 22 (e.g. duplication of the Ph chromosome), trisomy 8, i(17q), trisomy 19 and loss of the Y chromosome[1361]. The rate of transformation is low initially (approximate

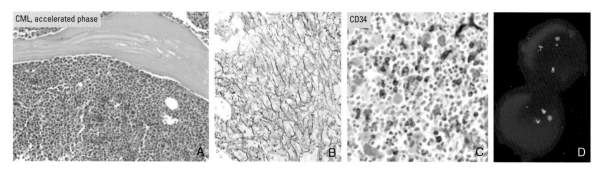

Figure 10.3   Chronic myeloid leukemia (CML), accelerated phase. A–B, histology showing hypercellular marrow with myeloid leftward shift (A) and diffuse reticulin fibrosis (B). The immunohistochemical staining with CD34 confirmed an increased number of blasts (C). D, positive *BCR–ABL* by fluorescence *in situ* hybridization

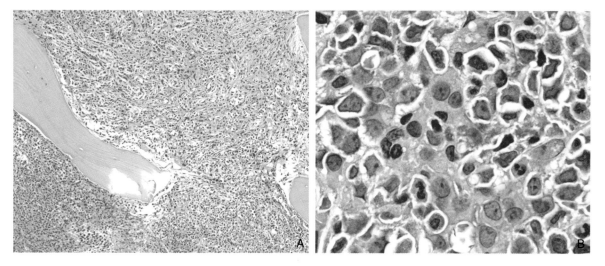

Figure 10.4   Chronic myeloid leukemia (CML) myeloid blast phase (acute myeloid leukemia evolving from CML). A, low magnification; B, high magnification. Bone marrow is virtually replaced by immature mononuclear cells

rate of 5% in the first year) and increases gradually to 20–25% in each year thereafter[1362,1363]. Signs and symptoms of accelerated phase include increasing blood basophilia to >20%, blasts in bone marrow or blood >10%, cytogenetic evolution, difficult to control WBC count, marrow fibrosis and thrombocytopenia $<100 \times 10^9$/l. Signs and laboratory features of blast crisis include blasts in marrow or blood >20%, clumps of blasts on marrow examination, and extramedullary myeloid tumor. The median survival of the blast phase is 2–6 months (long-term survival is uncommon)[1364–1366]. The

response to high-dose chemotherapy with allogeneic stem cell transplantation is poor[1365], owing to upregulation of anti-apoptotic signals and multidrug resistance (MDR). Despite the generally dismal prognosis of CML blast crisis when compared with *BCR–ABL*-negative acute leukemia, determination of blast lineage in transformed CML is clinically important. Patients with lymphoblastic transformation have a better response to chemotherapy and longer survival than patients with myeloblastic transformation[1367,1368]. Leukocyte alkaline phosphatase (LAP) is reduced in CML patients at diagnosis and

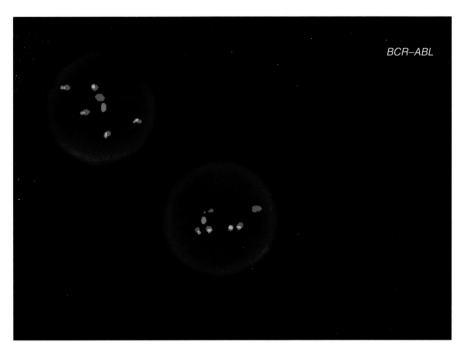

Figure 10.5   Multiple *BCR–ABL* fusion signals, suggesting chronic myeloid leukemia progression (FISH analysis)

the LAP values increase when CML transforms to more advanced disease (accelerated phase or blast crisis). Cytogenetic clonal evolution is a known poor prognostic factor in CML. The lack of cytogenetic response at 3 months appears to be a stronger independent poor prognostic factor for survival than clonal evolution for both chronic and accelerated phases. The presence of additional *BCR–ABL* copies (Figure 10.5) suggests disease progression and poor prognosis.

Disease monitoring

Imatinib can induce complete or nearly complete remission in up to 80% of patients[1369,1370]; 90% of patients with early-stage (chronic phase) CML and 60% of patients with advanced-stage CML (blast crisis) achieve a hematologic response to imatinib[1369,1371]. Mutations in the *BCR–ABL* kinase domain occur in over 90% of patients who relapse after an initial response[1372]. The response to treatment

is based on the hematologic, cytogenetic and molecular parameters. A hematologic remission indicates a return of peripheral blood cell counts and bone marrow morphology to normal, cytogenetic remission indicates the disappearance of the Ph chromosome and molecular remission is based on lack of a detectable *BCR–ABL* fusion transcript. Patients on imatinib who achieved at least some degree of cytogenetic response after 6 months had better survival; those with no cytogenetic response to imatinib had significantly worse survival. This suggests that cytogenetic responders obtain benefit from imatinib, but patients who show no cytogenetic response should be given alternative treatment[1373]. Resistance to imatinib can arise by multiple mechanisms including amplification or mutation of *BCR–ABL*. The acquisition of additional cytogenetic changes (clonal evolution) during treatment of CML with imatinib is currently regarded as an index of increasing resistance to imatinib. Cytogenetic clonal evolution is not an important factor for achieving a major or complete cytogenetic response with imatinib therapy, but it is an independent poor prognostic factor for survival in both chronic and accelerated phases of CML[1374]. Clonal evolution can be identified during treatment with imatinib in patients who are in complete hematologic remission. Patients with *de novo* clonal evolution in the absence of any other sign of disease progression had a significantly higher incidence of progression by 18 months than patients with non-clonal evolution[1375]. Acquisition of clonal evolution also increases the risk of subsequent disease progression in CML patients in complete hematologic remission on imatinib[1375]. Predictors for relapse after hematopoietic stem cell transplantation inlcude advanced disease stage and slow reduction of *BCR–ABL* transcripts at day 28 and day 56 following transplant. Lange *et al.* concluded that a complete clearance of *BCR–ABL* transcripts was achievable within 4 weeks from transplantation even after minimal conditioning, and that early kinetics of *BCR–ABL* transcripts significantly correlated with the probability of hematologic relapse.[1376] Sokal and Hasford scores did not predict survival after hematopoietic stem cell transplantation[1377]. Imatinib has significant activity against CML relapsing after allogeneic stem cell transplantation[1378]; the overall hematologic response rate was 84% (98% for patients relapsing in chronic phase). The complete cytogenetic response was 58% for patients in the chronic phase, 48% for the accelerated phase and 22% for patients in the blast phase. With imatinib treatment, 57% achieved full donor chimerism and 14% mixed chimerism[1378]. In advanced disease (accelerated phase and blast crisis) only a few patients respond to treatment on a molecular level (polymerase chain reaction (PCR) for *BCR–ABL* mRNA). In contrast to the *BCR–ABL* mRNA levels, the *WT1* mRNA levels are indicative of hematologic relapse[1379].

POLYCYTHEMIA VERA

PV is a chronic clonal myeloproliferative disorder characterized by an increase in the number of red blood cells and in the total blood volume, and often leukocytosis, thrombocytosis and splenomegaly. The natural history of PV includes hyperviscosity, expanded blood volume, thrombohemorrhagic complications and an increased lifetime risk of disease transformation into myelofibrosis with myeloid metaplasia, myelodysplasia (MDS) and AML. Although the majority of patients die from thrombosis or hemorrhage, up to 20% develop AML[1380]. The prognosis for untreated PV patients is quite poor. This differs from ET, in which the prognosis for asymptomatic patients is generally good. Proper treatments have been shown to reduce complications and significantly extend the life span. The median survival of untreated patients with PV was reported to be 18 months[1381], but with currently available treatment the median survival time can reach 10 years[1380,1382,1383]. Only age and hyperleukocytosis at diagnosis were found to have prognostic value in PV[1384]. Thrombotic complications are the major cause of morbidity and mortality in PV patients[1383,1385,1386]. Non-randomized studies have suggested that aggressive phlebotomy may improve survival in PV. The addition of cytoreductive therapy to phlebotomy in high-risk patients with PV may reduce the risk of recurrent thrombosis[1387]. Cytoreduction favorably affects the incidence of thrombotic events, but aggressive treatment seems to be associated with increased risk of neoplasm[1386,1388]. The increased risk of cancer in patients receiving myelosuppressive agents was seen approximately 6 years after diagnosis. The risk of MDS and acute leukemia is low in patients who have not been treated with cytotoxic agents, but increases following chemotherapy[1380,1382,1383]. AML can develop in approximately one-third of patients, either following marrow fibrosis and myeloid metaplasia or without preceding evidence of myelofibrosis. The prognosis of cases of PV that has transformed into acute leukemia is generally poor, because the majority of such cases are refractory to chemotherapy[1389]. The incidence of leukemia in patients treated with hydroxyurea appears to be low and similar to that observed in patients treated with phlebotomy alone[1390,1391].

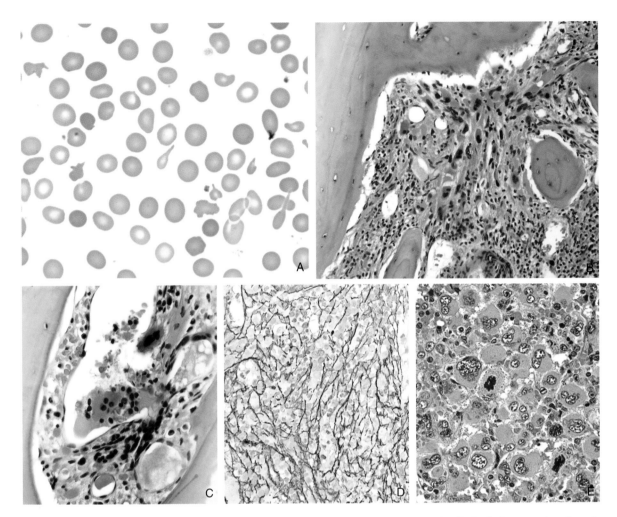

Figure 10.6 Chronic idiopathic myelofibrosis (CIMF). A, blood smear with irregular red cells (including tear-drop forms); B, histology with clusters of atypical megakaryocytes; C, high magnification showing intravascular hematopoiesis; D, diffuse reticulin fibrosis; E, myeloid metaplasia, spleen

ESSENTIAL THROMBOCYTHEMIA

ET is a clonal myeloproliferative disorder that involves a predominantly megakaryocytic lineage. It is characterized by sustained thrombocytosis (platelets $\geq 600 \times 10^9/l$) and megakaryocytosis with atypia and clustering in the bone marrow. It is an indolent disorder, characterized by long symptom-free intervals. Median survival times range between 10 and 15 years. Most cases are diagnosed in patients 50–60 years of age and therefore the life expectancy is near normal for most patients. Complications in the form of thrombotic or hemorrhagic episodes are

the major factors associated with morbidity and mortality. Progression to bone marrow fibrosis is rare[1392]. Transformation into MDS or acute leukemia (often acute myelomonocytic or megakaryoblastic) is less common than in PV and occurs in fewer than 5% of patients. Similarly to PV, the transformation to leukemia is linked to cytotoxic therapy[1393,1394].

CHRONIC IDIOPATHIC MYELOFIBROSIS

CIMF (Figure 10.6) is a clonal stem cell disorder characterized by the proliferation of megakaryocytes and granulocytic elements and deposition of excess collagen in the bone marrow. The clinical course of CIMF is variable, with some patients surviving for less than a year and others showing an indolent course. CIMF has a median survival of 3–7 years, and fewer than 20% of patients survive more than 10 years[173,1395–1397]. Hemoglobin level at diagnosis is one of the most important prognostic factors. Patients may be asymptomatic in the early stages, but later progress to marrow fibrosis, splenomegaly with pancytopenia leading to anemia, and other constitutional symptoms. Most of the care available is supportive and only palliates the constitutional symptoms. The prognosis of patients with CIMF is worse than the prognosis in patients with PV or ET[1397]. Most patients develop progressive splenic enlargement with portal hypertension and, eventually, symptoms of marrow failure. Infection, hemorrhage, cardiac failure and cerebrovascular accidents are the leading causes of death in patients with CIMF. Blast crisis (conversion into acute leukemia) has been reported in 5–30% of patients with CIMF[1395,1398–1401] and is characterized by abrupt onset and rapidly fatal course. The major causes of mortality and morbidity are bone marrow failure, thromboembolic complications, portal hypertension and transformation into acute leukemia.

A variety of clinical and laboratory parameters have been associated with inferior survival in CIMF. The prognosis is adversely affected by a short period of time (< 13 months) between first symptoms and diagnosis, age > 60 years, male sex, constitutional symptoms, hepatomegaly, markedly increased lactate dehydrogenase (LDH), anemia (hemoglobin < 10 g/dl), thrombocytopenia ($< 100 \times 10^9$/l), leukopenia ($< 3 \times 10^9$/l) or leukocytosis ($> 30 \times 10^9$/l),

abnormal karyotype, circulating blasts ($CD34^+$ count in blood) or erythroid progenitor cells, $> 10\%$ granulocyte precursors in the blood and hypercatabolic symptoms[173–176,1395,1396,1398,1399,1402–1407]. Favorable prognostic factors include lack of constitutional symptoms, hemoglobin ≥ 10 g/dl and absence of hepatomegaly. Younger patients have better survival than older patients[1398,1399,1408]. The median survival of patients aged 55 years or less is 128 months[1396]. In most young adults with CIMF the disease presents without adverse prognostic factors and may remain stable for years[1409]. Patients with any chromosomal abnormalities in general have a poorer prognosis, when compared with patients with a normal karyotype[1408], although some cytogenetic abnormalities (5q–, +8, 13q–, 20q–) may be associated with a better prognosis[1410]. Dupriez et al. proposed a score (the Lille scoring system) that was able to identify three distinct prognostic groups: (1) low-risk group (hemoglobin > 10 g/dl, WBC $4–30 \times 10^9$/l); (2) intermediate-risk group (hemoglobin < 10 g/dl or WBC $< 4 \times 10^9$/l or $> 30 \times 10^9$/l); and (3) high-risk group (hemoglobin < 10 g/dl and WBC $< 4 \times 10^9$/l or $> 30 \times 10^9$/l). The median survivals for these groups are 93 months, 26 months and 13 months, respectively[174].

Major indications for splenectomy in CIMF patients are transfusion-dependent anemia, symptomatic splenomegaly, portal hypertension and severe thrombocytopenia. Durable remissions in constitutional symptoms, transfusion-dependent anemia, portal hypertension and severe thrombocytopenia were achieved in 67%, 23%, 50% and 0% of patients, respectively[1411]. Presplenectomy thrombocytopenia may be a surrogate for advanced disease and is associated with an increased risk of blast transformation and inferior post-splenectomy survival[1411].

Abbreviations

ABC	activated B-cell like
AILT	angioimmunoblastic T-cell lymphoma
ALCL	anaplastic large cell lymphoma
ALK	anaplastic lymphoma kinase
ALL	acute lymphoblastic leukemia
AML	acute myeloid leukemia
APL	acute promyelocytic leukemia
ATCL	adult T-cell leukemia/lymphoma
ATRA	all-*trans*-retinoic acid
B-CLL	B-chronic lymphocytic leukemia
BCR	breakpoint cluster region gene
B-PLL	B-prolymphocytic leukemia
CHOP	cyclophosphamide + doxorubicin/ hydroxydoxorubicin + vincristine (Oncovin) + prednisone
CIMF	chronic idiopathic myelofibrosis
CML	chronic myeloid leukemia
CMML	chronic myelomonocytic leukemia
CR	complete remission
del	deletion
DLBCL	diffuse large B-cell lymphoma
EBER	Epstein–Barr virus early RNA
EBV	Epstein–Barr virus
ET	essential thrombocythemia
ETO	fusion gene associated with t(8;21) (ETO *for* eight-twenty one)
FAB	French–American–British (morphologic classification of acute leukemia)

FISH	fluorescence *in situ* hybridization
FL	follicular lymphoma
FLIPI	Follicular Lymphoma International Prognostic Index
GCB	germinal center B-cell like
HCL	hairy cell leukemia
HL	Hodgkin's lymphoma
HOX	homeobox gene
i	isochromosome
IgV_H	immunoglobulin heavy-chain variable gene
IL	interleukin
inv	inversion
IPI	International Prognostic Index (*lymphoma*)
IPSS	International Prognostic Scoring System (*MDS*)
ITD	internal tandem duplications
LDH	lactate dehydrogenase
LGL	large granular lymphocyte
L&H	lymphocyte and histiocyte cell (popcorn cell)
LyP	lymphomatoid papulosis
MALT	mucosa-associated lymphoid tissue
MC	mixed chimerism
MCL	mantle cell lymphoma
MDR	multidrug resistance
MDS	myelodysplastic syndrome
MGUS	monoclonal gammopathy of undetermined significance

MLL	mixed lineage leukemia gene (myeloid lymphoid leukemia gene)	RARS	refractory anemia with ringed sideroblasts
MM	multiple myeloma	RCMD	refractory cytopenia with multilineage dysplasia
MRD	minimal residual disease		
MZL	marginal zone lymphoma	RQ-PCR	real-time quantitative PCR
NHL	non-Hodgkin's lymphoma	R-S	Reed–Sternberg
NK	natural killer	RT-PCR	reverse transcriptase PCR
NLPHL	nodular lymphocyte-predominant Hodgkin's lymphoma	*RUNX1*	official name for *AML1* gene
		SLL	small lymphocytic lymphoma
NPM	nucleophosmin gene	SMZL	splenic marginal zone lymphoma
NS	nodular sclerosis	t	translocation
PCR	polymerase chain reaction	tAML	therapy-related AML
PEL	primary effusion lymphoma	T-ALL/LBL	precursor T-lymphoblastic leukemia/lymphoma
PLL	prolymphocytic leukemia		
PLZF	promyelocytic leukemia zinc finger gene	tAML	therapy-related AML
PML	promyelocytic leukemia gene	T-LGL	T-cell large granular lymphocyte leukemia
PTCL	peripheral T-cell lymphoma, unspecified		
		tMDS	therapy-related MDS
PV	polycythemia vera	*TP53*	official name for *p53* gene
RA	refractory anemia	T-PLL	T-cell prolymphocytic leukemia
RAEB	refractory anemia with excess blasts	WBC	white blood cell (count)
RARα	retinoic acid receptor α	ZAP-70	70-kDa zeta-associated protein

References

1. Anonymous. The International, Non-Hodgkin's Lymphoma, Prognostic Factors Project. A predictive model for aggressive non-Hodgkin's lymphoma. N Engl J Med 1993;329:987–94

2. Armitage JO, Weisenburger DD. New approach to classifying non-Hodgkin's lymphomas: clinical features of the major histologic subtypes. Non-Hodgkin's Lymphoma Classification Project. J Clin Oncol 1998;16:2780–95

3. Moller MB, Pedersen NT, Christensen BE. Factors predicting long-term survival in low-risk diffuse large B-cell lymphoma. Am J Hematol 2003;74:94–8

4. Coiffier B, et al. CHOP chemotherapy plus rituximab compared with CHOP alone in elderly patients with diffuse large-B-cell lymphoma. N Engl J Med 2002;346:235–42

5. Mounier N, et al. Rituximab plus CHOP (R-CHOP) overcomes bcl-2-associated resistance to chemotherapy in elderly patients with diffuse large B-cell lymphoma (DLBCL). Blood 2003;101:4279–84

6. Coiffier B, et al. Prognostic factors in follicular lymphomas. Semin Oncol 1993;20(Suppl 5):89–95

7. Hermans J, et al. International Prognostic Index for aggressive non-Hodgkin's lymphoma is valid for all malignancy grades. Blood 1995;86:1460–3

8. Lopez-Guillermo A, et al. Applicability of the International Index for aggressive lymphomas to patients with low-grade lymphoma. J Clin Oncol 1994;12:1343–8

9. Aviles A. The International Index is not useful in the classification of low-grade lymphoma. J Clin Oncol 1994;12:2766–8

10. Bastion Y, Coiffier B. Is the International Prognostic Index for Aggressive Lymphoma patients useful for follicular lymphoma patients? J Clin Oncol 1994;12:1340–2

11. Foussard C, et al. Is the International Prognostic Index for aggressive lymphomas useful for low-grade lymphoma patients? Applicability to stage III–IV patients. The GOELAMS Group, France. Ann Oncol 1997;8(Suppl 1):49–52

12. Nola M, et al. Prognostic factors influencing survival in patients with B-cell small lymphocytic lymphoma. Am J Hematol 2004;77:31–5

13. Solal-Celigny P, et al. Follicular lymphoma international prognostic index. Blood 2004;104:1258–65

14. Montoto S, et al. Predictive value of Follicular Lymphoma International Prognostic Index (FLIPI) in patients with follicular lymphoma at first progression. Ann Oncol 2004;15:1484–9

15. Raty R, et al. Ki-67 expression level, histological subtype, and the International Prognostic Index as outcome predictors in mantle cell lymphoma. Eur J Haematol 2002;69:11–20

16. Owen RG, et al. Waldenström macroglobulinemia. Development of diagnostic criteria and identification of prognostic factors. Am J Clin Pathol 2001;116: 420–8

17. Gisselbrecht C, et al. Prognostic significance of T-cell phenotype in aggressive non-Hodgkin's lymphomas. Groupe d'Etudes des Lymphomes de l'Adulte (GELA). Blood 1998;92:76–82

18. Arrowsmith ER, et al. Peripheral T-cell lymphomas: clinical features and prognostic factors of 92 cases

defined by the revised European American lymphoma classification. Leuk Lymphoma 2003;44:241–9

19. Ansell SM, et al. Predictive capacity of the International Prognostic Factor Index in patients with peripheral T-cell lymphoma. J Clin Oncol 1997;15: 2296–301

20. Savage KJ, et al. Characterization of peripheral T-cell lymphomas in a single North American institution by the WHO classification. Ann Oncol 2004; 15:1467–75

21. Intragumtornchai T, et al. Prognostic significance of the immunophenotype versus the International Prognostic Index in aggressive non-Hodgkin's lymphoma. Clin Lymphoma 2003;4:52–5

22. Falini B, et al. ALK+ lymphoma: clinico-pathological findings and outcome. Blood 1999;93:2697–706

23. Greenberg P, et al. International scoring system for evaluating prognosis in myelodysplastic syndromes. Blood 1997;89:2079–88

24. Verburgh E, et al. Additional prognostic value of bone marrow histology in patients subclassified according to the International Prognostic Scoring System for myelodysplastic syndromes. J Clin Oncol 2003;21:273–82

25. Sperr WR, et al. Survival analysis and AML development in patients with de novo myelodysplastic syndromes: comparison of six different prognostic scoring systems. Ann Hematol 2001;80:272–7

26. Vasconcelos Y, et al. Binet's staging system and VH genes are independent but complementary prognostic indicators in chronic lymphocytic leukemia. J Clin Oncol 2003;21:3928–32

27. Hasenclever D, Diehl V. A prognostic score for advanced Hodgkin's disease. International Prognostic Factors Project on Advanced Hodgkin's Disease. N Engl J Med 1998;339:1506–14

28. van der Velden VH, et al. Detection of minimal residual disease in hematologic malignancies by real-time quantitative PCR: principles, approaches, and laboratory aspects. Leukemia 2003;17:1013–34

29. Gabert J, et al. Standardization and quality control studies of 'real-time' quantitative reverse transcriptase polymerase chain reaction of fusion gene transcripts for residual disease detection in leukemia – a Europe Against Cancer program. Leukemia 2003;17:2318–57

30. Venditti A, et al. Multidimensional flow cytometry for detection of minimal residual disease in acute myeloid leukemia. Leuk Lymphoma 2003;44:445–50

31. San-Miguel JF, Vidriales MB, Orfao A. Immunological evaluation of minimal residual disease (MRD) in acute myeloid leukaemia (AML). Best Pract Res Clin Haematol 2002;15:105–18

32. Van Dongen JJM, Szczepanski T, et al. Detection of minimal residual disease in lymphoid malignancies. In Degos L, Linch DC, Lowenberg B, eds. Textbook of Malignant Hematology. London: Taylor & Francis, 2005:267–307

33. Esteve J, Villamor N, et al. Different clinical value of minimal residual disease after autologous and allogeneic stem cell transplantation for chronic lymphocytic leukemia. Blood 2002;99:1873–4

34. Maloum K, et al. Novel flow-cytometric analysis based on BCD5+ subpopulations for the evaluation of minimal residual disease in chronic lymphocytic leukaemia. Br J Haematol 2002;119:970–5

35. Rawstron AC, et al. Quantitation of minimal disease levels in chronic lymphocytic leukemia using a sensitive flow cytometric assay improves the prediction of outcome and can be used to optimize therapy. Blood 2001;98:29–35

36. Thiede C. Diagnostic chimerism analysis after allogeneic stem cell transplantation: new methods and markers. Am J Pharmacogenomics 2004;4:177–87

37. Thiede C, Bornhauser M, Ehninger G. Strategies and clinical implications of chimerism diagnostics after allogeneic hematopoietic stem cell transplantation. Acta Haematol 2004;112:16–23

38. van Dongen JJ, et al. Detection of minimal residual disease in acute leukemia by immunological marker analysis and polymerase chain reaction. Leukemia 1992;6(Suppl 1):47–59

39. van der Velden VH, et al. Detection of minimal residual disease in acute leukemia. J Biol Regul Homeost Agents 2004;18:146–54

40. Meyer C, et al. Diagnostic tool for the identification of MLL rearrangements including unknown partner genes. Proc Natl Acad Sci USA 2005;102:449–54

41. Khouri IF, et al. Long-term follow-up of patients with CLL treated with allogeneic hematopoietic transplantation. Cytotherapy 2002;4:217–21

42. Magnac C, et al. Detection of minimal residual disease in B chronic lymphocytic leukemia (CLL). Hematol Cell Ther 1999;41:13–18

43. Campana D, Coustan-Smith E. Minimal residual disease studies by flow cytometry in acute leukemia. Acta Haematol 2004;112:8–15

44. Bruggemann M, et al. Significance of minimal residual disease in lymphoid malignancies. Acta Haematol 2004;112:111–19

45. Peters RE, et al. Leukemia-associated changes identified by quantitative flow cytometry. III. B-cell gating in CD37/kappa/lambda clonality test. Leukemia 1994;8:1864–70

46. Brugiatelli M, et al. Immunologic and molecular evaluation of residual disease in B-cell chronic lymphocytic leukemia patients in clinical remission phase. Cancer 1989;63:1979–84

47. Bottcher S, et al. Comparative analysis of minimal residual disease detection using four-color flow cytometry, consensus IgH-PCR, and quantitative IgH PCR in CLL after allogeneic and autologous stem cell transplantation. Leukemia 2004;18:1637–45

48. Noy A, et al. Clonotypic polymerase chain reaction confirms minimal residual disease in CLL nodular PR: results from a sequential treatment CLL protocol. Blood 2001;97:1929–36

49. Brugiatelli M, et al. Long-term clinical outcome of B-cell chronic lymphocytic leukaemia patients in clinical remission phase evaluated at phenotypic level. Br J Haematol 1997;97:113–18

50. Rawstron AC, et al. Early prediction of outcome and response to alemtuzumab therapy in chronic lymphocytic leukemia. Blood 2004;103:2027–31

51. Cheson BD, et al. National Cancer Institute-sponsored Working Group guidelines for chronic lymphocytic leukemia: revised guidelines for diagnosis and treatment. Blood 1996;87:4990–7

52. Provan D, et al. Eradication of polymerase chain reaction-detectable chronic lymphocytic leukemia cells is associated with improved outcome after bone marrow transplantation. Blood 1996;88:2228–35

53. Moreton P, et al. Eradication of minimal residual disease in B-cell chronic lymphocytic leukemia after alemtuzumab therapy is associated with prolonged survival. J Clin Oncol 2005

54. Mandigers CM, et al. Lack of correlation between numbers of circulating t(14;18)-positive cells and response to first-line treatment in follicular lymphoma. Blood 2001;98:940–4

55. Lambrechts AC, et al. Clinical significance of t(14;18)-positive cells in the circulation of patients with stage III or IV follicular non-Hodgkin's lymphoma during first remission. J Clin Oncol 1994;12:1541–6

56. Lopez-Guillermo A, et al. The clinical significance of molecular response in indolent follicular lymphomas. Blood 1998;91:2955–60

57. Zwicky CS, et al. Eradication of polymerase chain reaction detectable immunoglobulin gene rearrangement in non-Hodgkin's lymphoma is associated with decreased relapse after autologous bone marrow transplantation. Blood 1996;88:3314–22

58. Jacquy C, et al. Peripheral blood stem cell contamination in mantle cell non-Hodgkin lymphoma: the case for purging? Bone Marrow Transplant 1999;23:681–6

59. Andersen NS, et al. Failure of immunologic purging in mantle cell lymphoma assessed by polymerase chain reaction detection of minimal residual disease. Blood 1997;90:4212–21

60. Howard OM, et al. Rituximab and CHOP induction therapy for newly diagnosed mantle-cell lymphoma: molecular complete responses are not predictive of progression-free survival. J Clin Oncol 2002;20:1288–94

61. Brugger W, et al. Rituximab consolidation after high-dose chemotherapy and autologous blood stem cell transplantation in follicular and mantle cell lymphoma: a prospective, multicenter phase II study. Ann Oncol 2004;15:1691–8

62. Lin P, et al. Flow cytometric immunophenotypic analysis of 306 cases of multiple myeloma. Am J Clin Pathol 2004;121:482–8

63. Barbui AM, et al. Negative selection of peripheral blood stem cells to support a tandem autologous transplantation programme in multiple myeloma. Br J Haematol 2002;116:202–10

64. Corradini P, et al. Molecular and clinical remissions in multiple myeloma: role of autologous and allogeneic transplantation of hematopoietic cells. J Clin Oncol 1999;17:208–15

65. Martinelli G, et al. Molecular remission after allogeneic or autologous transplantation of hematopoietic stem cells for multiple myeloma. J Clin Oncol 2000;18:2273–81

66. Bjorkstrand B, et al. Double high-dose chemoradiotherapy with autologous stem cell transplantation can induce molecular remissions in multiple myeloma. Bone Marrow Transplant 1995;15:367–71

67. Fenk R, et al. Levels of minimal residual disease detected by quantitative molecular monitoring herald relapse in patients with multiple myeloma. Haematologica 2004;89:557–66

68. Corradini P, et al. Molecular remission after myeloablative allogeneic stem cell transplantation predicts a better relapse-free survival in patients with multiple myeloma. Blood 2003;102:1927–9

69. Cavo M, et al. Molecular monitoring of minimal residual disease in patients in long-term complete remission after allogeneic stem cell transplantation for multiple myeloma. Blood 2000;96:355–7

70. Martinelli G, et al. Polymerase chain reaction-based detection of minimal residual disease in multiple myeloma patients receiving allogeneic stem cell transplantation. Haematologica 2000;85:930–4

71. Raab MS, et al. Molecular monitoring of tumour load kinetics predicts disease progression after non-myeloablative allogeneic stem cell transplantation in multiple myeloma. Ann Oncol 2005;16:611–17

72. San Miguel JF, et al. Early immunophenotypical evaluation of minimal residual disease in acute myeloid leukemia identifies different patient risk groups and may contribute to postinduction treatment stratification. Blood 2001;98:1746–51

73. Venditti A, et al. Level of minimal residual disease after consolidation therapy predicts outcome in acute myeloid leukemia. Blood 2000;96:3948–52

74. Venditti A, et al. Pretransplant minimal residual disease level predicts clinical outcome in patients with acute myeloid leukemia receiving high-dose chemotherapy and autologous stem cell transplantation. Leukemia 2003;17:2178–82

75. Lo-Coco F, et al. Molecular evaluation of residual disease as a predictor of relapse in acute promyelocytic leukaemia. Lancet 1992;340:1437–8

76. Burnett AK, et al. Presenting white blood cell count and kinetics of molecular remission predict prognosis in acute promyelocytic leukemia treated with all-trans retinoic acid: result of the randomized MRC trial. Blood 1999;93:4131–43

77. Grimwade D. The pathogenesis of acute promyelocytic leukaemia: evaluation of the role of molecular diagnosis and monitoring in the management of the disease. Br J Haematol 1999;106:591–613

78. Diverio D, et al. Monitoring of treatment outcome in acute promyelocytic leukemia by RT-PCR. Leukemia 1994;8:1105–7

79. Lo-Coco F, Breccia M, Diverio D. The importance of molecular monitoring in acute promyelocytic leukaemia. Best Pract Res Clin Haematol 2003; 16:503–20

80. Mitterbauer M, et al. Molecular disease eradication is a prerequisite for long-term remission in patients with t(8;21) positive acute myeloid leukemia: a single center study. Leuk Lymphoma 2004;45:971–7

81. Miyamoto T, Weissman IL, Akashi K. AML1/ETO-expressing nonleukemic stem cells in acute myelogenous leukemia with 8;21 chromosomal translocation. Proc Natl Acad Sci USA 2000;97:7521–6

82. Szczepanski T, et al. Minimal residual disease in leukaemia patients. Lancet Oncol 2001;2:409–17

83. O'Reilly J, et al. Correlation of bone marrow minimal residual disease and apparent isolated extramedullary relapse in childhood acute lymphoblastic leukaemia. Leukemia 1995;9:624–7

84. Neale GA, et al. Comparative analysis of flow cytometry and polymerase chain reaction for the detection of minimal residual disease in childhood acute lymphoblastic leukemia. Leukemia 2004;18:934–8

85. Neale GA, et al. Detection of minimal residual disease in T-cell acute lymphoblastic leukemia using polymerase chain reaction predicts impending relapse. Blood 1991;78:739–47

86. Malec M, et al. Analysis of minimal residual disease in childhood acute lymphoblastic leukemia: comparison between RQ-PCR analysis of Ig/TcR gene rearrangements and multicolor flow cytometric immunophenotyping. Leukemia 2004;18:1630–6

87. van der Velden VH, et al. Minimal residual disease levels in bone marrow and peripheral blood are comparable in children with T cell acute lymphoblastic leukemia (ALL), but not in precursor-B-ALL. Leukemia 2002;16:1432–6

88. Yamada M, et al. Minimal residual disease in childhood B-lineage lymphoblastic leukemia. Persistence of leukemic cells during the first 18 months of treatment. N Engl J Med 1990;323:448–55

89. Gruhn B, et al. Minimal residual disease after intensive induction therapy in childhood acute lymphoblastic leukemia predicts outcome. Leukemia 1998;12:675–81

90. van Dongen JJ, et al. Prognostic value of minimal residual disease in acute lymphoblastic leukaemia in childhood. Lancet 1998;352:1731–8

91. Brisco MJ, et al. Outcome prediction in childhood acute lymphoblastic leukaemia by molecular quantification of residual disease at the end of induction. Lancet 1994;343:196–200

92. Cave H, et al. Clinical significance of minimal residual disease in childhood acute lymphoblastic leukemia. European Organization for Research and Treatment of Cancer–Childhood Leukemia Cooperative Group. N Engl J Med 1998;339:591–8

93. Nyvold C, et al. Precise quantification of minimal residual disease at day 29 allows identification of children with acute lymphoblastic leukemia and an excellent outcome. Blood 2002;99:1253–8

94. Knechtli CJ, et al. Minimal residual disease status before allogeneic bone marrow transplantation is an important determinant of successful outcome for children and adolescents with acute lymphoblastic leukemia. Blood 1998;92:4072–9

95. Sanchez J, et al. Clinical value of immunological monitoring of minimal residual disease in acute lymphoblastic leukaemia after allogeneic transplantation. Br J Haematol 2002;116:686–94

96. Knechtli CJ, et al. Minimal residual disease status as a predictor of relapse after allogeneic bone marrow transplantation for children with acute lymphoblastic leukaemia. Br J Haematol 1998;102:860–71

97. Hooijkaas H, et al. Terminal deoxynucleotidyl transferase (TdT)-positive cells in cerebrospinal fluid and development of overt CNS leukemia: a 5-year follow-up study in 113 children with a TdT-positive leukemia or non-Hodgkin's lymphoma. Blood 1989;74:416–22

98. Subira D, et al. Flow cytometry and the study of central nervous disease in patients with acute leukaemia. Br J Haematol 2001;112:381–4

99. Foroni L, Hoffbrand AV. Molecular analysis of minimal residual disease in adult acute lymphoblastic leukaemia. Best Pract Res Clin Haematol 2002;15:71–90

100. Amiel A, et al. Clinical detection of BCR-abl fusion by in situ hybridization in chronic myelogenous leukemia. Cancer Genet Cytogenet 1993;65:32–4

101. Bentz M, et al. Detection of chimeric BCR–ABL genes on bone marrow samples and blood smears in chronic myeloid and acute lymphoblastic leukemia by in situ hybridization. Blood 1994;83:1922–8

102. el-Rifai W, et al. Minimal residual disease after allogeneic bone marrow transplantation for chronic myeloid leukaemia: a metaphase-FISH study. Br J Haematol 1996;92:365–9

103. San Miguel J, Gonzalez M, Orfao A. Detection of minimal residual disease in myeloid malignancies. In Degos L, Linch DC, Lowenberg B, eds. Textbook of Malignant Hematology, 2nd edn. London: Taylor & Francis, 2005:308–25

104. Olavarria E, et al. Early detection of BCR–ABL transcripts by quantitative reverse transcriptase-polymerase chain reaction predicts outcome after allogeneic stem cell transplantation for chronic myeloid leukemia. Blood 2001;97:1560–5

105. Radich JP, et al. The significance of bcr-abl molecular detection in chronic myeloid leukemia patients 'late,' 18 months or more after transplantation. Blood 2001;98:1701–7

106. Engelhard M, et al. Subclassification of diffuse large B-cell lymphomas according to the Kiel classification: distinction of centroblastic and immunoblastic lymphomas is a significant prognostic risk factor. Blood 1997;89:2291–7

107. Diebold J, et al. Diffuse large B-cell lymphoma: a clinicopathologic analysis of 444 cases classified according to the updated Kiel classification. Leuk Lymphoma 2002;43:97–104

108. Cairo MS, et al. Burkitt's and Burkitt-like lymphoma in children and adolescents: a review of the Children's Cancer Group experience. Br J Haematol 2003;120:660–70

109. Bowman WP, et al. Improved survival for children with B-cell acute lymphoblastic leukemia and stage IV small noncleaved-cell lymphoma: a pediatric oncology group study. J Clin Oncol 1996;14:1252–61

110. Fenaux P, et al. Burkitt cell acute leukaemia (L3 ALL) in adults: a report of 18 cases. Br J Haematol 1989; 71:371–6

111. Soussain C, et al. Small noncleaved cell lymphoma and leukemia in adults. A retrospective study of 65 adults treated with the LMB pediatric protocols. Blood 1995;85:664–74

112. Phekoo KJ, et al. A population study to define the incidence and survival of multiple myeloma in a National Health Service Region in UK. Br J Haematol 2004;127:299–304

113. Leith CP, et al. Acute myeloid leukemia in the elderly: assessment of multidrug resistance (MDR1) and cytogenetics distinguishes biologic subgroups with remarkably distinct responses to standard chemotherapy. A Southwest Oncology Group study. Blood 1997;89:3323–9

114. Leith CP, et al. Frequency and clinical significance of the expression of the multidrug resistance proteins MDR1/P-glycoprotein, MRP1, and LRP in acute myeloid leukemia: a Southwest Oncology Group Study. Blood 1999;94:1086–99

115. Grimwade D, et al. The importance of diagnostic cytogenetics on outcome in AML: analysis of 1,612 patients entered into the MRC AML 10 trial. The Medical Research Council Adult and Children's Leukaemia Working Parties. Blood 1998;92:2322–33

116. Grimwade D, et al. The predictive value of hierarchical cytogenetic classification in older adults with acute myeloid leukemia (AML): analysis of 1065 patients entered into the United Kingdom Medical Research Council AML11 trial. Blood 2001;98:1312–20

117. Schoch C, et al. The influence of age on prognosis of de novo acute myeloid leukemia differs according to cytogenetic subgroups. Haematologica 2004;89: 1082–90

118. Rossi G, et al. Cytogenetic analogy between myelodysplastic syndrome and acute myeloid leukemia of elderly patients. Leukemia 2000;14:636–41

119. Byrd JC, et al. Pretreatment cytogenetic abnormalities are predictive of induction success, cumulative incidence of relapse, and overall survival in adult patients with de novo acute myeloid leukemia: results from Cancer and Leukemia Group B (CALGB 8461). Blood 2002;100:4325–36

120. Frohling S, et al. Prognostic significance of activating FLT3 mutations in younger adults (16 to 60 years) with acute myeloid leukemia and normal cytogenetics: a study of the AML Study Group Ulm. Blood 2002;100:4372–80

121. Abu-Duhier FM, et al. FLT3 internal tandem duplication mutations in adult acute myeloid leukaemia define a high-risk group. Br J Haematol 2000;111: 190–5

122. Kiyoi H, et al. Prognostic implication of FLT3 and N-RAS gene mutations in acute myeloid leukemia. Blood 1999;93:3074–80

123. Bassan R, et al. Adult acute lymphoblastic leukaemia. Crit Rev Oncol Hematol 2004;50:223–61

124. Swan F Jr, et al. A new serologic staging system for large-cell lymphomas based on initial beta 2-microglobulin and lactate dehydrogenase levels. J Clin Oncol 1989;7:1518–27

125. Litam P, et al. Prognostic value of serum beta-2 microglobulin in low-grade lymphoma. Ann Intern Med 1991;114:855–60

126. Marti RM, et al. Sézary syndrome and related variants of classic cutaneous T-cell lymphoma. A descriptive and prognostic clinicopathologic study of 29 cases. Leuk Lymphoma 2003;44:59–69

127. Rajkumar SV, Greipp PR. Prognostic factors in multiple myeloma. Hematol Oncol Clin North Am 1999;13:1295–314, xi

128. Rajkumar SV, et al. Beta2-microglobulin and bone marrow plasma cell involvement predict complete responders among patients undergoing blood cell transplantation for myeloma. Bone Marrow Transplant 1999;23:1261–6

129. Durie BG, et al. Prognostic value of pretreatment serum beta 2 microglobulin in myeloma: a Southwest Oncology Group Study. Blood 1990;75:823–30

130. Merlini G, et al. Prognostic factors in symptomatic Waldenström's macroglobulinemia. Semin Oncol 2003;30:211–15

131. Dhodapkar MV, et al. Prognostic factors and response to fludarabine therapy in patients with Waldenström macroglobulinemia: results of United States intergroup trial (Southwest Oncology Group S9003). Blood 2001;98:41–8

132. Garcia-Sanz R, et al. Waldenström macroglobulinaemia: presenting features and outcome in a series with 217 cases. Br J Haematol 2001;115:575–82

133. Chronowski GM, et al. An elevated serum beta-2-microglobulin level is an adverse prognostic factor for overall survival in patients with early-stage Hodgkin disease. Cancer 2002;95:2534–8

134. Bairey O, et al. Serum CA 125 as a prognostic factor in non-Hodgkin's lymphoma. Leuk Lymphoma 2003;44:1733–8

135. Zidan J, et al. Serum CA 125: a tumor marker for monitoring response to treatment and follow-up in patients with non-Hodgkin's lymphoma. Oncologist 2004;9:417–21

136. Kutluk T, et al. Serum CA 125 levels in children with non-Hodgkin's lymphoma. Pediatr Hematol Oncol 1999;16:311–19

137. Aydin F, et al. Correlation of serum IL-2, IL-6 and IL-10 levels with International Prognostic Index in patients with aggressive non-Hodgkin's lymphoma. Am J Clin Oncol 2002;25:570–2

138. Lai R, et al. Prognostic value of plasma interleukin-6 levels in patients with chronic lymphocytic leukemia. Cancer 2002;95:1071–5

139. Ferrajoli A, et al. The clinical significance of tumor necrosis factor-alpha plasma level in patients having chronic lymphocytic leukemia. Blood 2002;100: 1215–19

140. Goto H, et al. Serum-soluble interleukin-2 receptor (sIL-2R) level determines clinical outcome in patients with aggressive non-Hodgkin's lymphoma: in combination with the International Prognostic Index. J Cancer Res Clin Oncol 2005;131:73–9

141. Janik JE, et al. Elevated serum-soluble interleukin-2 receptor levels in patients with anaplastic large cell lymphoma. Blood 2004;104:3355–7

142. Yamamura M, et al. Circulating interleukin-6 levels are elevated in adult T-cell leukaemia/lymphoma patients and correlate with adverse clinical features and survival. Br J Haematol 1998;100: 129–34

143. Lauta VM. A review of the cytokine network in multiple myeloma: diagnostic, prognostic, and therapeutic implications. Cancer 2003;97:2440–52

144. Alexandrakis MG, et al. Serum level of interleukin-16 in multiple myeloma patients and its relationship to disease activity. Am J Hematol 2004;75:101–6

145. Alexandrakis MG, et al. Interleukin-18 in multiple myeloma patients: serum levels in relation to response to treatment and survival. Leuk Res 2004; 28:259–66

146. Seymour JF, et al. Clinical correlates of elevated serum levels of interleukin 6 in patients with untreated Hodgkin's disease. Am J Med 1997;102:21–8

147. Vener C, et al. Soluble cytokine levels correlate with the activity and clinical stage of Hodgkin's disease at diagnosis. Leuk Lymphoma 2000;37:333–9

148. Salgami EV, et al. High pretreatment interleukin-10 is an independent predictor of poor failure-free survival in patients with Hodgkin's lymphoma. Haematologia (Budap) 2002;32:377–87

149. Bohlen H, et al. Poor clinical outcome of patients with Hodgkin's disease and elevated interleukin-10 serum levels. Clinical significance of interleukin-10 serum levels for Hodgkin's disease. Ann Hematol 2000;79:110–13

150. Wu S, et al. Cytokine/cytokine receptor gene expression in childhood acute lymphoblastic leukemia. Cancer 2005;103:1054–63

151. Littlewood T, Mandelli F. The effects of anemia in hematologic malignancies: more than a symptom. Semin Oncol 2002;29(Suppl 8):40–4

152. Ludwig H. Anemia of hematologic malignancies: what are the treatment options? Semin Oncol 2002;29(Suppl 8):45–54

153. Binet JL, et al. A new prognostic classification of chronic lymphocytic leukemia derived from a multivariate survival analysis. Cancer 1981;48:198–206

154. Mandelli F, et al. Prognosis in chronic lymphocytic leukemia: a retrospective multicentric study from the GIMEMA group. J Clin Oncol 1987;5:398–406

155. Montserrat E, Bosch F, Rozman C. B-cell chronic lymphocytic leukemia: recent progress in biology, diagnosis, and therapy. Ann Oncol 1997;8(Suppl 1): 93–101

156. Montserrat E, Rozman C. Chronic lymphocytic leukaemia: prognostic factors and natural history. Baillières Clin Haematol 1993;6:849–66

157. Orfao A, et al. B-cell chronic lymphocytic leukaemia: prognostic value of the immunophenotype and the clinico-haematological features. Am J Hematol 1989;31:26–31

158. Rozman C, et al. Prognosis of chronic lymphocytic leukemia: a multivariate survival analysis of 150 cases. Blood 1982;59:1001–5

159. Egerer G, et al. Use of erythropoietin in patients with multiple myeloma. Onkologie 2003;26:80–4

160. Mittelman M. The implications of anemia in multiple myeloma. Clin Lymphoma 2003;4(Suppl 1):S23–9

161. Matzner Y, Benbassat J, Polliack A. Prognostic factors in multiple myeloma: a retrospective study using conventional statistical methods and a computer program. Acta Haematol 1978;60:257–68

162. Hannisdal E, et al. Prognostic factors in multiple myeloma in a population-based trial. Eur J Haematol 1990;45:198–202

163. San Miguel JF, Sanchez J, Gonzalez M. Prognostic factors and classification in multiple myeloma. Br J Cancer 1989;59:113–18

164. Seiden MV, Anderson KC. Multiple myeloma. Curr Opin Oncol 1994;6:41–9

165. Tsuchiya J, et al. Ten-year survival and prognostic factors in multiple myeloma. Japan Myeloma Study Group. Br J Haematol 1994;87:832–4

166. San Miguel JF, et al. A new staging system for multiple myeloma based on the number of S-phase plasma cells. Blood 1995;85:448–55

167. Aul C, et al. Evaluating the prognosis of patients with myelodysplastic syndromes. Ann Hematol 2002;81:485–97

168. Aul C, et al. Primary myelodysplastic syndromes: analysis of prognostic factors in 235 patients and proposals for an improved scoring system. Leukemia 1992;6:52–9

169. Sanz GF, Sanz MA, Greenberg PL. Prognostic factors and scoring systems in myelodysplastic syndromes. Haematologica 1998;83:358–68

170. Oguma S, et al. Factors influencing survival in Philadelphia chromosome positive chronic myelocytic leukemia. Cancer 1982;50:2928–34

171. Cortes J, et al. Erythropoietin is effective in improving the anemia induced by imatinib mesylate therapy in patients with chronic myeloid leukemia in chronic phase. Cancer 2004;100:2396–402

172. Yoong Y, et al. Clinical correlates of submicroscopic deletions involving the ABL–BCR translocation region in chronic myeloid leukemia. Eur J Haematol 2005;74:124–7

173. Visani G, et al. Myelofibrosis with myeloid metaplasia: clinical and haematological parameters predicting survival in a series of 133 patients. Br J Haematol 1990;75:4–9

174. Dupriez B, et al. Prognostic factors in agnogenic myeloid metaplasia: a report on 195 cases with a new scoring system. Blood 1996;88:1013–18

175. Reilly JT. Idiopathic myelofibrosis: pathogenesis, natural history and management. Blood Rev 1997;11:233–42

176. Rupoli S, et al. Primary myelofibrosis: a detailed statistical analysis of the clinicopathological variables influencing survival. Ann Hematol 1994;68:205–12

177. Bouafia F, et al. Profiles and prognostic values of serum LDH isoenzymes in patients with haematopoietic malignancies. Bull Cancer 2004;91:E229–40

178. Stein RS, et al. Large-cell lymphomas: clinical and prognostic features. J Clin Oncol 1990;8:1370–9

179. Seidemann K, et al. Primary mediastinal large B-cell lymphoma with sclerosis in pediatric and adolescent patients: treatment and results from three therapeutic studies of the Berlin–Frankfurt–Munster Group. J Clin Oncol 2003;21:1782–9

180. Sandlund JT, et al. CNS involvement in children with newly diagnosed non-Hodgkin's lymphoma. J Clin Oncol 2000;18:3018–24

181. Kondo E, et al. Assessment of prognostic factors in follicular lymphoma patients. Int J Hematol 2001;73:363–8

182. Gascoyne RD, et al. Prognostic significance of anaplastic lymphoma kinase (ALK) protein expression in adults with anaplastic large cell lymphoma. Blood 1999;93:3913–21

183. Gallamini A, et al. Peripheral T-cell lymphoma unspecified (PTCL-U): a new prognostic model from a retrospective multicentric clinical study. Blood 2004;103:2474–9

184. Suguro M, et al. High serum lactate dehydrogenase level predicts short survival after vincristine–doxorubicin–dexamethasone (VAD) salvage for refractory multiple myeloma. Am J Hematol 2000; 65:132–5

185. Pui CH, et al. Serum lactic dehydrogenase level has prognostic value in childhood acute lymphoblastic leukemia. Blood 1985;66:778–82

186. Pui CH, et al. Cytogenetic features and serum lactic dehydrogenase level predict a poor treatment outcome for children with pre-B-cell leukemia. Blood 1986;67:1688–92

187. Wimazal F, et al. Prognostic value of lactate dehydrogenase activity in myelodysplastic syndromes. Leuk Res 2001;25:287–94

188. Haferlach T, et al. Morphologic dysplasia in de novo acute myeloid leukemia (AML) is related to unfavorable cytogenetics but has no independent prognostic relevance under the conditions of intensive induction therapy: results of a multiparameter analysis from the German AML Cooperative Group studies. J Clin Oncol 2003;21:256–65

189. Last KW, et al. Presentation serum selenium predicts for overall survival, dose delivery, and first treatment response in aggressive non-Hodgkin's lymphoma. J Clin Oncol 2003;21:2335–41

190. Martin AR, et al. Prognostic value of cellular proliferation and histologic grade in follicular lymphoma. Blood 1995;85:3671–8

191. McLaughlin P, et al. Stage III follicular lymphoma: durable remissions with a combined chemotherapy–radiotherapy regimen. J Clin Oncol 1987;5:867–74

192. Bartlett NL, et al. Follicular large-cell lymphoma: intermediate or low grade? J Clin Oncol 1994;12:1349–57

193. Miller TP, et al. Follicular lymphomas: do histologic subtypes predict outcome? Hematol Oncol Clin North Am 1997;11:893–900

194. Chau I, et al. Outcome of follicular lymphoma grade 3: is anthracycline necessary as front-line therapy? Br J Cancer 2003;89:36–42

195. Rodriguez J, et al. Follicular large cell lymphoma: an aggressive lymphoma that often presents with favorable prognostic features. Blood 1999;93:2202–7

196. Glas AM, et al. Gene expression profiling in follicular lymphoma to assess clinical aggressiveness and to guide the choice of treatment. Blood 2005;105:301–7

197. Brittinger G, et al. Clinical and prognostic relevance of the Kiel classification of non-Hodgkin lymphomas results of a prospective multicenter study by the Kiel Lymphoma Study Group. Hematol Oncol 1984;2:269–306

198. Salar A, et al. Diffuse large B-cell lymphoma: is morphologic subdivision useful in clinical management? Eur J Haematol 1998;60:202–8

199. Alizadeh AA, et al. Distinct types of diffuse large B-cell lymphoma identified by gene expression profiling. Nature 2000;403:503–11

200. Simonitsch-Klupp I, et al. Diffuse large B-cell lymphomas with plasmablastic/plasmacytoid features are associated with TP53 deletions and poor clinical outcome. Leukemia 2004;18:146–55

201. Feller AC, Diebold J. Histopathology of Nodal and Extranodal non-Hodgkin's Lymphomas, 3rd edn. Berlin: Springer-Verlag, 2004

202. Ascani S, et al. Peripheral T-cell lymphomas. Clinicopathologic study of 168 cases diagnosed according to the R.E.A.L. Classification. Ann Oncol 1997;8:583–92

203. Matolcsy A. High-grade transformation of low-grade non-Hodgkin's lymphomas: mechanisms of tumor progression. Leuk Lymphoma 1999;34:251–9

204. Warnke RA. Tumor progression in malignant lymphomas. Bull Cancer 1991;78:181–6

205. Muller-Hermelink HK, et al. Pathology of lymphoma progression. Histopathology 2001;38:285–306

206. Jares P, et al. Expression of retinoblastoma gene product (pRb) in mantle cell lymphomas. Correlation with cyclin D1 (PRAD1/CCND1) mRNA levels and proliferative activity. Am J Pathol 1996;148:1591–600

207. Kiviniemi M, et al. Cell cycle regulators p27 and pRb in lymphomas – correlation with histology and proliferative activity. Br J Cancer 2000;83:1161–7

208. Du M, et al. The accumulation of p53 abnormalities is associated with progression of mucosa-associated lymphoid tissue lymphoma. Blood 1995;86:4587–93

209. Lo Coco F, et al. p53 mutations are associated with histologic transformation of follicular lymphoma. Blood 1993;82:2289–95

210. Sander CA, et al. p53 mutation is associated with progression in follicular lymphomas. Blood 1993;82: 1994–2004

211. Hernandez L, et al. p53 gene mutations and protein overexpression are associated with aggressive variants of mantle cell lymphomas. Blood 1996;87:3351–9

212. Tsimberidou AM, Keating MJ. Richter syndrome. Cancer 2005;103:216–28

213. Mulligan SP, et al. Splenic lymphoma with villous lymphocytes: natural history and response to therapy in 50 cases. Br J Haematol 1991;78:206–9

214. Oscier D, Owen R, Johnson S. Splenic marginal zone lymphoma. Blood Rev 2005;19:39–51

215. Elenitoba-Johnson KS, et al. Homozygous deletions at chromosome 9p21 involving p16 and p15 are associated with histologic progression in follicle center lymphoma. Blood 1998;91:4677–85

216. El Shabrawi-Caelen L, Kerl H, Cerroni L. Lymphomatoid papulosis: reappraisal of clinicopathologic presentation and classification into subtypes A, B, and C. Arch Dermatol 2004;140:441–7

217. Willemze R, Beljaards RC. Spectrum of primary cutaneous CD30 (Ki-1)-positive lymphoproliferative disorders. A proposal for classification and guidelines for management and treatment. J Am Acad Dermatol 1993;28:973–80

218. Willemze R, et al. EORTC classification for primary cutaneous lymphomas: a proposal from the Cutaneous Lymphoma Study Group of the European Organization for Research and Treatment of Cancer. Blood 1997;90:354–71

219. McCarty MJ, et al. Lymphomatoid papulosis associated with Ki-1-positive anaplastic large cell lymphoma. A report of two cases and a review of the literature. Cancer 1994;74:3051–8

220. Chott A, et al. The dominant T cell clone is present in multiple regressing skin lesions and associated T cell lymphomas of patients with lymphomatoid papulosis. J Invest Dermatol 1996;106:696–700

221. Huang JZ, et al. Diffuse large B-cell lymphoma arising in nodular lymphocyte predominant hodgkin lymphoma. A report of 21 cases from the Nebraska Lymphoma Study Group. Leuk Lymphoma 2003; 44:1903–10

222. Hansmann ML, et al. Nodular paragranuloma can transform into high-grade malignant lymphoma of B type. Hum Pathol 1989;20:1169–75

223. Fan Z, et al. Characterization of variant patterns of nodular lymphocyte predominant Hodgkin lymphoma with immunohistologic and clinical correlation. Am J Surg Pathol 2003;27:1346–56

224. Miettinen M, Franssila KO, Saxen E. Hodgkin's disease, lymphocytic predominance nodular. Increased risk for subsequent non-Hodgkin's lymphomas. Cancer 1983;51:2293–300

225. Jaffe ES, Harris NL, Stein H, Vardiman JW (eds). World Health Organization Classification of Tumours. Pathology and Genetics of Tumors of Haematopoietic and Lymphoid Tissues. Lyon: IARC Press, 2001

226. Germing U, et al. Validation of the WHO proposals for a new classification of primary myelodysplastic syndromes: a retrospective analysis of 1600 patients. Leuk Res 2000;24:983–92

227. Hornsten P, et al. Myelodysplastic syndromes – a population-based study on transformation and survival. Acta Oncol 1995;34:473–8

228. Chang KL, et al. Primary myelodysplasia occurring in adults under 50 years old: a clinicopathologic study of 52 patients. Leukemia 2002;16:623–31

229. Sato N, et al. Transformation of myelodysplastic syndrome to acute lymphoblastic leukemia: a case report and review of the literature. Int J Hematol 2004;79:147–51

230. Moehler TM, et al. Angiogenesis in hematologic malignancies. Ann Hematol 2001;80:695–705

231. Kumar S, et al. Bone marrow angiogenesis and circulating plasma cells in multiple myeloma. Br J Haematol 2003;122:272–4

232. Alexandrakis MG, et al. The relation between bone marrow angiogenesis and the proliferation index Ki-67 in multiple myeloma. J Clin Pathol 2004;57:856–60

233. Sezer O, et al. Bone marrow microvessel density is a prognostic factor for survival in patients with multiple myeloma. Ann Hematol 2000;79:574–7

234. Schreiber S, et al. Multiple myeloma with deletion of chromosome 13q is characterized by increased bone marrow neovascularization. Br J Haematol 2000;110: 605–9

235. Rajkumar SV, et al. Prognostic value of bone marrow angiogenesis in multiple myeloma. Clin Cancer Res 2000;6:3111–16

236. Molica S, et al. Prognostic value of enhanced bone marrow angiogenesis in early B-cell chronic lymphocytic leukemia. Blood 2002;100:3344–51

237. Kini AR, Kay NE, Peterson LC. Increased bone marrow angiogenesis in B cell chronic lymphocytic leukemia. Leukemia 2000;14:1414–18

238. Salven P, et al. Simultaneous elevation in the serum concentrations of the angiogenic growth factors VEGF and bFGF is an independent predictor of poor prognosis in non-Hodgkin lymphoma: a single-institution study of 200 patients. Blood 2000;96:3712–18

239. Shaun N, Thomas B. Cell cycle regulation. In Degos L, Linch DC, Lowenberg B, eds. Textbook of Malignant Hematology, 2nd edn. London: Taylor & Francis, 2005

240. Witzig TE, et al. S-phase fraction by the labeling index as a predictive factor for progression and survival in low grade non-Hodgkin's lymphoma. Cancer 1995;76:1059–64

241. Miller TP, et al. Prognostic significance of the Ki-67-associated proliferative antigen in aggressive non-Hodgkin's lymphomas: a prospective Southwest Oncology Group trial. Blood 1994;83:1460–6

242. Grogan TM, et al. Independent prognostic significance of a nuclear proliferation antigen in diffuse large cell lymphomas as determined by the monoclonal antibody Ki-67. Blood 1988;71:1157–60

243. Gerdes J. Ki-67 and other proliferation markers useful for immunohistological diagnostic and prognostic evaluations in human malignancies. Semin Cancer Biol 1990;1:199–206

244. Holte H, et al. Prognostic value of lymphoma-specific S-phase fraction compared with that of other cell proliferation markers. Acta Oncol 1999;38:495–503

245. Mochen C, et al. MIB-1 and S-phase cell fraction predict survival in non-Hodgkin's lymphomas. Cell Prolif 1997;30:37–47

246. Saito B, et al. Efficacy of rituximab plus chemotherapy in follicular lymphoma depends on Ki-67 expression. Pathol Int 2004;54:667–74

247. Shiozawa E, et al. Disappearance of CD21-positive follicular dendritic cells preceding the transformation of follicular lymphoma: immunohistological study of the transformation using CD21, p53, Ki-67, and P-glycoprotein. Pathol Res Pract 2003;199:293–302

248. Nakamura S, et al. A clinicopathologic study of 233 cases with special reference to evaluation with the MIB-1 index. Cancer 1995;76:1313–24

249. Bosch F, et al. Mantle cell lymphoma: presenting features, response to therapy, and prognostic factors. Cancer 1998;82:567–75

250. Ek S, et al. Increased expression of Ki-67 in mantle cell lymphoma is associated with de-regulation of several cell cycle regulatory components, as identified by global gene expression analysis. Haematologica 2004;89:686–95

251. Izban KF, et al. Multiparameter immunohistochemical analysis of the cell cycle proteins cyclin D1, Ki-67, p21WAF1, p27KIP1, and p53 in mantle cell lymphoma. Arch Pathol Lab Med 2000;124:1457–62

252. Drach J, et al. The biological and clinical significance of the Ki-67 growth fraction in multiple myeloma. Hematol Oncol 1992;10:125–34

253. Alexandrakis MG, et al. Ki-67 proliferation index: correlation with prognostic parameters and outcome in multiple myeloma. Am J Clin Oncol 2004;27:8–13

254. Morente MM, et al. Adverse clinical outcome in Hodgkin's disease is associated with loss of retinoblastoma protein expression, high Ki67 proliferation index, and absence of Epstein–Barr virus-latent membrane protein 1 expression. Blood 1997;90:2429–36

255. Garcia JF, et al. Hodgkin and Reed–Sternberg cells harbor alterations in the major tumor suppressor pathways and cell-cycle checkpoints: analyses using tissue microarrays. Blood 2003;101:681–9

256. Imamura J, Miyoshi I, Koeffler HP. p53 in hematologic malignancies. Blood 1994;84:2412–21

257. Hermine O, et al. Prognostic significance of bcl-2 protein expression in aggressive non-Hodgkin's lymphoma. Groupe d'Etude des Lymphomes de l'Adulte (GELA). Blood 1996;87:265–72

258. Campos L, et al. High expression of bcl-2 protein in acute myeloid leukemia cells is associated with poor response to chemotherapy. Blood 1993;81:3091–6

259. Rathmell JC, Thompson CB. The central effectors of cell death in the immune system. Annu Rev Immunol 1999;17:781–828

260. Adida C, et al. Anti-apoptosis gene, survivin, and prognosis of neuroblastoma. Lancet 1998;351:882–3

261. Adida C, et al. Prognostic significance of survivin expression in diffuse large B-cell lymphomas. Blood 2000;96:1921–5

262. Joza N, et al. Essential role of the mitochondrial apoptosis-inducing factor in programmed cell death. Nature 2001;410:549–54

263. Li PF, Dietz R, von Harsdorf R. p53 regulates mitochondrial membrane potential through reactive oxygen species and induces cytochrome C-independent apoptosis blocked by Bcl-2. Embo J 1999;18:6027–36

264. Muzio M, et al. FLICE, a novel FADD-homologous ICE/CED-3-like protease, is recruited to the CD95 (Fas/APO-1) death-inducing signaling complex. Cell 1996;85:817–27

265. Hakem R, et al. Differential requirement for caspase 9 in apoptotic pathways in vivo. Cell 1998;94:339–52

266. Muris JJ, et al. Immunohistochemical profiling of caspase signaling pathways predicts clinical response to chemotherapy in primary nodal diffuse large B-cell lymphomas. Blood 2005;105:2916–23

267. Korkolopoulou P, et al. Prognostic relevance of apoptotic cell death in non-Hodgkin's lymphomas: a multivariate survival analysis including Ki67 and p53 oncoprotein expression. Histopathology 1998;33:240–7

268. Hoyer KK, et al. An anti-apoptotic role for galectin-3 in diffuse large B-cell lymphomas. Am J Pathol 2004;164:893–902

269. Karin M, Lin A. NF-kappaB at the crossroads of life and death. Nat Immunol 2002;3:221–7

270. Bai M, et al. Cluster analysis of apoptosis-associated bcl2 family proteins in diffuse large B-cell lymphomas. Relations with the apoptotic index, the proliferation profile and the B-cell differentiation immunophenotypes. Anticancer Res 2004;24:3081–8

271. Bai M, et al. Diffuse large B-cell lymphomas with germinal center B-cell-like differentiation immunophenotypic profile are associated with high apoptotic index, high expression of the proapoptotic proteins bax, bak and bid and low expression of the antiapoptotic protein bcl-xl. Mod Pathol 2004;17:847–56

272. Gascoyne RD, et al. Prognostic significance of Bcl-2 protein expression and Bcl-2 gene rearrangement in diffuse aggressive non-Hodgkin's lymphoma. Blood 1997;90:244–51

273. Houldsworth J, et al. REL proto-oncogene is frequently amplified in extranodal diffuse large cell lymphoma. Blood 1996;87:25–9

274. Rao PH, et al. Chromosomal and gene amplification in diffuse large B-cell lymphoma. Blood 1998;92:234–40

275. Joos S, et al. Primary mediastinal (thymic) B-cell lymphoma is characterized by gains of chromosomal material including 9p and amplification of the REL gene. Blood 1996;87:1571–8

276. Reed CJ. Apoptosis and cancer: strategies for integrating programmed cell death. Semin Hematol 2000;37(Suppl 7):9–16

277. Danilov AV, et al. Differential control of G0 programme in chronic lymphocytic leukaemia: a novel prognostic factor. Br J Haematol 2005;128:472–81

278. Zhao WL, et al. Prognostic significance of bcl-xL gene expression and apoptotic cell counts in follicular lymphoma. Blood 2004;103:695–7

279. Tsujimoto Y, et al. Involvement of the bcl-2 gene in human follicular lymphoma. Science 1985;228:1440–3

280. Akagi T, et al. A novel gene, MALT1 at 18q21, is involved in t(11;18)(q21;q21) found in low-grade B-cell lymphoma of mucosa-associated lymphoid tissue. Oncogene 1999;18:5785–94

281. Dierlamm J, et al. The apoptosis inhibitor gene API2 and a novel 18q gene, MLT, are recurrently rearranged in the t(11;18)(q21;q21)p6ssociated with mucosa-associated lymphoid tissue lymphomas. Blood 1999;93:3601–9

282. Morgan JA, et al. Breakpoints of the t(11;18)(q21;q21) in mucosa-associated lymphoid tissue (MALT) lymphoma lie within or near the previously undescribed gene MALT1 in chromosome 18. Cancer Res 1999;59:6205–13

283. Stoffel A, Le Beau MM. The API2/MALT1 fusion product may lead to germinal center B cell lymphomas by suppression of apoptosis. Hum Hered 2001;51:1–7

284. Roy N, et al. The c-IAP-1 and c-IAP-2 proteins are direct inhibitors of specific caspases. Embo J 1997;16:6914–25

285. Hosokawa Y, et al. Antiapoptotic function of apoptosis inhibitor 2-MALT1 fusion protein involved in t(11;18) (q21;q21) mucosa-associated lymphoid tissue lymphoma. Cancer Res 2004;64:3452–7

286. Ohara T, et al. Eradication therapy of Helicobacter pylori directly induces apoptosis in inflammation-related immunocytes in the gastric mucosa – possible mechanism for cure of peptic ulcer disease and MALT lymphoma with a low-grade malignancy. Hepatogastroenterology 2003;50:607–9

287. ten Berge RL, et al. Expression levels of apoptosis-related proteins predict clinical outcome in anaplastic large cell lymphoma. Blood 2002;99:4540–6

288. O'Connor OA. The emerging role of bortezomib in the treatment of indolent non-Hodgkin's and mantle cell lymphomas. Curr Treat Options Oncol 2004;5:269–81

289. Oancea M, et al. Apoptosis of multiple myeloma. Int J Hematol 2004;80:224–31

290. Mattioli M, et al. Gene expression profiling of plasma cell dyscrasias reveals molecular patterns associated with distinct IGH translocations in multiple myeloma. Oncogene 2005

291. Chaidos AI, et al. Incidence of apoptosis and cell proliferation in multiple myeloma: correlation with bcl-2 protein expression and serum levels of inter-leukin-6 (IL-6) and soluble IL-6 receptor. Eur J Haematol 2002;69:90–4

292. Hideshima T, et al. The proteasome inhibitor PS-341 inhibits growth, induces apoptosis, and overcomes drug resistance in human multiple myeloma cells. Cancer Res 2001;61:3071–6

293. Cheson BD. Hematologic malignancies: new developments and future treatments. Semin Oncol 2002; 29(Suppl 13):33–45

294. Chanan-Khan AA. Bcl-2 antisense therapy in multiple myeloma. Oncology (Huntingt) 2004;18(Suppl 10): 21–4

295. Hattori Y, Iguchi T. Thalidomide for the treatment of multiple myeloma. Congenit Anom (Kyoto) 2004; 44:125–36

296. Mathas S, et al. c-FLIP mediates resistance of Hodgkin/Reed–Sternberg cells to death receptor-induced apoptosis. J Exp Med 2004;199:1041–52

297. Thomas RK, et al. Constitutive expression of c-FLIP in Hodgkin and Reed–Sternberg cells. Am J Pathol 2002;160:1521–8

298. Suárez L, et al. CD34+ cells from acute myeloid leukemia, myelodysplastic syndromes, and normal bone marrow display different apoptosis and drug resistance-associated phenotypes. Clin Cancer Res 2004;10:7599–606

299. Bincoletto C, et al. Haematopoietic response and bcl-2 expression in patients with acute myeloid leukaemia. Eur J Haematol 1999;62:38–42

300. Del Poeta G, et al. Amount of spontaneous apoptosis detected by Bax/Bcl-2 ratio predicts outcome in acute myeloid leukemia (AML). Blood 2003;101:2125–31

301. Kohler T, et al. High Bad and Bax mRNA expression correlate with negative outcome in acute myeloid leukemia (AML). Leukemia 2002;16:22–9

302. Smith BD, et al. Inhibited apoptosis and drug resis-tance in acute myeloid leukaemia. Br J Haematol 1998;102:1042–9

303. Tamm I, et al. High expression levels of X-linked inhibitor of apoptosis protein and survivin correlate with poor overall survival in childhood de novo acute myeloid leukemia. Clin Cancer Res 2004;10:3737–44

304. Tamm I, et al. Expression and prognostic significance of IAP-family genes in human cancers and myeloid leukemias. Clin Cancer Res 2000;6:1796–803

305. Adida C, et al. Expression and prognostic significance of survivin in de novo acute myeloid leukaemia. Br J Haematol 2000;111:196–203

306. Carter BZ, et al. Caspase-independent cell death in AML: caspase inhibition in vitro with pan-caspase inhibitors or in vivo by XIAP or Survivin does not affect cell survival or prognosis. Blood 2003;102:4179–86

307. Holleman A, et al. Gene-expression patterns in drug-resistant acute lymphoblastic leukemia cells and response to treatment. N Engl J Med 2004;351: 533–42

308. Prokop A, et al. Relapse in childhood acute lym-phoblastic leukemia is associated with a decrease of the Bax/Bcl-2 ratio and loss of spontaneous caspase-3 processing in vivo. Leukemia 2000;14:1606–13

309. Davis RE, Greenberg PL. Bcl-2 expression by myeloid precursors in myelodysplastic syndromes: relation to disease progression. Leuk Res 1998;22: 767–77

310. Rajapaksa R, et al. Altered oncoprotein expression and apoptosis in myelodysplastic syndrome marrow cells. Blood, 1996;88:4275–87

311. Parker JE, et al. 'Low-risk' myelodysplastic syndrome is associated with excessive apoptosis and an increased ratio of pro- versus anti-apoptotic bcl-2-related proteins. Br J Haematol 1998;103:1075–82

312. Tsoplou P, et al. Apoptosis in patients with myelodysplastic syndromes: differential involvement of marrow cells in 'good' versus 'poor' prognosis patients and correlation with apoptosis-related genes. Leukemia 1999;13:1554–63

313. Ribeiro E, et al. Flow cytometric analysis of the expression of Fas/Fasl in bone marrow CD34+ cells in myelodysplastic syndromes: relation to disease progression. Leuk Lymphoma 2004;45:309–13

314. Yamamoto K, et al. Expression of IAP family proteins in myelodysplastic syndromes transforming to overt leukemia. Leuk Res 2004;28:1203–11

315. Jones RJ. Biology and treatment of chronic myeloid leukemia. Curr Opin Oncol 1997;9:3–7

316. Bedi A, et al. Inhibition of apoptosis by BCR-ABL in chronic myeloid leukemia. Blood 1994;83:2038–44

317. Di Bacco A, et al. Molecular abnormalities in chronic myeloid leukemia: deregulation of cell growth and apoptosis. Oncologist 2000;5:405–15

318. Stuppia L, et al. p53 loss and point mutations are associated with suppression of apoptosis and progression of CML into myeloid blastic crisis. Cancer Genet Cytogenet 1997;98:28–35

319. Schnittger S, et al. Analysis of FLT3 length mutations in 1003 patients with acute myeloid leukemia: correlation to cytogenetics, FAB subtype, and prognosis in the AMLCG study and usefulness as a marker for the detection of minimal residual disease. Blood 2002;100:59–66

320. Golub TR, et al. Molecular classification of cancer: class discovery and class prediction by gene expression monitoring. Science 1999;286:531–7

321. Haferlach T, Kern W, et al. Gene expression profiling in leukemias using microarrays. In Degos L, Linch DC, Lowenberg B, eds. Textbook of Malignant Hematology, 2nd edn. London: Taylor & Francis, 2005:254–65

322. Michiels S, Koscielny S, Hill C. Prediction of cancer outcome with microarrays: a multiple random validation strategy. Lancet 2005;365:488–92

323. Dybkaer K, et al. Molecular diagnosis and outcome prediction in diffuse large B-cell lymphoma and other subtypes of lymphoma. Clin Lymphoma 2004;5:19–28

324. Siebert R, et al. Molecular features of B-cell lymphoma. Curr Opin Oncol 2001;13:316–24

325. Rosenwald A, Staudt LM. Gene expression profiling of diffuse large B-cell lymphoma. Leuk Lymphoma 2003;(Suppl 3):S41–7

326. Rosenwald A, et al. The use of molecular profiling to predict survival after chemotherapy for diffuse large-B-cell lymphoma. N Engl J Med 2002;346:1937–47

327. Kersten MJ, et al. Beyond the International Prognostic Index: new prognostic factors in follicular lymphoma and diffuse large-cell lymphoma. A meeting report of the Second International Lunenburg Lymphoma Workshop. Hematol J 2004;5:202–8

328. Kuttler F, et al. Relationship between expression of genes involved in cell cycle control and apoptosis in diffuse large B cell lymphoma: a preferential survivin–cyclin B link. Leukemia 2002;16:726–35

329. Hans CP, et al. Confirmation of the molecular classification of diffuse large B-cell lymphoma by immunohistochemistry using a tissue microarray. Blood 2004;103:275–82

330. Glas AM, et al. Gene expression profiling in follicular lymphoma to assess clinical aggressiveness and to guide the choice of treatment. Blood 2004

331. Elenitoba-Johnson KS, et al. Involvement of multiple signaling pathways in follicular lymphoma transformation: p38-mitogen-activated protein kinase as a target for therapy. Proc Natl Acad Sci USA, 2003;100:7259–64

332. Dave SS, et al. Prediction of survival in follicular lymphoma based on molecular features of tumor-infiltrating immune cells. N Engl J Med 2004;351:2159–69

333. Aalto Y, et al. Distinct gene expression profiling in chronic lymphocytic leukemia with 11q23 deletion. Leukemia 2001;15:1721–8

334. Rosenwald A, et al. Relation of gene expression phenotype to immunoglobulin mutation genotype in B cell chronic lymphocytic leukemia. J Exp Med 2001;194:1639–47

335. Durig J, et al. Expression of ribosomal and translation-associated genes is correlated with a favorable clinical course in chronic lymphocytic leukemia. Blood 2003;101:2748–55

336. Stankovic T, et al. Microarray analysis reveals that TP53- and ATM-mutant B-CLLs share a defect in activating proapoptotic responses after DNA damage but are distinguished by major differences in activating prosurvival responses. Blood 2004;103: 291–300

337. Zhan F, et al. Global gene expression profiling of multiple myeloma, monoclonal gammopathy of undetermined significance, and normal bone marrow plasma cells. Blood 2002;99:1745–57

338. Fonseca R, et al. Genetics and cytogenetics of multiple myeloma: a workshop report. Cancer Res 2004; 64:1546–58

339. Chesi M, et al. The t(4;14) translocation in myeloma dysregulates both FGFR3 and a novel gene, MMSET, resulting in IgH/MMSET hybrid transcripts. Blood 1998;92:3025–34

340. Shaughnessy J Jr, et al. Cyclin D3 at 6p21 is dysregulated by recurrent chromosomal translocations to immunoglobulin loci in multiple myeloma. Blood 2001;98:217–23

341. Hideshima T, et al. Advances in biology of multiple myeloma: clinical applications. Blood 2004;104: 607–18

342. Bergsagel PL, et al. Cyclin D dysregulation: an early and unifying pathogenic event in multiple myeloma. Blood 2005;106:296–303

343. Schoch C, et al. Acute myeloid leukemias with reciprocal rearrangements can be distinguished by specific gene expression profiles. Proc Natl Acad Sci USA 2002;99:10008–13

344. Yagi T, et al. Identification of a gene expression signature associated with pediatric AML prognosis. Blood 2003;102:1849–56

345. Steinbach D, et al. BCRP gene expression is associated with a poor response to remission induction therapy in childhood acute myeloid leukemia. Leukemia 2002;16:1443–7

346. Valk PJ, et al. Prognostically useful gene-expression profiles in acute myeloid leukemia. N Engl J Med 2004;350:1617–28

347. Gutierrez NC, et al. Gene expression profile reveals deregulation of genes with relevant functions in the different subclasses of acute myeloid leukemia. Leukemia 2005;19:402–9

348. Drabkin HA, et al. Quantitative HOX expression in chromosomally defined subsets of acute myelogenous leukemia. Leukemia 2002;16:186–95

349. Thompson A, et al. Global down-regulation of HOX gene expression in PML−RARalpha+ acute promyelocytic leukemia identified by small-array real-time PCR. Blood 2003;101:1558–65

350. Roche J, et al. Hox expression in AML identifies a distinct subset of patients with intermediate cytogenetics. Leukemia 2004;18:1059–63

351. Debernardi S, et al. Genome-wide analysis of acute myeloid leukemia with normal karyotype reveals a unique pattern of homeobox gene expression distinct from those with translocation-mediated fusion events. Genes Chromosomes Cancer 2003;37:149–58

352. Kern W, et al. Correlation of protein expression and gene expression in acute leukemia. Cytometry B Clin Cytom 2003;55:29–36

353. Armstrong SA, et al. MLL translocations specify a distinct gene expression profile that distinguishes a unique leukemia. Nat Genet 2002;30:41–7

354. Moos PJ, et al. Identification of gene expression profiles that segregate patients with childhood leukemia. Clin Cancer Res 2002;8:3118–30

355. Yeoh EJ, et al. Classification, subtype discovery, and prediction of outcome in pediatric acute lymphoblastic leukemia by gene expression profiling. Cancer Cell 2002;1:133–43

356. Ferrando AA, et al. Gene expression signatures define novel oncogenic pathways in T cell acute lymphoblastic leukemia. Cancer Cell 2002;1:75–87

357. Ferrando AA, Look AT. Gene expression profiling in T-cell acute lymphoblastic leukemia. Semin Hematol 2003;40:274–80

358. Pellagatti A, et al. Gene expression profiling in the myelodysplastic syndromes using cDNA microarray technology. Br J Haematol 2004;125:576–83

359. Miyazato A, et al. Identification of myelodysplastic syndrome-specific genes by DNA microarray analysis with purified hematopoietic stem cell fraction. Blood 2001;98:422–7

360. Bader P, et al. How and when should we monitor chimerism after allogeneic stem cell transplantation? Bone Marrow Transplant 2005;35:107–19

361. Jolkowska J, et al. Hematopoietic chimerism after allogeneic stem cell transplantation: a comparison of quantitative analysis by automated DNA sizing and fluorescent in situ hybridization. BMC Blood Disord 2005;5:1

362. Alizadeh M, et al. Quantitative assessment of hematopoietic chimerism after bone marrow transplantation by real-time quantitative polymerase chain reaction. Blood 2002;99:4618–25

363. Wekerle T, Sykes M. Mixed chimerism as an approach for the induction of transplantation tolerance. Transplantation 1999;68:459–67

364. Mackinnon S, et al. Minimal residual disease is more common in patients who have mixed T-cell chimerism after bone marrow transplantation for chronic myelogenous leukemia. Blood 1994;83:3409–16

365. Mattsson J, et al. T cell mixed chimerism is significantly correlated to a decreased risk of acute graft-versus-host disease after allogeneic stem cell transplantation. Transplantation 2001;71:433–9

366. Bader P, et al. Serial and quantitative analysis of mixed hematopoietic chimerism by PCR in patients with acute leukemias allows the prediction of relapse after allogeneic BMT. Bone Marrow Transplant 1998;21:487–95

367. Ramirez M, et al. Chimerism after allogeneic hematopoietic cell transplantation in childhood acute lymphoblastic leukemia. Bone Marrow Transplant 1996;18:1161–5

368. Jimenez-Velasco A, et al. Reliable quantification of hematopoietic chimerism after allogeneic transplantation for acute leukemia using amplification by real-time PCR of null alleles and insertion/deletion polymorphisms. Leukemia 2005;19:336–43

369. Bader P, et al. Monitoring of donor cell chimerism for the detection of relapse and early immunotherapeutic intervention in acute lymphoblastic leukemias. Ann Hematol 2002;81(Suppl 2):S25–7

370. Bader P, et al. Mixed hematopoietic chimerism after allogeneic bone marrow transplantation: the impact of quantitative PCR analysis for prediction of relapse and graft rejection in children. Bone Marrow Transplant 1997;19:697–702

371. Bader P, et al. Children with myelodysplastic syndrome (MDS) and increasing mixed chimaerism after allogeneic stem cell transplantation have a poor outcome which can be improved by pre-emptive immunotherapy. Br J Haematol 2005;128:649–58

372. Bader P, et al. Increasing mixed chimerism is an important prognostic factor for unfavorable outcome in children with acute lymphoblastic leukemia after allogeneic stem-cell transplantation: possible role for pre-emptive immunotherapy? J Clin Oncol 2004;22:1696–705

373. Michallet AS, et al. Impact of chimaerism analysis and kinetics on allogeneic haematopoietic stem cell transplantation outcome after conventional and reduced-intensity conditioning regimens. Br J Haematol 2005;128:676–89

374. Formankova R, et al. Prediction and reversion of post-transplant relapse in patients with chronic myeloid leukemia using mixed chimerism and residual disease detection and adoptive immunotherapy. Leuk Res 2000;24:339–47

375. Socie G, et al. Studies on hemopoietic chimerism following allogeneic bone marrow transplantation in the molecular biology era. Leuk Res 1995;19:497–504

376. Suttorp M, et al. Monitoring of chimerism after allogeneic bone marrow transplantation with unmanipulated marrow by use of DNA polymorphisms. Leukemia 1993;7:679–87

377. Koss LG, et al. Flow cytometric measurements of DNA and other cell components in human tumors: a critical appraisal. Hum Pathol 1989;20:528–48

378. Czerniak B, et al. Flow cytometry in clinical oncology: cell cycle and DNA ploidy in assessing tumor behavior. Mater Med Pol 1989;21:3–9

379. Ott G, et al. Blastoid variants of mantle cell lymphoma: frequent bcl-1 rearrangements at the major translocation cluster region and tetraploid chromosome clones. Blood 1997;89:1421–9

380. Debes-Marun CS, et al. Chromosome abnormalities clustering and its implications for pathogenesis and prognosis in myeloma. Leukemia 2003;17:427–36

381. Fassas AB, et al. Both hypodiploidy and deletion of chromosome 13 independently confer poor prognosis in multiple myeloma. Br J Haematol 2002;118:1041–7

382. Smadja NV, et al. Hypodiploidy is a major prognostic factor in multiple myeloma. Blood 2001;98:2229–38

383. Garcia-Sanz R, et al. Prognostic implications of DNA aneuploidy in 156 untreated multiple myeloma patients. Castelano-Leones (Spain) Cooperative Group for the Study of Monoclonal Gammopathies. Br J Haematol 1995;90:106–12

384. Garcia-Sanz R, et al. Primary plasma cell leukemia: clinical, immunophenotypic, DNA ploidy, and cytogenetic characteristics. Blood 1999;93:1032–7

385. Wang S, et al. Flow cytometric DNA ploidy analysis of peripheral blood from patients with sezary syndrome: detection of aneuploid neoplastic T cells in the blood is associated with large cell transformation in tissue. Am J Clin Pathol 2004;122:774–82

386. Secker-Walker LM, Lawler SD, Hardisty RM. Prognostic implications of chromosomal findings in acute lymphoblastic leukaemia at diagnosis. Br Med J 1978;2:1529–30

387. Williams DL, et al. Prognostic importance of chromosome number in 136 untreated children with acute lymphoblastic leukemia. Blood 1982;60:864–71

388. Bloomfield CD, et al. Chromosomal abnormalities identify high-risk and low-risk patients with acute lymphoblastic leukemia. Blood 1986;67:415–20

389. Pui CH, Crist WM, Look AT. Biology and clinical significance of cytogenetic abnormalities in childhood acute lymphoblastic leukemia. Blood 1990;76:1449–63

390. Kaspers GJ, et al. Favorable prognosis of hyperdiploid common acute lymphoblastic leukemia may be explained by sensitivity to antimetabolites and other drugs: results of an in vitro study. Blood 1995;85:751–6

391. Look AT, et al. Prognostic importance of blast cell DNA content in childhood acute lymphoblastic leukemia. Blood 1985;65:1079–86

392. Raimondi SC. Current status of cytogenetic research in childhood acute lymphoblastic leukemia. Blood 1993;81:2237–51

393. Trueworthy R, et al. Ploidy of lymphoblasts is the strongest predictor of treatment outcome in B-progenitor cell acute lymphoblastic leukemia of childhood: a Pediatric Oncology Group study. J Clin Oncol 1992;10:606–13

394. Pui CH, et al. Hypodiploidy is associated with a poor prognosis in childhood acute lymphoblastic leukemia. Blood 1987;70:247–53

395. Pui CH, et al. Near-triploid and near-tetraploid acute lymphoblastic leukemia of childhood. Blood 1990;76:590–6

396. Zemanova Z, et al. Prognostic value of structural chromosomal rearrangements and small cell clones with high hyperdiploidy in children with acute lymphoblastic leukemia. Leuk Res 2005;29:273–81

397. Heerema NA, et al. Hypodiploidy with less than 45 chromosomes confers adverse risk in childhood acute lymphoblastic leukemia: a report from the children's cancer group. Blood 1999;94:4036–45

398. Raimondi SC, et al. Reassessment of the prognostic significance of hypodiploidy in pediatric patients with acute lymphoblastic leukemia. Cancer 2003;98:2715–22

399. Anonymous. Cytogenetic abnormalities in adult acute lymphoblastic leukemia: correlations with hematologic findings outcome. A Collaborative Study of the Groupe Francais de Cytogenetique Hematologique. Blood 1996;87:3135–42

400. Secker-Walker LM, et al. Cytogenetics adds independent prognostic information in adults with acute lymphoblastic leukaemia on MRC trial UKALL XA. MRC Adult Leukaemia Working Party. Br J Haematol 1997;96:601–10

401. Callen DF, et al. Acute lymphoblastic leukemia with a hypodiploid karyotype with less than 40 chromosomes: the basis for division into two subgroups. Leukemia 1989;3:749–52

402. Charrin C, et al. A report from the LALA-94 and LALA-SA groups on hypodiploidy with 30 to 39 chromosomes and near-triploidy: 2 possible expressions of a sole entity conferring poor prognosis in adult acute lymphoblastic leukemia (ALL). Blood 2004;104:2444–51

403. Giagounidis AA, et al. The 5q– syndrome. Hematology 2004;9:271–7

404. Giagounidis AA, et al. Clinical, morphological, cytogenetic, and prognostic features of patients with myelodysplastic syndromes and del(5q) including band q31. Leukemia 2004;18:113–19

405. Side LE, et al. RAS, FLT3, and TP53 mutations in therapy-related myeloid malignancies with abnormalities of chromosomes 5 and 7. Genes Chromosomes Cancer 2004;39:217–23

406. Johansson B, Mertens F, Mitelman F. Cytogenetic deletion maps of hematologic neoplasms: circumstantial evidence for tumor suppressor loci. Genes Chromosomes Cancer 1993;8:205–18

407. Tilly H, et al. Prognostic value of chromosomal abnormalities in follicular lymphoma. Blood 1994; 84:1043–9

408. Viardot A, et al. Clinicopathologic correlations of genomic gains and losses in follicular lymphoma. J Clin Oncol 2002;20:4523–30

409. Stilgenbauer S, et al. Incidence and clinical significance of 6q deletions in B cell chronic lymphocytic leukemia. Leukemia 1999;13:1331–4

410. Cuneo A, et al. Chronic lymphocytic leukemia with 6q– shows distinct hematological features and intermediate prognosis. Leukemia 2004;18:476–83

411. Fischer TC, et al. Genomic aberrations and survival in cutaneous T cell lymphomas. J Invest Dermatol 2004;122:579–86

412. Wong KF, Chan JK, Kwong YL. Identification of del(6)(q21q25) as a recurring chromosomal abnormality in putative NK cell lymphoma/leukaemia. Br J Haematol 1997;98:922–6

413. Tien HF, et al. Clonal chromosomal abnormalities as direct evidence for clonality in nasal T/natural killer cell lymphomas. Br J Haematol 1997;97:621–5

414. Heerema NA, et al. Clinical significance of deletions of chromosome arm 6q in childhood acute lymphoblastic leukemia: a report from the Children's Cancer Group. Leuk Lymphoma 2000;36:467–78

415. Mancini M, et al. Partial deletions of long arm of chromosome 6: biologic and clinical implications in adult acute lymphoblastic leukemia. Leukemia 2002;16:2055–61

416. Tosi S, et al. Delineation of multiple deleted regions in 7q in myeloid disorders. Genes Chromosomes Cancer 1999;25:384–92

417. Brozek I, et al. Cytogenetic analysis and clinical significance of chromosome 7 aberrations in acute leukaemia. J Appl Genet 2003;44:401–12

418. Baldus C, et al. MDR-1 expression and deletions of chromosomes 7 and 5(Q) separately indicate adverse prognosis in AML. Leuk Lymphoma 2001;40:613–23

419. Velloso ER, et al. Deletions of the long arm of chromosome 7 in myeloid disorders: loss of band 7q32 implies worst prognosis. Br J Haematol 1996;92: 574–81

420. Baranger L, et al. Monosomy-7 in childhood hemopoietic disorders. Leukemia 1990;4:345–9

421. McKenna RW. Myelodysplasia and myeloproliferative disorders in children. Am J Clin Pathol 2004;122 (Suppl):S58–69

422. Evans JP, et al. Childhood monosomy 7 revisited. Br J Haematol 1988;69:41–5

423. Trobaugh-Lotrario AD, et al. Monosomy 7 associated with pediatric acute myeloid leukemia (AML) and myelodysplastic syndrome (MDS): successful management by allogeneic hematopoietic stem cell transplant (HSCT). Bone Marrow Transplant 2004

424. Passmore SJ, et al. Paediatric myelodysplastic syndromes and juvenile myelomonocytic leukaemia in the UK: a population-based study of incidence and survival. Br J Haematol 2003;121:758–67

425. Trobaugh-Lotrario AD, et al. Monosomy 7 associated with pediatric acute myeloid leukemia (AML) and myelodysplastic syndrome (MDS): successful management by allogeneic hematopoietic stem cell transplant (HSCT). Bone Marrow Transplant 2005;35: 143–9

426. Frohling S, et al. Acute myeloid leukemia with deletion 9q within a noncomplex karyotype is associated with CEBPA loss-of-function mutations. Genes Chromosomes Cancer 2005;42:427–32

427. Leroy H, et al. CEBPA point mutations in hematological malignancies. Leukemia 2005;19:329–34

428. Marcucci G, Mrozek K, Bloomfield CD. Molecular heterogeneity and prognostic biomarkers in adults with acute myeloid leukemia and normal cytogenetics. Curr Opin Hematol 2005;12:68–75

429. Andreasson P, et al. Cytogenetic and FISH studies of a single center consecutive series of 152 childhood acute lymphoblastic leukemias. Eur J Haematol 2000;65:40–51

430. Dohner H, et al. 11q deletions identify a new subset of B-cell chronic lymphocytic leukemia characterized by extensive nodal involvement and inferior prognosis. Blood 1997;89:2516–22

431. Dickinson JD, et al. Unique gene expression and clinical characteristics are associated with the 11q23 deletion in chronic lymphocytic leukaemia. Br J Haematol 2005;128:460–71

432. Cuneo A, et al. 13q14 deletion in non-Hodgkin's lymphoma: correlation with clinicopathologic features. Haematologica 1999;84:589–93

433. Dohner H, et al. Cytogenetic and molecular cytogenetic analysis of B cell chronic lymphocytic leukemia: specific chromosome aberrations identify prognostic subgroups of patients and point to loci of candidate genes. Leukemia 1997;11(Suppl 2):S19–24

434. Dohner H, et al. Genomic aberrations and survival in chronic lymphocytic leukemia. N Engl J Med 2000; 343:1910–16

435. Chena C, et al. Interphase cytogenetic analysis in Argentinean B-cell chronic lymphocytic leukemia patients: association of trisomy 12 and del(13q14). Cancer Genet Cytogenet 2003;146:154–60

436. Sawyer JR, et al. Cytogenetic findings in 200 patients with multiple myeloma. Cancer Genet Cytogenet 1995;82:41–9

437. Tricot G, et al. Poor prognosis in multiple myeloma is associated only with partial or complete deletions of chromosome 13 or abnormalities involving 11q and not with other karyotype abnormalities. Blood 1995;86:4250–6

438. Desikan R, et al. Results of high-dose therapy for 1000 patients with multiple myeloma: durable complete remissions and superior survival in the absence of chromosome 13 abnormalities. Blood 2000;95: 4008–10

439. Fassas AB, Tricot G. Chromosome 13 deletion/ hypodiploidy and prognosis in multiple myeloma patients. Leuk Lymphoma 2004;45:1083–91

440. Kaufmann H, et al. Both chromosome 13 abnormalities by metaphase cytogenetics and deletion of 13q by interphase FISH only are prognostically relevant in multiple myeloma. Eur J Haematol 2003;71:179–83

441. Castro PD, Liang JC, Nagarajan L. Deletions of chromosome 5q13.3 and 17p loci cooperate in myeloid neoplasms. Blood 2000;95:2138–43

442. Watson N, et al. 17p– syndrome arising from a novel dicentric translocation in a patient with acute myeloid leukemia. Cancer Genet Cytogenet 2000;118:159–62

443. Hoglund M, et al. Identification of cytogenetic subgroups and karyotypic pathways of clonal evolution in follicular lymphomas. Genes Chromosomes Cancer 2004;39:195–204

444. Geisler CH, et al. In B-cell chronic lymphocytic leukaemia chromosome 17 abnormalities and not trisomy 12 are the single most important cytogenetic abnormalities for the prognosis: a cytogenetic and immunophenotypic study of 480 unselected newly diagnosed patients. Leuk Res 1997;21:1011–23

445. Byrd JC, et al. Interphase cytogenetic abnormalities in chronic lymphocytic leukemia may predict response to rituximab. Cancer Res 2003;63:36–8

446. Kurtin PJ, et al. Hematologic disorders associated with deletions of chromosome 20q: a clinicopathologic study of 107 patients. Am J Clin Pathol 1996; 106:680–8

447. Belhadj K, et al. Hepatosplenic gammadelta T-cell lymphoma is a rare clinicopathologic entity with poor outcome: report on a series of 21 patients. Blood 2003;102:4261–9

448. Fioretos T, et al. Isochromosome 17q in blast crisis of chronic myeloid leukemia and in other hematologic malignancies is the result of clustered breakpoints in 17p11 and is not associated with coding TP53 mutations. Blood 1999;94:225–32

449. Liu P, et al. Fusion between transcription factor CBF beta/PEBP2 beta and a myosin heavy chain in acute myeloid leukemia. Science 1993;261:1041–4

450. Loffler H, Gassmann W, Haferlach T. AML M1 and M2 with eosinophilia and AML M4Eo: diagnostic and clinical aspects. Leuk Lymphoma 1995; 18(Suppl 1):61–3

451. Marlton P, et al. Cytogenetic and clinical correlates in AML patients with abnormalities of chromosome 16. Leukemia 1995;9:965–71

452. Levine EG, Bloomfield CD. Cytogenetics of non-Hodgkin's lymphoma. J Natl Cancer Inst Monogr 1990:7–12

453. Yunis JJ, et al. bcl-2 and other genomic alterations in the prognosis of large-cell lymphoma. N Engl J Med 1989;320:1047–54

454. Elliott MA, et al. The prognostic significance of trisomy 8 in patients with acute myeloid leukemia. Leuk Lymphoma 2002;43:583–6

455. de Botton S, et al. Additional chromosomal abnormalities in patients with acute promyelocytic leukaemia (APL) do not confer poor prognosis: results of APL 93 trial. Br J Haematol 2000;111:801–6

456. Cuneo A, et al. Cytogenetic profile of lymphoma of follicle mantle lineage: correlation with clinicobiologic features. Blood 1999;93:1372–80

457. Han T, et al. Prognostic importance of cytogenetic abnormalities in patients with chronic lymphocytic leukemia. N Engl J Med 1984;310:288–92

458. Foon KA, Rai KR, Gale RP. Chronic lymphocytic leukemia: new insights into biology and therapy. Ann Intern Med 1990;113:525–39

459. Bea S, et al. Clinicopathologic significance and prognostic value of chromosomal imbalances in diffuse large B-cell lymphomas. J Clin Oncol 2004;22:3498–506

460. Krugmann J, et al. Unfavourable prognosis of patients with trisomy 18q21 detected by fluorescence in situ hybridisation in t(11;18) negative, surgically resected, gastrointestinal B cell lymphomas. J Clin Pathol 2004;57:360–4

461. Michaux L, et al. Translocation t(1;6)(p35.3;p25.2): a new recurrent aberration in 'unmutated' B-CLL. Leukemia 2005;19:77–82

462. Willis TG, et al. Bcl10 is involved in t(1;14)(p22;q32) of MALT B cell lymphoma and mutated in multiple tumor types. Cell 1999;96:35–45

463. Zhang Q, et al. Inactivating mutations and overexpression of BCL10, a caspase recruitment domain-containing gene, in MALT lymphoma with t(1;14) (p22;q32). Nat Genet 1999;22:63–8

464. Ye H, et al. BCL10 expression in normal and neoplastic lymphoid tissue. Nuclear localization in MALT lymphoma. Am J Pathol 2000;157:1147–54

465. Ohshima K, et al. Bcl10 expression, rearrangement and mutation in MALT lymphoma: correlation with expression of nuclear factor-kappaB. Int J Oncol 2001;19:283–9

466. Maes B, et al. BCL10 mutation does not represent an important pathogenic mechanism in gastric MALT-type lymphoma, and the presence of the API2-MLT fusion is associated with aberrant nuclear BCL10 expression. Blood 2002;99:1398–404

467. Liu H, et al. T(11;18)(q21;q21) is associated with advanced mucosa-associated lymphoid tissue lymphoma that expresses nuclear BCL10. Blood 2001;98:1182–7

468. Wotherspoon AC, et al. Low-grade primary B-cell lymphoma of the lung. An immunohistochemical, molecular, and cytogenetic study of a single case. Am J Clin Pathol 1990;94:655–60

469. Crist WM, et al. Poor prognosis of children with pre-B acute lymphoblastic leukemia is associated with the t(1;19)(q23;p13): a Pediatric Oncology Group study. Blood 1990;76:117–22

470. Raimondi SC, et al. Cytogenetics of pre-B-cell acute lymphoblastic leukemia with emphasis on prognostic implications of the t(1;19). J Clin Oncol 1990;8: 1380–8

471. Bernstein J, et al. Nineteen cases of the t(1;22) (p13;q13) acute megakaryblastic leukaemia of infants/children and a review of 39 cases: report from a t(1;22) study group. Leukemia 2000;14:216–18

472. Delsol G, et al. A new subtype of large B-cell lymphoma expressing the ALK kinase and lacking the 2;5 translocation. Blood 1997;89:1483–90

473. Gascoyne RD, et al. ALK-positive diffuse large B-cell lymphoma is associated with clathrin–ALK rearrangements: report of 6 cases. Blood 2003;102:2568–73

474. Kwong YL. Translocation (3;5)(q21;q34) in erythroleukemia: a molecular and in situ hybridization study. Cancer Genet Cytogenet 1998;103:15–19

475. Shi G, et al. 3p21 is a recurrent treatment-related breakpoint in myelodysplastic syndrome and acute myeloid leukemia. Cytogenet Cell Genet 1996;74: 295–9

476. Zent C, Rowley JD, Nucifora G. Rearrangements of the AML1/CBFA2 gene in myeloid leukemia with the 3;21 translocation: in vitro and in vivo studies. Leukemia 1997;11(Suppl 3):273–8

477. Drabkin HA, Erickson P. Down syndrome and leukemia, an update. Prog Clin Biol Res 1995;393: 169–76

478. Behm FG, et al. Rearrangement of the MLL gene confers a poor prognosis in childhood acute lymphoblastic leukemia, regardless of presenting age. Blood 1996; 87:2870–7

479. Heerema NA, et al. Cytogenetic studies of infant acute lymphoblastic leukemia: poor prognosis of infants with t(4;11) – a report of the Children's Cancer Group. Leukemia, 1999;13:679–86

480. Cimino G, et al. Clinico-biologic features and treatment outcome of adult pro-B-ALL patients enrolled in the GIMEMA 0496 study: absence of the

ALL1/AF4 and of the BCR/ABL fusion genes correlates with a significantly better clinical outcome. Blood 2003;102:2014–20

481. Chang H, et al. The t(4;14) is associated with poor prognosis in myeloma patients undergoing autologous stem cell transplant. Br J Haematol 2004;125: 64–8

482. von Lindern M, et al. The translocation (6;9), associated with a specific subtype of acute myeloid leukemia, results in the fusion of two genes, dek and can, and the expression of a chimeric, leukemia-specific dek–can mRNA. Mol Cell Biol 1992;12: 1687–97

483. Soekarman D, et al. The translocation (6;9) (p23;q34) shows consistent rearrangement of two genes and defines a myeloproliferative disorder with specific clinical features. Blood 1992;79:2990–7

484. Au WY, et al. The spectrum of lymphoma with 8q24 aberrations: a clinical, pathological and cytogenetic study of 87 consecutive cases. Leuk Lymphoma 2004;45:519–28

485. Velloso ER, et al. Translocation t(8;16)(p11;p13) in acute non-lymphocytic leukemia: report on two new cases and review of the literature. Leuk Lymphoma 1996;21:137–42

486. Harris NL, et al. World Health Organization classification of neoplastic diseases of the hematopoietic and lymphoid tissues: report of the Clinical Advisory Committee meeting – Airlie House, Virginia, November 1997. J Clin Oncol 1999;17:3835–49

487. Khoury H, et al. Acute myelogenous leukemia with t(8;21) – identification of a specific immunophenotype. Leuk Lymphoma 2003;44:1713–18

488. Erickson PF, et al. The ETO portion of acute myeloid leukemia t(8;21) fusion transcript encodes a highly evolutionarily conserved, putative transcription factor. Cancer Res 1994;54:1782–6

489. Andrieu V, et al. Molecular detection of t(8;21)/AML1-ETO in AML M1/M2: correlation with cytogenetics, morphology and immunophenotype. Br J Haematol 1996;92:855–65

490. Byrd JC, Weiss RB. Recurrent granulocytic sarcoma. An unusual variation of acute myelogenous leukemia associated with 8;21 chromosomal translocation and blast expression of the neural cell adhesion molecule. Cancer 1994;73:2107–12

491. Bloomfield CD, et al. Frequency of prolonged remission duration after high-dose cytarabine intensification in acute myeloid leukemia varies by cytogenetic subtype. Cancer Res 1998;58:4173–9

492. Schoch C, et al. Fifty-one patients with acute myeloid leukemia and translocation t(8;21)(q22;q22): an additional deletion in 9q is an adverse prognostic factor. Leukemia 1996;10:1288–95

493. Leroy H, et al. Prognostic value of real-time quantitative PCR (RQ-PCR) in AML with t(8;21). Leukemia 2005;19:367–72

494. Rubnitz JE, et al. Favorable impact of the t(9;11) in childhood acute myeloid leukemia. J Clin Oncol 2002;20:2302–9

495. Offit K, et al. t(9;14)(p13;q32) denotes a subset of low-grade non-Hodgkin's lymphoma with plasmacytoid differentiation. Blood 1992;80:2594–9

496. Cook JR, et al. Lack of PAX5 rearrangements in lymphoplasmacytic lymphomas: reassessing the reported association with t(9;14). Hum Pathol 2004;35:447–54

497. Huntly BJ, et al. Derivative chromosome 9 deletions in chronic myeloid leukemia: poor prognosis is not associated with loss of ABL–BCR expression, elevated BCR–ABL levels, or karyotypic instability. Blood 2002;99:4547–53

498. Lundan T, et al. Allogeneic stem cell transplantation reverses the poor prognosis of CML patients with deletions in derivative chromosome 9. Leukemia 2005;19:138–40

499. Gleissner B, et al. Leading prognostic relevance of the BCR–ABL translocation in adult acute B-lineage lymphoblastic leukemia: a prospective study of the German Multicenter Trial Group and confirmed polymerase chain reaction analysis. Blood 2002;99:1536–43

500. Suryanarayan K, et al. Consistent involvement of the bcr gene by 9;22 breakpoints in pediatric acute leukemias. Blood 1991;77:324–30

501. Brisco MJ, et al. Effect of the Philadelphia chromosome on minimal residual disease in acute lymphoblastic leukemia. Leukemia 1997;11:1497–500

502. Troussard X, et al. Cyclin D1 expression in patients with multiple myeloma. Hematol J 2000;1:181–5

503. Pruneri G, et al. Immunohistochemical analysis of cyclin D1 shows deregulated expression in multiple myeloma with the t(11;14). Am J Pathol 2000;156: 1505–13

504. Panani AD, et al. Cytogenetic data as a prognostic factor in multiple myeloma patients: involvement of 1p12 region an adverse prognostic factor. Anticancer Res 2004;24:4141–6

505. Bosch F, et al. Increased expression of the PRAD-1/CCND1 gene in hairy cell leukaemia. Br J Haematol 1995;91:1025–30

506. Melnick A, Licht JD. Deconstructing a disease: RARalpha, its fusion partners, and their roles in the pathogenesis of acute promyelocytic leukemia. Blood 1999;93:3167–215

507. Licht JD, et al. Clinical and molecular characterization of a rare syndrome of acute promyelocytic leukemia associated with translocation (11;17). Blood 1995;85:1083–94

508. Grimwade D, et al. Characterization of acute promyelocytic leukemia cases lacking the classic t(15;17): results of the European Working Party. Groupe Francais de Cytogenetique Hematologique, Groupe de Francais d'Hematologie Cellulaire, UK Cancer Cytogenetics Group and BIOMED 1 European Community-Concerted Action 'Molecular Cytogenetic Diagnosis in Haematological Malignancies'. Blood 2000;96:1297–308

509. Streubel B, et al. T(14;18)(q32;q21) involving IGH and MALT1 is a frequent chromosomal aberration in MALT lymphoma. Blood 2003;101:2335–9

510. Isaacson PG, Du MQ. Gastrointestinal lymphoma: where morphology meets molecular biology. J Pathol 2005;205:255–74

511. Liu H, et al. t(11;18) is a marker for all stage gastric MALT lymphomas that will not respond to H. pylori eradication. Gastroenterology 2002;122:1286–94

512. Streubel B, et al. Translocation t(11;18)(q21;q21) is not predictive of response to chemotherapy with 2CdA in patients with gastric MALT lymphoma. Oncology 2004;66:476–80

513. Raynaud SD, et al. Cytogenetic abnormalities associated with the t(12;21): a collaborative study of 169 children with t(12;21)-positive acute lymphoblastic leukemia. Leukemia 1999;13:1325–30

514. Wang ZG, et al. Role of PML in cell growth and the retinoic acid pathway. Science 1998;279:1547–51

515. Wang ZG, et al. PML is essential for multiple apoptotic pathways. Nat Genet 1998;20:266–72

516. Grimwade D, et al. Impact of karyotype on treatment outcome in acute myeloid leukemia. Ann Hematol 2004;83(Suppl 1):S45–8

517. Reiter A, Lengfelder E, Grimwade D. Pathogenesis, diagnosis and monitoring of residual disease in acute promyelocytic leukaemia. Acta Haematol 2004;112:55–67

518. Pettitt AR, et al. p53 dysfunction in B-cell chronic lymphocytic leukemia: inactivation of ATM as an alternative to TP53 mutation. Blood 2001;98:814–22

519. Stankovic T, et al. Ataxia telangiectasia mutated-deficient B-cell chronic lymphocytic leukemia occurs in pregerminal center cells and results in defective damage response and unrepaired chromosome damage. Blood 2002;99:300–9

520. Starostik P, et al. Deficiency of the ATM protein expression defines an aggressive subgroup of B-cell chronic lymphocytic leukemia. Cancer Res 1998;58:4552–7

521. Bullrich F, et al. ATM mutations in B-cell chronic lymphocytic leukemia. Cancer Res 1999;59:24–7

522. Lossos IS, et al. Mutation of the ATM gene is not involved in the pathogenesis of either follicle center lymphoma or its transformation to higher-grade lymphoma. Leuk Lymphoma 2002;43:1079–85

523. Soverini S, et al. Cyclin D1 overexpression is a favorable prognostic variable for newly diagnosed multiple myeloma patients treated with high-dose chemotherapy and single or double autologous transplantation. Blood 2003;102:1588–94

524. Markovic O, et al. Immunohistochemical analysis of cyclin D1 and p53 in multiple myeloma: relationship to proliferative activity and prognostic significance. Med Oncol 2004;21:73–80

525. Rasmussen T, Knudsen LM, Johnsen HE. Frequency and prognostic relevance of cyclin D1 dysregulation in multiple myeloma. Eur J Haematol 2001;67:296–301

526. Hoechtlen-Vollmar W, et al. Amplification of cyclin D1 gene in multiple myeloma: clinical and prognostic relevance. Br J Haematol 2000;109:30–8

527. Specht K, et al. Different mechanisms of cyclin D1 overexpression in multiple myeloma revealed by fluorescence in situ hybridization and quantitative analysis of mRNA levels. Blood 2004;104:1120–6

528. Vasef MA, et al. Cyclin D1 protein in multiple myeloma and plasmacytoma: an immunohisto-chemical study using fixed, paraffin-embedded tissue sections. Mod Pathol 1997;10:927–32

529. Reed JC. Bcl-2 family proteins: regulators of apoptosis and chemoresistance in hematologic malignancies. Semin Hematol 1997;34(Suppl 5):9–19

530. Tang SC, et al. Clinical significance of bcl-2–MBR gene rearrangement and protein expression in diffuse large-cell non-Hodgkin's lymphoma: an analysis of 83 cases. J Clin Oncol 1994;12:149–54

531. Kramer MH, et al. Clinical significance of bcl2 and p53 protein expression in diffuse large B-cell lymphoma: a population-based study. J Clin Oncol 1996;14:2131–8

532. Rantanen S, et al. Causes and consequences of BCL2 overexpression in diffuse large B-cell lymphoma. Leuk Lymphoma 2001;42:1089–98

533. Monni O, et al. BCL2 overexpression associated with chromosomal amplification in diffuse large B-cell lymphoma. Blood 1997;90:1168–74

534. Piris MA, et al. p53 and bcl-2 expression in high-grade B-cell lymphomas: correlation with survival time. Br J Cancer 1994;69:337–41

535. Villuendas R, et al. Different bcl-2 protein expression in high-grade B-cell lymphomas derived from lymph node or mucosa-associated lymphoid tissue. Am J Pathol 1991;139:989–93

536. Skinnider BF, et al. Bcl-6 and Bcl-2 protein expression in diffuse large B-cell lymphoma and follicular lymphoma: correlation with 3q27 and 18q21 chromosomal abnormalities. Hum Pathol 1999;30:803–8

537. Gascoyne RD. Pathologic prognostic factors in diffuse aggressive non-Hodgkin's lymphoma. Hematol Oncol Clin North Am 1997;11:847–62

538. Hill ME, et al. Prognostic significance of BCL-2 expression and bcl-2 major breakpoint region rearrangement in diffuse large cell non-Hodgkin's lymphoma: a British National Lymphoma Investigation Study. Blood 1996; 88:1046–51

539. Sanchez E, et al. Clinical outcome in diffuse large B-cell lymphoma is dependent on the relationship between different cell-cycle regulator proteins. J Clin Oncol 1998;16:1931–9

540. Barrans SL, et al. Germinal center phenotype and bcl-2 expression combined with the International Prognostic Index improves patient risk stratification in diffuse large B-cell lymphoma. Blood 2002;99: 1136–43

541. Colomo L, et al. Clinical impact of the differentiation profile assessed by immunophenotyping in patients with diffuse large B-cell lymphoma. Blood 2003;101: 78–84

542. Maartense E, et al. Lack of prognostic significance of BCL2 and p53 protein overexpression in elderly patients with diffuse large B-cell non-Hodgkin's lymphoma: results from a population-based non-Hodgkin's lymphoma registry. Leuk Lymphoma 2004;45:101–7

543. Ghia P, et al. Unbalanced expression of bcl-2 family proteins in follicular lymphoma: contribution of CD40 signaling in promoting survival. Blood 1998; 91:244–51

544. Rassidakis GZ, et al. BCL-2 family proteins in peripheral T-cell lymphomas: correlation with tumour apoptosis and proliferation. J Pathol 2003;200:240–8

545. Villalva C, et al. Bcl-2 expression in anaplastic large cell lymphoma. Am J Pathol 2001;158:1889–90

546. Rassidakis GZ, et al. BCL-2 expression in Hodgkin and Reed–Sternberg cells of classical Hodgkin disease predicts a poorer prognosis in patients treated with ABVD or equivalent regimens. Blood 2002;100: 3935–41

547. Vassallo J, et al. The prognostic relevance of apoptosis-related proteins in classical Hodgkin's lymphomas. Leuk Lymphoma 2003;44:483–8

548. Coustan-Smith E, et al. Clinical relevance of BCL-2 overexpression in childhood acute lymphoblastic leukemia. Blood 1996;87:1140–6

549. Dent AL, Vasanwala FH, Toney LM. Regulation of gene expression by the proto-oncogene BCL-6. Crit Rev Oncol Hematol 2002;41:1–9

550. Shaffer AL, et al. BCL-6 represses genes that function in lymphocyte differentiation, inflammation, and cell cycle control. Immunity 2000;13:199–212

551. Onizuka T, et al. BCL-6 gene product, a 92- to 98-kD nuclear phosphoprotein, is highly expressed in germinal center B cells and their neoplastic counterparts. Blood 1995;86:28–37

552. Flenghi L, et al. Monoclonal antibodies PG-B6a and PG-B6p recognize, respectively, a highly conserved

and a formol-resistant epitope on the human BCL-6 protein amino-terminal region. Am J Pathol 1996; 148:1543–55

553. Falini B, et al. Distinctive expression pattern of the BCL-6 protein in nodular lymphocyte predominance Hodgkin's disease. Blood 1996;87:465–71

554. Dogan A, et al. CD10 and BCL-6 expression in paraffin sections of normal lymphoid tissue and B-cell lymphomas. Am J Surg Pathol 2000;24:846–52

555. Artiga MJ, et al. A short mutational hot spot in the first intron of BCL-6 is associated with increased BCL-6 expression and with longer overall survival in large B-cell lymphomas. Am J Pathol 2002;160: 1371–80

556. Phan RT, Dalla-Favera R. The BCL6 proto-oncogene suppresses p53 expression in germinal-centre B cells. Nature 2004;432:635–9

557. Offit K, et al. Rearrangement of the bcl-6 gene as a prognostic marker in diffuse large-cell lymphoma. N Engl J Med 1994;331:74–80

558. Lossos IS, et al. Expression of a single gene, BCL-6, strongly predicts survival in patients with diffuse large B-cell lymphoma. Blood 2001;98:945–51

559. Akasaka T, et al. Nonimmunoglobulin (non-Ig)/ BCL6 gene fusion in diffuse large B-cell lymphoma results in worse prognosis than Ig/BCL6. Blood 2000;96:2907–9

560. Melnick A. Reprogramming specific gene expression pathways in B-cell lymphomas. Cell Cycle 2005:4

561. Polo JM, et al. Specific peptide interference reveals BCL6 transcriptional and oncogenic mechanisms in B-cell lymphoma cells. Nat Med 2004;10:1329–35

562. Akasaka T, Lossos IS, Levy R. BCL6 gene transloca-tion in follicular lymphoma: a harbinger of eventual transformation to diffuse aggressive lymphoma. Blood 2003;102:1443–8

563. Sarsotti E, et al. Bcl-6 mutation status provides clini-cally valuable information in early-stage B-cell chronic lymphocytic leukemia. Leukemia 2004;18: 743–6

564. Sahota SS, et al. Somatic mutation of bcl-6 genes can occur in the absence of V(H) mutations in chronic lymphocytic leukemia. Blood 2000;95:3534–40

565. Ye H, et al. MALT lymphoma with t(14;18) (q32;q21)/IGH-MALT1 is characterized by strong cytoplasmic MALT1 and BCL10 expression. J Pathol 2005;205:293–301

566. Chevallier N, et al. The ETO protein of t(8;21) AML is a corepressor for the Bcl-6 B-cell lymphoma oncoprotein. Blood, 2003

567. Chevallier N, et al. ETO protein of t(8;21) AML is a corepressor for Bcl-6 B-cell lymphoma oncoprotein. Blood 2004;103:1454–63

568. Lossos IS, et al. Prediction of survival in diffuse large-B-cell lymphoma based on the expression of six genes. N Engl J Med 2004;350:1828–37

569. Stirewalt DL, et al. FLT3, RAS, and TP53 mutations in elderly patients with acute myeloid leukemia. Blood 2001;97:3589–95

570. Birg F, et al. The expression of FMS, KIT and FLT3 in hematopoietic malignancies. Leuk Lymphoma 1994;13:223–7

571. Birg F, et al. Expression of the FMS/KIT-like gene FLT3 in human acute leukemias of the myeloid and lymphoid lineages. Blood 1992;80:2584–93

572. Carow CE, et al. Expression of the hematopoietic growth factor receptor FLT3 (STK-1/Flk2) in human leukemias. Blood 1996;87:1089–96

573. Stacchini A, et al. Expression of type III receptor tyrosine kinases FLT3 and KIT and responses to their ligands by acute myeloid leukemia blasts. Leukemia 1996;10:1584–91

574. Brown P, et al. FLT3 inhibition selectively kills child-hood acute lymphoblastic leukemia cells with high levels of FLT3 expression. Blood 2005;105:812–20

575. Gilliland DG, Griffin JD. The roles of FLT3 in hematopoiesis and leukemia. Blood 2002;100: 1532–42

576. Kussick SJ, et al. A distinctive nuclear morphology in acute myeloid leukemia is strongly associated with loss of HLA-DR expression and FLT3 internal tandem duplication. Leukemia 2004;18:1591–8

577. Kondo M, et al. Prognostic value of internal tandem duplication of the FLT3 gene in childhood acute myelogenous leukemia. Med Pediatr Oncol 1999;33: 525–9

578. Chillon MC, et al. FLT3-activating mutations are associated with poor prognostic features in AML at diagnosis but they are not an independent prognostic factor. Hematol J 2004;5:239–46

579. Ozeki K, et al. Biologic and clinical significance of the FLT3 transcript level in acute myeloid leukemia. Blood 2004;103:1901–8

580. Thiede C, et al. Analysis of FLT3-activating mutations in 979 patients with acute myelogenous leukemia: association with FAB subtypes and identification of subgroups with poor prognosis. Blood 2002;99:4326–35

581. Whitman SP, et al. Absence of the wild-type allele predicts poor prognosis in adult de novo acute myeloid leukemia with normal cytogenetics and the internal tandem duplication of FLT3: a cancer and leukemia group B study. Cancer Res 2001;61:7233–9

582. Meshinchi S, et al. Prevalence and prognostic significance of Flt3 internal tandem duplication in pediatric acute myeloid leukemia. Blood 2001;97:89–94

583. Shih LY, et al. Acquisition of FLT3 or N-ras mutations is frequently associated with progression of myelodysplastic syndrome to acute myeloid leukemia. Leukemia 2004;18:466–75

584. Shih LY, et al. Internal tandem duplication of fms-like tyrosine kinase 3 is associated with poor outcome in patients with myelodysplastic syndrome. Cancer 2004;101:989–98

585. Katoh M, Katoh M. Human FOX gene family [Review]. Int J Oncol 2004;25:1495–500

586. Barrans SL, et al. Strong expression of FOXP1 identifies a distinct subset of diffuse large B-cell lymphoma (DLBCL) patients with poor outcome. Blood 2004;104:2933–5

587. Banham AH, et al. Expression of the FOXP1 transcription factor is strongly associated with inferior survival in patients with diffuse large B-cell lymphoma. Clin Cancer Res 2005;11:1065–72

588. Lacronique V, et al. A TEL-JAK2 fusion protein with constitutive kinase activity in human leukemia. Science 1997;278:1309–12

589. Peeters P, et al. Fusion of TEL, the ETS-variant gene 6 (ETV6), to the receptor-associated kinase JAK2 as a result of t(9;12) in a lymphoid and t(9;15;12) in a myeloid leukemia. Blood 1997;90:2535–40

590. Baxter EJ, Scott LM. Acquired mutation of the tyrosine kinase JAK2 in human myeloproliferative disorders. Lancet 2005;365:1054–61

591. Johnstone RW, Cretney E, Smyth MJ. P-glycoprotein protects leukemia cells against caspase-dependent, but not caspase-independent, cell death. Blood 1999;93:1075–85

592. Juranka PF, Zastawny RL, Ling V. P-glycoprotein: multidrug-resistance and a superfamily of membrane-associated transport proteins. Faseb J 1989;3: 2583–92

593. Wood P, et al. P-glycoprotein expression on acute myeloid leukaemia blast cells at diagnosis predicts response to chemotherapy and survival. Br J Haematol 1994;87:509–14

594. Musto P, et al. High risk of early resistant relapse for leukaemic patients with presence of multidrug resistance associated P-glycoprotein positive cells in complete remission. Br J Haematol 1991;77:50–3

595. Guerci A, et al. Predictive value for treatment outcome in acute myeloid leukemia of cellular daunorubicin accumulation and P-glycoprotein expression simultaneously determined by flow cytometry. Blood 1995;85:2147–53

596. Zochbauer S, et al. P-glycoprotein expression as unfavorable prognostic factor in acute myeloid leukemia. Leukemia 1994;8:974–7

597. Steinbach D, et al. Contrary to adult patients, expression of the multidrug resistance gene (MDR1) fails to define a poor prognostic group in childhood AML. Leukemia 2003;17:470–1

598. Schaich M, et al. MDR1 and MRP1 gene expression are independent predictors for treatment outcome in adult acute myeloid leukaemia. Br J Haematol 2005;128:324–32

599. Schaich M, et al. Association of specific cytogenetic aberrations with mdr1 gene expression in adult myeloid leukemia and its implication in treatment outcome. Haematologica 2002;87:455–64

600. List AF, et al. Benefit of cyclosporine modulation of drug resistance in patients with poor-risk acute myeloid leukemia: a Southwest Oncology Group study. Blood 2001;98:3212–20

601. List AF, et al. Cyclosporine inhibition of P-glycoprotein in chronic myeloid leukemia blast phase. Blood 2002; 100:1910–12

602. van den Heuvel-Eibrink MM, Sonneveld P, Pieters R. The prognostic significance of membrane transport-associated multidrug resistance (MDR) proteins in leukemia. Int J Clin Pharmacol Ther 2000;38: 94–110

603. el Rouby S, et al. p53 gene mutation in B-cell chronic lymphocytic leukemia is associated with drug resistance and is independent of MDR1/MDR3 gene expression. Blood 1993;82:3452–9

604. Yamaguchi M, et al. Frequent expression of P-glycoprotein/MDR1 by nasal T-cell lymphoma cells. Cancer 1995;76:2351–6

605. Grier DG, et al. The pathophysiology of HOX genes and their role in cancer. J Pathol 2005;205:154–71

606. Schoch C, et al. AML with 11q23/MLL abnormalities as defined by the WHO classification: incidence, partner chromosomes, FAB subtype, age distribution, and prognostic impact in an unselected series of 1897 cytogenetically analyzed AML cases. Blood 2003; 102:2395–402

607. Hilden JM, Kersey JH. The MLL (11q23) and AF-4 (4q21) genes disrupted in t(4;11) acute leukemia: molecular and clinical studies. Leuk Lymphoma 1994;14:189–95

608. Harrison CJ. The detection and significance of chromosomal abnormalities in childhood acute lymphoblastic leukaemia. Blood Rev 2001;15:49–59

609. Pui CH, et al. Improved outcome for children with acute lymphoblastic leukemia: results of Total Therapy Study XIIIB at St Jude Children's Research Hospital. Blood 2004;104:2690–6

610. Falini B, et al. A monoclonal antibody (MUM1p) detects expression of the MUM1/IRF4 protein in a subset of germinal center B cells, plasma cells, and activated T cells. Blood 2000;95:2084–92

611. Tsuboi K, et al. MUM1/IRF4 expression as a frequent event in mature lymphoid malignancies. Leukemia 2000;14:449–56

612. Natkunam Y, et al. Analysis of MUM1/IRF4 protein expression using tissue microarrays and immunohistochemistry. Mod Pathol 2001;14:686–94

613. Hans CP, et al. Confirmation of the molecular classification of diffuse large B-cell lymphoma by immunohistochemistry using a tissue microarray. Blood 2003

614. Boxer LM, Dang CV. Translocations involving c-myc and c-myc function. Oncogene 2001;20:5595–610

615. Taub R, et al. Translocation of the c-myc gene into the immunoglobulin heavy chain locus in human Burkitt lymphoma and murine plasmacytoma cells. Proc Natl Acad Sci USA 1982;79:7837–41

616. Kramer MH, et al. Clinical relevance of BCL2, BCL6, and MYC rearrangements in diffuse large B-cell lymphoma. Blood 1998;92:3152–62

617. Chang CC, et al. Expression of c-Myc and p53 correlates with clinical outcome in diffuse large B-cell lymphomas. Am J Clin Pathol 2000;113:512–18

618. Pagnano KB, et al. p53, Mdm2, and c-Myc overexpression is associated with a poor prognosis in aggressive non-Hodgkin's lymphomas. Am J Hematol 2001;67:84–92

619. Nagy B, et al. Abnormal expression of apoptosis-related genes in haematological malignancies: overexpression of MYC is poor prognostic sign in mantle cell lymphoma. Br J Haematol 2003;120: 434–41

620. Morris SW, et al. Fusion of a kinase gene, ALK, to a nucleolar protein gene, NPM, in non-Hodgkin's lymphoma. Science 1994;263:1281–4

621. Redner RL, et al. The t(5;17) variant of acute promyelocytic leukemia expresses a nucleophosmin–retinoic acid receptor fusion. Blood 1996;87:882–6

622. Yoneda-Kato N, et al. The t(3;5)(q25.1;q34) of myelodysplastic syndrome and acute myeloid leukemia produces a novel fusion gene, NPM–MLF1. Oncogene 1996;12:265–75

623. Falini B, et al. Cytoplasmic nucleophosmin in acute myelogenous leukemia with a normal karyotype. N Engl J Med 2005;352:254–66

624. Maier H, Hagman J. Roles of EBF and Pax-5 in B lineage commitment and development. Semin Immunol 2002;14:415–22

625. Busslinger M, Urbanek P. The role of BSAP (Pax-5) in B-cell development. Curr Opin Genet Dev 1995; 5:595–601

626. Iida S, et al. The t(9;14)(p13;q32) chromosomal translocation associated with lymphoplasmacytoid lymphoma involves the PAX-5 gene. Blood 1996;88: 4110–7

627. Amakawa R, Ohno H, Fukuhara S. t(9;14)(p13;q32) involving the PAX-5 gene: a unique subtype of 14q32 translocation in B cell non-Hodgkin's lymphoma. Int J Hematol 1999;69:65–9

628. Morrison AM, et al. Deregulated PAX-5 transcription from a translocated IgH promoter in marginal zone lymphoma. Blood 1998;92:3865–78

629. Gurrieri C, et al. Mutations of the PML tumor suppressor gene in acute promyelocytic leukemia. Blood 2004;103:2358–62

630. Radich JP, et al. N-ras mutations in adult de novo acute myelogenous leukemia: prevalence and clinical significance. Blood 1990;76:801–7

631. Neubauer A, et al. Prognostic importance of mutations in the ras proto-oncogenes in de novo acute myeloid leukemia. Blood 1994;83:1603–11

632. Coghlan DW, et al. The incidence and prognostic significance of mutations in codon 13 of the N-ras gene in acute myeloid leukemia. Leukemia 1994;8:1682–7

633. Rasmussen T, et al. Possible roles for activating RAS mutations in the MGUS to MM transition and in the intramedullary to extramedullary transition in some plasma cell tumors. Blood 2005;105:317–23

634. Godbout R, et al. Somatic inactivation of genes on chromosome 13 is a common event in retinoblastoma. Nature 1983;304:451–3

635. Zhu YM, et al. Abnormalities of retinoblastoma gene expression in hematological malignancies. Leuk Lymphoma 1995;18:61–7

636. Jamal R, et al. The retinoblastoma gene (rb1) in acute myeloid leukaemia: analysis of gene rearrangements, protein expression and comparison of disease outcome. Br J Haematol 1996;94:342–51

637. Sanchez-Beato M, et al. Anomalous retinoblastoma protein expression in Sternberg–Reed cells in Hodgkin's disease: a comparative study with p53 and Ki67 expression. Br J Cancer 1996;74:1056–62

638. Krug U, Ganser A, Koeffler HP. Tumor suppressor genes in normal and malignant hematopoiesis. Oncogene 2002;21:3475–95

639. Tsai T, et al. Tumor suppressor gene alteration in adult acute lymphoblastic leukemia (ALL). Analysis of retinoblastoma (Rb) and p53 gene expression in lymphoblasts of patients with de novo, relapsed, or refractory ALL treated in Southwest Oncology Group studies. Leukemia 1996;10:1901–10

640. Rassidakis GZ, et al. Retinoblastoma protein is frequently absent or phosphorylated in anaplastic large-cell lymphoma. Am J Pathol 2004;164:2259–67

641. Sauerbrey A, et al. Expression of the retinoblastoma tumor suppressor gene (RB-1) in acute leukemia. Leuk Lymphoma 1998;28:275–83

642. Miyoshi H, et al. t(8;21) breakpoints on chromosome 21 in acute myeloid leukemia are clustered within a limited region of a single gene, AML1. Proc Natl Acad Sci USA 1991;88:10431–4

643. Zhang Y, et al. PRDX4, a member of the peroxiredoxin family, is fused to AML1 (RUNX1) in an acute myeloid leukemia patient with a t(X;21)(p22;q22). Genes Chromosomes Cancer 2004;40:365–70

644. Ramsey H, Christopherson K, Hromas R. Forced expression of AML1–AMP19, a fusion transcript generated from a radiation-associated t(19;21) leukemia, blocks myeloid differentiation. Leuk Res 2004;28:863–8

645. Mitani K, et al. Generation of the AML1-EVI-1 fusion gene in the t(3;21)(q26;q22) causes blastic crisis in chronic myelocytic leukemia. Embo J 1994;13:504–10

646. Golub TR, et al. Fusion of the TEL gene on 12p13 to the AML1 gene on 21q22 in acute lymphoblastic leukemia. Proc Natl Acad Sci USA 1995;92:4917–21

647. Steensma DP, et al. Somatic point mutations in RUNX1/CBFA2/AML1 are common in high-risk myelodysplastic syndrome, but not in myelofibrosis with myeloid metaplasia. Eur J Haematol 2005;74:47–53

648. Taketani T, et al. AML1/RUNX1 mutations are infrequent, but related to AML-M0, acquired trisomy 21, and leukemic transformation in pediatric hematologic malignancies. Genes Chromosomes Cancer 2003;38:1–7

649. Asakura K, et al. TEL/AML1 overcomes drug resistance through transcriptional repression of multidrug resistance-1 gene expression. Mol Cancer Res 2004;2:339–47

650. Attarbaschi A, et al. Incidence and relevance of secondary chromosome abnormalities in childhood TEL/AML1+ acute lymphoblastic leukemia: an interphase FISH analysis. Leukemia 2004;18:1611–16

651. Ramakers-van Woerden NL, et al. TEL/AML1 gene fusion is related to in vitro drug sensitivity for L-asparaginase in childhood acute lymphoblastic leukemia. Blood 2000;96:1094–9

652. Lane DP. Cancer. p53, guardian of the genome. Nature 1992;358:15–16

653. Lowe SW, et al. p53-dependent apoptosis modulates the cytotoxicity of anticancer agents. Cell 1993;74:957–67

654. Vogelstein B, Kinzler KW. p53 function and dysfunction. Cell 1992;70:523–6

655. Soussi T, Beroud C. Assessing TP53 status in human tumours to evaluate clinical outcome. Nat Rev Cancer 2001;1:233–40

656. Aguilar-Santelises M, et al. Bcl-2, Bax and p53 expression in B-CLL in relation to in vitro survival and clinical progression. Int J Cancer 1996;69:114–19

657. Dohner H, et al. p53 gene deletion predicts for poor survival and non-response to therapy with purine analogs in chronic B-cell leukemias. Blood 1995;85:1580–9

658. Sturm I, et al. Mutation of p53 and consecutive selective drug resistance in B-CLL occurs as a consequence of prior DNA-damaging chemotherapy. Cell Death Differ 2003;10:477–84

659. Wattel E, et al. p53 mutations are associated with resistance to chemotherapy and short survival in hematologic malignancies. Blood 1994;84:3148–57

660. Lozanski G, et al. Alemtuzumab is an effective therapy for chronic lymphocytic leukemia with p53 mutations and deletions. Blood 2004;103:3278–81

661. Carter A, et al. Detection of p53 dysfunction by flow cytometry in chronic lymphocytic leukaemia. Br J Haematol 2004;127:425–8

662. Baldini L, et al. Poor prognosis in non-villous splenic marginal zone cell lymphoma is associated with p53 mutations. Br J Haematol 1997;99:375–8

663. Greiner TC, et al. p53 mutations in mantle cell lymphoma are associated with variant cytology and predict a poor prognosis. Blood 1996;87:4302–10

664. Sanchez-Beato M, et al. Overall survival in aggressive B-cell lymphomas is dependent on the accumulation of alterations in p53, p16, and p27. Am J Pathol 2001;159:205–13

665. Moller MB, et al. Aberrations of the p53 pathway components p53, MDM2 and CDKN2A appear independent in diffuse large B cell lymphoma. Leukemia 1999;13:453–9

666. Ichikawa A, et al. Mutations of the p53 gene as a prognostic factor in aggressive B-cell lymphoma. N Engl J Med 1997;337:529–34

667. Ichikawa A. Prognostic and predictive significance of p53 mutation in aggressive B-cell lymphoma. Int J Hematol 2000;71:211–20

668. Kerbauy F, et al. Detection and possible prognostic relevance of p53 gene mutations in diffuse large B-cell lymphoma. An analysis of 51 cases and review of the literature. Leuk Lymphoma 2004;45:2071–8

669. Chang H, et al. p53 gene deletion detected by fluorescence in situ hybridization is an adverse prognostic factor for patients with multiple myeloma following autologous stem cell transplantation. Blood 2005;105:358–60

670. Pescarmona E, et al. p53 over-expression identifies a subset of nodal peripheral T-cell lymphomas with a distinctive biological profile and poor clinical outcome. J Pathol 2001;195:361–6

671. Stevenson F, et al. Insight into the origin and clonal history of B-cell tumors as revealed by analysis of immunoglobulin variable region genes. Immunol Rev 1998;162:247–59

672. Oscier DG, et al. Multivariate analysis of prognostic factors in CLL: clinical stage, IGVH gene mutational status, and loss or mutation of the p53 gene are independent prognostic factors. Blood 2002;100:1177–84

673. Hamblin TJ, et al. Immunoglobulin V genes and CD38 expression in CLL. Blood 2000;95:2455–7

674. Kienle D, et al. VH mutation status and VDJ rearrangement structure in mantle cell lymphoma: correlation with genomic aberrations, clinical characteristics, and outcome. Blood 2003;102:3003–9

675. Galimberti S, et al. Significant co-expression of WT1 and MDR1 genes in acute myeloid leukemia patients at diagnosis. Eur J Haematol 2004;72:45–51

676. Karnan S, et al. Analysis of chromosomal imbalances in de novo CD5-positive diffuse large-B-cell lymphoma detected by comparative genomic hybridization. Genes Chromosomes Cancer 2004;39:77–81

677. Kita K, et al. Clinical importance of CD7 expression in acute myelocytic leukemia. The Japan Cooperative Group of Leukemia/Lymphoma. Blood 1993;81:2399–405

678. Jensen AW, et al. Solitary expression of CD7 among T-cell antigens in acute myeloid leukemia: identification of a group of patients with similar T-cell receptor beta and delta rearrangements and course of disease suggestive of poor prognosis. Blood 1991;78:1292–300

679. Consolini R, et al. Clinical relevance of CD10 expression in childhood ALL. The Italian Association for

Pediatric Hematology and Oncology (AIEOP). Haematologica 1998;83:967–73

680. Bai M, et al. Increased expression of the bcl6 and CD10 proteins is associated with increased apoptosis and proliferation in diffuse large B-cell lymphomas. Mod Pathol 2003;16:471–80

681. Bilalovic N, et al. Expression of bcl-6 and CD10 protein is associated with longer overall survival and time to treatment failure in follicular lymphoma. Am J Clin Pathol 2004;121:34–42

682. Ohshima K, et al. CD10 and Bcl10 expression in diffuse large B-cell lymphoma: CD10 is a marker of improved prognosis. Histopathology 2001;39:156–62

683. Zhang X, et al. Comparison of genetic aberrations in CD10+ diffused large B-cell lymphoma and follicular lymphoma by comparative genomic hybridization and tissue-fluorescence in situ hybridization. Cancer Sci 2004;95:809–14

684. Jardin F, et al. Follicular lymphoma without t(14;18) and with BCL-6 rearrangement: a lymphoma subtype with distinct pathological, molecular and clinical characteristics. Leukemia 2002;16:2309–17

685. Kurec AS, et al. Significance of aberrant immunophenotypes in childhood acute lymphoid leukemia. Cancer 1991;67:3081–6

686. Pui CH, et al. Characterization of childhood acute leukemia with multiple myeloid and lymphoid markers at diagnosis and at relapse. Blood 1991;78:1327–37

687. Wiersma SR, et al. Clinical importance of myeloid-antigen expression in acute lymphoblastic leukemia of childhood. N Engl J Med 1991;324:800–8

688. Uckun FM, et al. Clinical features and treatment outcome of children with myeloid antigen positive acute lymphoblastic leukemia: a report from the Children's Cancer Group. Blood 1997;90:28–35

689. Pui CH, et al. Myeloid-associated antigen expression lacks prognostic value in childhood acute lymphoblastic leukemia treated with intensive multiagent chemotherapy. Blood 1990;75:198–202

690. Hamann PR, et al. Gemtuzumab ozogamicin, a potent and selective anti-CD33 antibody–calicheamicin conjugate for treatment of acute myeloid leukemia. Bioconjug Chem 2002;13:47–58

691. Tomblyn MR, Tallman MS. New developments in antibody therapy for acute myeloid leukemia. Semin Oncol 2003;30:502–8

692. Lo-Coco F, et al. Gemtuzumab ozogamicin (Mylotarg) as a single agent for molecularly relapsed acute promyelocytic leukemia. Blood 2004;104:1995–9

693. Hiddemann W, Dreyling M, Unterhalt M. Rituximab plus chemotherapy in follicular and mantle cell lymphomas. Semin Oncol 2003; 30(Suppl 2):16–20

694. Coiffier B. Rituximab in the treatment of diffuse large B-cell lymphomas. Semin Oncol 2002;29(Suppl 2): 30–5

695. Hofmeister JK, Cooney D, Coggeshall KM. Clustered CD20 induced apoptosis: src-family kinase, the proximal regulator of tyrosine phosphorylation, calcium influx, and caspase 3-dependent apoptosis. Blood Cells Mol Dis 2000;26:133–43

696. Golay J, et al. Rituximab-mediated antibody-dependent cellular cytotoxicity against neoplastic B cells is stimulated strongly by interleukin-2. Haematologica 2003;88:1002–12

697. Golay J, et al. Biologic response of B lymphoma cells to anti-CD20 monoclonal antibody rituximab in vitro: CD55 and CD59 regulate complement-mediated cell lysis. Blood 2000;95:3900–8

698. Harjunpaa A, Junnikkala S, Meri S. Rituximab (anti-CD20) therapy of B-cell lymphomas: direct complement killing is superior to cellular effector mechanisms. Scand J Immunol 2000;51:634–41

699. Golay J, et al. CD20 levels determine the in vitro susceptibility to rituximab and complement of B-cell chronic lymphocytic leukemia: further regulation by CD55 and CD59. Blood 2001;98:3383–9

700. Weng WK, Levy R. Two immunoglobulin G fragment C receptor polymorphisms independently predict response to rituximab in patients with follicular lymphoma. J Clin Oncol 2003;21: 3940–7

701. Bohen SP, et al. Variation in gene expression patterns in follicular lymphoma and the response to rituximab. Proc Natl Acad Sci USA 2003;100:1926–30

702. Ghobrial I, et al. Prognostic factors in patients with post-transplant lymphoproliferative disorders (PTLD) in the rituximab era. Leuk Lymphoma 2005;46:191–6

703. Portlock CS, et al. Adverse prognostic significance of CD20 positive Reed–Sternberg cells in classical Hodgkin's disease. Br J Haematol 2004;125:701–8

704. Robillard N, et al. CD20 is associated with a small mature plasma cell morphology and t(11;14) in multiple myeloma. Blood 2003;102:1070–1

705. Ruiz-Arguelles GJ, San Miguel JF. Cell surface markers in multiple myeloma. Mayo Clin Proc 1994;69:684–90

706. San Miguel JF, et al. Immunophenotypic heterogeneity of multiple myeloma: influence on the biology and clinical course of the disease. Castellano-Leones (Spain) Cooperative Group for the Study of Monoclonal Gammopathies. Br J Haematol 1991;77:185–90

707. Stefanato CM, Tallini G, Crotty PL. Histologic and immunophenotypic features prior to transformation in patients with transformed cutaneous T-cell lymphoma: is CD25 expression in skin biopsy samples predictive of large cell transformation in cutaneous T-cell lymphoma? Am J Dermatopathol 1998;20:1–6

708. Jones D, et al. Degree of CD25 expression in T-cell lymphoma is dependent on tissue site: implications for targeted therapy. Clin Cancer Res 2004;10:5587–94

709. Mey U, et al. Advances in the treatment of hairy-cell leukaemia. Lancet Oncol 2003;4:86–94

710. Lauria F, Forconi F. Towards the pharmacotherapy of hairy cell leukaemia. Expert Opin Pharmacother 2004;5:1523–33

711. Falini B, et al. CD30 (Ki-1) molecule: a new cytokine receptor of the tumor necrosis factor receptor superfamily as a tool for diagnosis and immunotherapy. Blood 1995;85:1–14

712. Gardner LJ, et al. CD30 expression in follicular lymphoma. Arch Pathol Lab Med 2001;125:1036–41

713. de Bruin PC, et al. CD30 expression in normal and neoplastic lymphoid tissue: biological aspects and clinical implications. Leukemia 1995;9:1620–7

714. Miettinen M. CD30 distribution. Immunohistochemical study on formaldehyde-fixed, paraffin-embedded Hodgkin's and non-Hodgkin's lymphomas. Arch Pathol Lab Med 1992;116:1197–201

715. Al-Shamkhani A. The role of CD30 in the pathogenesis of haematopoietic malignancies. Curr Opin Pharmacol 2004;4:355–9

716. Borchmann P, et al. Monoclonal antibody-based immunotherapy of Hodgkin's lymphoma. Curr Opin Invest Drugs 2004;5:1262–7

717. Hombach A, Heuser C, Abken H. Simultaneous targeting of IL2 and IL12 to Hodgkin's lymphoma cells enhances activation of resting NK cells and tumor cell lysis. Int J Cancer 2005;115:241–7

718. Ciolli S, et al. CD34 expression fails to predict the outcome in adult acute myeloid leukemia. Haematologica 1993;78:151–5

719. Damle RN, et al. IgV gene mutation status and CD38 expression as novel prognostic indicators in chronic lymphocytic leukemia. Blood 1999;94:1840–7

720. Del Poeta G, et al. Clinical significance of CD38 expression in chronic lymphocytic leukemia. Blood 2001;98:2633–9

721. Hamblin TJ, et al. Unmutated IgV(H) genes are associated with a more aggressive form of chronic lymphocytic leukemia. Blood 1999;94:1848–54

722. Hamblin TJ, et al. CD38 expression and immunoglobulin variable region mutations are independent prognostic variables in chronic lymphocytic leukemia, but CD38 expression may vary during the course of the disease. Blood 2002;99:1023–9

723. Krober A, et al. V(H) mutation status, CD38 expression level, genomic aberrations, and survival in chronic lymphocytic leukemia. Blood 2002;100:1410–16

724. Drillenburg P, et al. CD44 expression predicts disease outcome in localized large B cell lymphoma. Leukemia 1999;13:1448–55

725. Villamor N, Montserrat E, Colomer D. Mechanism of action and resistance to monoclonal antibody therapy. Semin Oncol 2003;30:424–33

726. Dearden CE, Matutes E, Catovsky D. Alemtuzumab in T-cell malignancies. Med Oncol 2002;19(Suppl):S27–32

727. Cao TM, Coutre SE. T-cell prolymphocytic leukemia: update and focus on alemtuzumab (Campath-1H). Hematology 2003;8:1–6

728. Pangalis GA, et al. Campath-1H (anti-CD52) monoclonal antibody therapy in lymphoproliferative disorders. Med Oncol 2001;18:99–107

729. Dearden CE, Foss FM. Peripheral T-cell lymphomas: diagnosis and management. Hematol Oncol Clin North Am 2003;17:1351–66

730. Dearden CE, et al. High remission rate in T-cell prolymphocytic leukemia with CAMPATH-1H. Blood 2001;98:1721–6

731. Enblad G, et al. A pilot study of alemtuzumab (anti-CD52 monoclonal antibody) therapy for patients with relapsed or chemotherapy-refractory peripheral T-cell lymphomas. Blood 2004;103:2920–4

732. Baer MR, et al. Expression of the neural cell adhesion molecule CD56 is associated with short remission duration and survival in acute myeloid leukemia with t(8;21)(q22;q22). Blood 1997;90:1643–8

733. Murray CK, et al. CD56 expression in acute promyelocytic leukemia: a possible indicator of poor treatment outcome? J Clin Oncol 1999;17:293–7

734. Suzuki R, et al. Prognostic significance of CD56 expression for ALK-positive and ALK-negative anaplastic large-cell lymphoma of T/null cell phenotype. Blood 2000;96:2993–3000

735. Salhany KE, et al. Subcutaneous panniculitis-like T-cell lymphoma: clinicopathologic, immunophenotypic, and genotypic analysis of alpha/beta and gamma/delta subtypes. Am J Surg Pathol 1998;22:881–93

736. Takeshita M, et al. Clinicopathologic analysis of 22 cases of subcutaneous panniculitis-like CD56– or CD56+ lymphoma and review of 44 other reported cases. Am J Clin Pathol 2004;121:408–16

737. Van Camp B, et al. Plasma cells in multiple myeloma express a natural killer cell-associated antigen: CD56 (NKH-1; Leu-19). Blood 1990;76:377–82

738. Mathew P, et al. Clinicopathological correlates of CD56 expression in multiple myeloma: a unique entity? Br J Haematol 1995;90:459–61

739. Oyama T, et al. Senile EBV + B-cell lymphoproliferative disorders: a clinicopathologic study of 22 patients. Am J Surg Pathol 2003;27:16–26

740. Ansell SM, et al. Epstein–Barr virus infection in Richter's transformation. Am J Hematol 1999;60:99–104

741. Dutton A, et al. Expression of the cellular FLICE-inhibitory protein (c-FLIP) protects Hodgkin's lymphoma cells from autonomous Fas-mediated death. Proc Natl Acad Sci USA 2004;101:6611–16

742. Uherova P, et al. Expression of c-FLIP in classic and nodular lymphocyte-predominant Hodgkin lymphoma. Appl Immunohistochem Mol Morphol 2004;12:105–10

743. Valnet-Rabier MB, et al. c-Flip protein expression in Burkitt's lymphomas is associated with a poor clinical outcome. Br J Haematol 2005;128:767–73

744. Medeiros LJ, et al. Major histocompatibility complex class I and class II antigen expression in diffuse large cell and large cell immunoblastic lymphomas. Absence of a correlation between antigen expression and clinical outcome. Am J Pathol 1993;143:1086–97

745. Darom A, et al. HLA-DR antigen and bax protein expression in patients with primary non-Hodgkin's gastric lymphoma. Hybrid Hybridomics 2004;23:87–92

746. Miller TP, et al. HLA-DR (Ia) immune phenotype predicts outcome for patients with diffuse large cell lymphoma. J Clin Invest 1988;82:370–2

747. Rimsza LM, et al. Loss of MHC class II gene and protein expression in diffuse large B cell lymphoma is related to decreased tumor immunosurveillance and poor patient survival irrespective of other prognostic factors: A follow-up study from the Leukemia and Lymphoma Molecular Profiling Project. Blood 2004

748. Ambrosini G, Adida C, Altieri DC. A novel anti-apoptosis gene, survivin, expressed in cancer and lymphoma. Nat Med 1997;3:917–21

749. Martinez A, et al. Nuclear survivin expression in mantle cell lymphoma is associated with cell proliferation and survival. Am J Pathol 2004;164:501–10

750. Nakayama K, Kamihira S. Survivin an important determinant for prognosis in adult T-cell leukemia: a novel biomarker in practical hemato-oncology. Leuk Lymphoma 2002;43:2249–55

751. Schlette EJ, et al. Survivin expression predicts poorer prognosis in anaplastic large-cell lymphoma. J Clin Oncol 2004;22:1682–8

752. Crespo M, et al. ZAP-70 expression as a surrogate for immunoglobulin-variable-region mutations in chronic lymphocytic leukemia. N Engl J Med 2003;348:1764–75

753. Orchard JA, et al. ZAP-70 expression and prognosis in chronic lymphocytic leukaemia. Lancet 2004;363:105–11

754. Durig J, et al. ZAP-70 expression is a prognostic factor in chronic lymphocytic leukemia. Leukemia 2003;17:2426–34

755. Rassenti LZ, et al. ZAP-70 compared with immunoglobulin heavy-chain gene mutation status as a predictor of disease progression in chronic lymphocytic leukemia. N Engl J Med 2004;351:893–901

756. Carreras J, et al. Immunohistochemical analysis of ZAP-70 expression in B-cell lymphoid neoplasms. J Pathol 2005;205:507–13

757. Montillo M, et al. Chronic lymphocytic leukemia: novel prognostic factors and their relevance for risk-adapted therapeutic strategies. Haematologica 2005;90:391–9

758. Giles FJ, et al. A prognostic model for survival in chronic lymphocytic leukaemia based on p53 expression. Br J Haematol 2003;121:578–85

759. Lin K, et al. Relationship between p53 dysfunction, CD38 expression, and IgV(H) mutation in chronic lymphocytic leukemia. Blood 2002;100:1404–9

760. Montserrat E. Treatment options in chronic lymphocytic leukemia. Hematol J 2004;5(Suppl 1):S2–9

761. Zinzani PL, et al. Fludarabine in patients with advanced and/or resistant B-chronic lymphocytic leukemia. Eur J Haematol 1993;51:93–7

762. Montserrat E, et al. Fludarabine in resistant or relapsing B-cell chronic lymphocytic leukemia: the Spanish Group experience. Leuk Lymphoma 1996;21:467–72

763. Bosch F, et al. Fludarabine, cyclophosphamide and mitoxantrone in the treatment of resistant or relapsed chronic lymphocytic leukaemia. Br J Haematol 2002; 119:976–84

764. Montserrat E. Rituximab in chronic lymphocytic leukemia. Semin Oncol 2003;30(Suppl 2):34–9

765. Keating MJ. Chronic lymphocytic leukemia. Semin Oncol 1999;26(Suppl 14):107–14

766. Hallek M, et al. Serum beta(2)-microglobulin and serum thymidine kinase are independent predictors of progression-free survival in chronic lymphocytic leukemia and immunocytoma. Leuk Lymphoma 1996;22:439–47

767. Ibrahim S, et al. CD38 expression as an important prognostic factor in B-cell chronic lymphocytic leukemia. Blood 2001;98:181–6

768. Molica S, et al. Clinico-prognostic implications of simultaneous increased serum levels of soluble CD23 and beta2-microglobulin in B-cell chronic lymphocytic leukemia. Eur J Haematol 1999;62:117–22

769. Knauf WU, et al. Serum levels of soluble CD23, but not soluble CD25, predict disease progression in early stage B-cell chronic lymphocytic leukemia. Leuk Lymphoma 1997;27:523–32

770. Apostolopoulos A, Symeonidis A, Zoumbos N. Prognostic significance of immune function parameters in patients with chronic lymphocytic leukaemia. Eur J Haematol 1990;44:39–44

771. Keating MJ, et al. Long-term follow-up of patients with chronic lymphocytic leukemia (CLL) receiving fludarabine regimens as initial therapy. Blood 1998; 92:1165–71

772. Matutes E, et al. Trisomy 12 defines a group of CLL with atypical morphology: correlation between cytogenetic, clinical and laboratory features in 544 patients. Br J Haematol 1996;92:382–8

773. Geisler CH, Philip P, Hansen MM. B-cell chronic lymphocytic leukaemia: clonal chromosome abnormalities and prognosis in 89 cases. Eur J Haematol 1989;43:397–403

774. Oscier DG, et al. Atypical lymphocyte morphology: an adverse prognostic factor for disease progression in stage A CLL independent of trisomy 12. Br J Haematol 1997;98:934–9

775. Rozman C, et al. Bone marrow histologic pattern – the best single prognostic parameter in chronic lymphocytic leukemia: a multivariate survival analysis of 329 cases. Blood 1984;64:642–8

776. Mauro FR, et al. Prognostic value of bone marrow histology in chronic lymphocytic leukemia. A study of 335 untreated cases from a single institution. Haematologica 1994;79:334–41

777. Oudat R, et al. Significance of the levels of bone marrow lymphoid infiltrate in chronic lymphocytic leukemia patients with nodular partial remission. Leukemia 2002;16:632–5

778. Capello D, et al. Distribution and pattern of BCL-6 mutations throughout the spectrum of B-cell neoplasia. Blood 2000;95:651–9

779. Maloum K, et al. Expression of unmutated VH genes is a detrimental prognostic factor in chronic lymphocytic leukemia. Blood 2000;96:377–9

780. Fais F, et al. Chronic lymphocytic leukemia B cells express restricted sets of mutated and unmutated antigen receptors. J Clin Invest 1998;102: 1515–25

781. Thornton PD, et al. Characterisation of TP53 abnormalities in chronic lymphocytic leukaemia. Hematol J 2004;5:47–54

782. Tobin G, et al. Somatically mutated IgV(H)3-21 genes characterize a new subset of chronic lymphocytic leukemia. Blood 2002;99:2262–4

783. Tobin G, et al. Chronic lymphocytic leukemias utilizing the VH3-21 gene display highly restricted Vlambda2-14 gene use and homologous CDR3s: implicating recognition of a common antigen epitope. Blood 2003;101:4952–7

784. Iwashima M, et al. Sequential interactions of the TCR with two distinct cytoplasmic tyrosine kinases. Science 1994;263:1136–9

785. Chen L, et al. Expression of ZAP-70 is associated with increased B-cell receptor signaling in chronic lymphocytic leukemia. Blood 2002;100:4609–14

786. Wiestner A, et al. ZAP-70 expression identifies a chronic lymphocytic leukemia subtype with unmutated immunoglobulin genes, inferior clinical outcome, and distinct gene expression profile. Blood 2003;101:4944–51

787. Nuckel H, et al. HLA-G expression is associated with an unfavorable outcome and immunodeficiency in chronic lymphocytic leukemia. Blood 2005;105: 1694–8

788. Geisler CH, et al. Prognostic importance of flow cytometric immunophenotyping of 540 consecutive patients with B-cell chronic lymphocytic leukemia. Blood 1991;78:1795–802

789. Bea S, et al. Genetic imbalances in progressed B-cell chronic lymphocytic leukemia and transformed large-cell lymphoma (Richter's syndrome). Am J Pathol 2002;161:957–68

790. Juliusson G, et al. Prognostic subgroups in B-cell chronic lymphocytic leukemia defined by specific chromosomal abnormalities. N Engl J Med 1990; 323:720–4

791. Criel A, et al. Trisomy 12 is uncommon in typical chronic lymphocytic leukaemias. Br J Haematol 1994;87:523–8

792. O'Connor SJ, et al. The relationship between typical and atypical B-cell chronic lymphocytic leukemia. A comparative genomic hybridization-based study. Am J Clin Pathol 2000;114:448–58

793. Criel A, Michaux L, De Wolf-Peeters C. The concept of typical and atypical chronic lymphocytic leukaemia. Leuk Lymphoma 1999;33:33–45

794. Bigoni R, et al. Chromosome aberrations in atypical chronic lymphocytic leukemia: a cytogenetic and interphase cytogenetic study. Leukemia 1997;11:1933–40

795. Stilgenbauer S, Lichter P, Dohner H. Genetic features of B-cell chronic lymphocytic leukemia. Rev Clin Exp Hematol 2000;4:48–72

796. Stilgenbauer S, et al. Genetics of chronic lymphocytic leukemia: genomic aberrations and V(H) gene mutation status in pathogenesis and clinical course. Leukemia 2002;16:993–1007

797. Neilson JR, et al. Deletions at 11q identify a subset of patients with typical CLL who show consistent disease progression and reduced survival. Leukemia 1997;11:1929–32

798. Criel A, et al. Further characterization of morphologically defined typical and atypical CLL: a clinical, immunophenotypic, cytogenetic and prognostic study on 390 cases. Br J Haematol 1997;97:383–91

799. Matutes E. Trisomy 12 in chronic lymphocytic leukaemia. Leuk Res 1996;20:375–7

800. Hernandez JM, et al. Cytogenetic analysis of B cell chronic lymphoid leukemias classified according to morphologic and immunophenotypic (FAB) criteria. Leukemia 1995;9:2140–6

801. Juliusson G, Gahrton G. Chromosome aberrations in B-cell chronic lymphocytic leukemia. Pathogenetic and clinical implications. Cancer Genet Cytogenet 1990;45:143–60

802. Escudier SM, et al. Fluorescent in situ hybridization and cytogenetic studies of trisomy 12 in chronic lymphocytic leukemia. Blood 1993;81:2702–7

803. Auer RL, et al. The sequential analysis of trisomy 12 in B-cell chronic lymphocytic leukaemia. Br J Haematol 1999;104:742–4

804. Robertson LE, et al. Richter's syndrome: a report on 39 patients. J Clin Oncol 1993;11:1985–9

805. Kjeldsberg CR, Marty J. Prolymphocytic transformation of chronic lymphocytic leukemia. Cancer 1981;48:2447–57

806. Enno A, et al. 'Prolymphocytoid' transformation of chronic lymphocytic leukaemia. Br J Haematol 1979;41:9–18

807. Pugh WC, Manning JT, Butler JJ. Paraimmunoblastic variant of small lymphocytic lymphoma/leukemia. Am J Surg Pathol 1988;12:907–17

808. Ohno T, et al. Origin of the Hodgkin/Reed–Sternberg cells in chronic lymphocytic leukemia with 'Hodgkin's transformation'. Blood 1998;91:1757–61

809. Williams J, et al. Chronic lymphocytic leukemia with coexistent Hodgkin's disease. Implications for the origin of the Reed–Sternberg cell. Am J Surg Pathol 1991;15:33–42

810. Brecher M, Banks PM. Hodgkin's disease variant of Richter's syndrome. Report of eight cases. Am J Clin Pathol 1990;93:333–9

811. Momose H, et al. Chronic lymphocytic leukemia/small lymphocytic lymphoma with Reed–Sternberg-like cells and possible transformation to Hodgkin's disease. Mediation by Epstein–Barr virus. Am J Surg Pathol 1992;16:859–67

812. Kanzler H, et al. Hodgkin and Reed–Sternberg-like cells in B-cell chronic lymphocytic leukemia represent the outgrowth of single germinal-center B-cell-derived clones: potential precursors of Hodgkin and Reed–Sternberg cells in Hodgkin's disease. Blood 2000;95:1023–31

813. Tsimberidou AM, Keating MJ. Richter syndrome: biology, incidence, and therapeutic strategies. Cancer 2005;103:216–28

814. Wiernik PH. Second neoplasms in patients with chronic lymphocytic leukemia. Curr Treat Options Oncol 2004;5:215–23

815. Harousseau JL, et al. Malignant lymphoma supervening in chronic lymphocytic leukemia and related disorders. Richter's syndrome: a study of 25 cases. Cancer 1981;48:1302–8

816. Travis LB, et al. Second cancers following non-Hodgkin's lymphoma. Cancer 1991;67:2002–9

817. Torelli UL, et al. Simultaneously increased expression of the c-Myc and mu chain genes in the acute blastic transformation of a chronic lymphocytic leukaemia. Br J Haematol 1987;65:165–70

818. Pangalis GA, et al. B-chronic lymphocytic leukemia, small lymphocytic lymphoma, and lymphoplasmacytic lymphoma, including Waldenström's macroglobulinemia: a clinical, morphologic, and biologic spectrum of similar disorders. Semin Hematol 1999;36:104–14

819. Han T, et al. Prognostic significance of karyotypic abnormalities in B cell chronic lymphocytic leukemia: an update. Semin Hematol 1987;24:257–63

820. Oscier D, et al. Karyotypic evolution in B-cell chronic lymphocytic leukaemia. Genes Chromosomes Cancer 1991;3:16–20

821. Fegan C, et al. Karyotypic evolution in CLL: identification of a new sub-group of patients with deletions of 11q and advanced or progressive disease. Leukemia 1995;9:2003–8

822. Palestro G, et al. Cell proliferation, bcl-2, c-myc, p53 and apoptosis as indicators of different aggressiveness in small lymphocytic lymphoma (SLL). Eur J Haematol 1997;59:148–54

823. Hercher C, et al. A multicentric study of 41 cases of B-prolymphocytic leukemia: two evolutive forms. Leuk Lymphoma 2001;42:981–7

824. Shvidel L, et al. B-cell prolymphocytic leukemia: a survey of 35 patients emphasizing heterogeneity, prognostic factors and evidence for a group with an indolent course. Leuk Lymphoma 1999;33:169–79

825. Lens D, et al. p53 abnormalities in B-cell prolymphocytic leukemia. Blood 1997;89:2015–23

826. Goodman GR, Bethel KJ, Saven A. Hairy cell leukemia: an update. Curr Opin Hematol 2003;10:258–66

827. Platanias LC, Golomb HM. Hairy cell leukaemia. Baillières Clin Haematol 1993;6:887–98

828. Frassoldati A, et al. Hairy cell leukemia: a clinical review based on 725 cases of the Italian Cooperative Group (ICGHCL). Italian Cooperative Group for Hairy Cell Leukemia. Leuk Lymphoma 1994;13:307–16

829. Federico M, et al. Hairy cell leukemia: the Italian Cooperative Group experience. Leukemia 1992;6(Suppl 4):147–8

830. Goodman GR, et al. Extended follow-up of patients with hairy cell leukemia after treatment with cladribine. J Clin Oncol 2003;21:891–6

831. Jehn U, et al. An update: 12-year follow-up of patients with hairy cell leukemia following treatment with 2-chlorodeoxyadenosine. Leukemia 2004;18:1476–81

832. Vardiman JW, Golomb HM. Autopsy findings in hairy cell leukemia. Semin Oncol 1984;11:370–80

833. Malik ST, et al. Hairy cell leukemia – mediastinal involvement. A report of two cases and review of the literature. Hematol Oncol 1989;7:303–6

834. Kampmeier P, et al. Increased incidence of second neoplasms in patients treated with interferon alpha 2b for hairy cell leukemia: a clinicopathologic assessment. Blood 1994;83:2931–8

835. Rice L, et al. Granulomatous infections complicating hairy cell leukemia. Cancer 1982;49:1924–8

836. Jacobs RH, Vokes EE, Golomb HM. Second malignancies in hairy cell leukemia. Cancer 1985;56:1462–7

837. Flinn IW, et al. Long-term follow-up of remission duration, mortality, and second malignancies in hairy cell leukemia patients treated with pentostatin. Blood 2000;96:2981–6

838. Horning SJ. Natural history of and therapy for the indolent non-Hodgkin's lymphomas. Semin Oncol 1993;20(Suppl 5):75–88

839. Yuen AR, et al. Long-term survival after histologic transformation of low-grade follicular lymphoma. J Clin Oncol 1995;13:1726–33

840. Soubeyran P, et al. Follicular lymphomas – a review of treatment modalities. Crit Rev Oncol Hematol 2000; 35:13–32

841. Gallagher CJ, et al. Follicular lymphoma: prognostic factors for response and survival. J Clin Oncol 1986; 4:1470–80

842. Soubeyran P, et al. Low-grade follicular lymphomas: analysis of prognosis in a series of 281 patients. Eur J Cancer 1991;27:1606–13

843. Bastion Y, et al. Follicular lymphomas: assessment of prognostic factors in 127 patients followed for 10 years. Ann Oncol 1991;2(Suppl 2):123–9

844. Decaudin D, et al. Low-grade stage III–IV follicular lymphoma: multivariate analysis of prognostic factors in 484 patients – a study of the groupe d'Etude des lymphomes de l'Adulte. J Clin Oncol 1999;17: 2499–505

845. Cameron DA, et al. Identification of prognostic groups in follicular lymphoma. The Scotland and Newcastle Lymphoma Group Therapy Working Party. Leuk Lymphoma 1993;10:89–99

846. Federico M, et al. Prognosis of follicular lymphoma: a predictive model based on a retrospective analysis of 987 cases. Intergruppo Italiano Linfomi. Blood 2000;95:783–9

847. Maartense E, et al. Age-related differences among patients with follicular lymphoma and the importance of prognostic scoring systems: analysis from a population-based non-Hodgkin's lymphoma registry. Ann Oncol 2002;13:1275–84

848. Advani R, Rosenberg SA, Horning SJ. Stage I and II follicular non-Hodgkin's lymphoma: long-term follow-up of no initial therapy. J Clin Oncol 2004; 22:1454–9

849. Toze CL, et al. Long-term disease-free survival of patients with advanced follicular lymphoma after allogeneic bone marrow transplantation. Br J Haematol 2004;127:311–21

850. Canioni D, et al. Bone marrow histological patterns can predict survival of patients with grade 1 or 2 follicular lymphoma: a study from the Groupe d'Etude des Lymphomes Folliculaires. Br J Haematol 2004;126:364–71

851. Goodlad JR, et al. Primary cutaneous follicular lymphoma: a clinicopathologic and molecular study of 16 cases in support of a distinct entity. Am J Surg Pathol 2002;26:733–41

852. Goodlad JR, et al. Extranodal follicular lymphoma: a clinicopathological and genetic analysis of 15 cases arising at non-cutaneous extranodal sites. Histopathology 2004;44:268–76

853. Shia J, et al. Primary follicular lymphoma of the gastrointestinal tract: a clinical and pathologic study of 26 cases. Am J Surg Pathol 2002;26:216–24

854. Hans CP, et al. A significant diffuse component predicts for inferior survival in grade 3 follicular lymphoma, but cytologic subtypes do not predict survival. Blood 2003;101:2363–7

855. Hsi ED, et al. A clinicopathologic evaluation of follicular lymphoma grade 3A versus grade 3B reveals no survival differences. Arch Pathol Lab Med 2004; 128:863–8

856. Katzenberger T, et al. Cytogenetic alterations affecting BCL6 are predominantly found in follicular lymphomas grade 3B with a diffuse large B-cell component. Am J Pathol 2004;165:481–90

857. Llanos M, et al. Prognostic significance of Ki-67 nuclear proliferative antigen, bcl-2 protein, and p53 expression in follicular and diffuse large B-cell lymphoma. Med Oncol 2001;18:15–22

858. Yunis JJ, et al. Distinctive chromosomal abnormalities in histologic subtypes of non-Hodgkin's lymphoma. N Engl J Med 1982;307:1231–6

859. Horsman DE, et al. Analysis of secondary chromosomal alterations in 165 cases of follicular lymphoma with t(14;18). Genes Chromosomes Cancer 2001;30: 375–82

860. Lestou VS, et al. Multicolour fluorescence in situ hybridization analysis of t(14;18)-positive follicular lymphoma and correlation with gene expression data and clinical outcome. Br J Haematol 2003;122:745–59

861. Hubbard SM, et al. Histologic progression in non-Hodgkin's lymphoma. Blood 1982;59:258–64

862. Horning SJ, Rosenberg SA. The natural history of initially untreated low-grade non-Hodgkin's lymphomas. N Engl J Med 1984;311:1471–5

863. Bastion Y, et al. Incidence, predictive factors, and outcome of lymphoma transformation in follicular lymphoma patients. J Clin Oncol 1997;15:1587–94

864. Ersboll J, et al. Follicular low-grade non-Hodgkin's lymphoma: long-term outcome with or without tumor progression. Eur J Haematol 1989;42:155–63

865. Acker B, et al. Histologic conversion in the non-Hodgkin's lymphomas. J Clin Oncol 1983;1:11–16

866. Lee JT, Innes DJ Jr, Williams ME. Sequential bcl-2 and c-myc oncogene rearrangements associated with the clinical transformation of non-Hodgkin's lymphoma. J Clin Invest 1989;84:1454–9

867. Natkunam Y, et al. Blastic/blastoid transformation of follicular lymphoma: immunohistologic and molecular analyses of five cases. Am J Surg Pathol 2000;24:525–34

868. de Jong D, et al. Activation of the c-myc oncogene in a precursor-B-cell blast crisis of follicular lymphoma, presenting as composite lymphoma. N Engl J Med 1988;318:1373–8

869. Kroft SH, et al. Precursor B-lymphoblastic transformation of grade I follicle center lymphoma. Am J Clin Pathol 2000;113:411–18

870. Nagy M, et al. Genetic instability is associated with histological transformation of follicle center lymphoma. Leukemia 2000;14:2142–8

871. Yunis JJ, et al. Multiple recurrent genomic defects in follicular lymphoma. A possible model for cancer. N Engl J Med 1987;316:79–84

872. Armitage JO, et al. Correlation of secondary cytogenetic abnormalities with histologic appearance in non-Hodgkin's lymphomas bearing t(14;18)(q32;q21). J Natl Cancer Inst 1988;80:576–80

873. Richardson ME, et al. Intermediate- to high-grade histology of lymphomas carrying t(14;18) is associated with additional nonrandom chromosome changes. Blood 1987;70:444–7

874. Yano T, et al. MYC rearrangements in histologically progressed follicular lymphomas. Blood 1992;80: 758–67

875. Lossos IS, Levy R. Higher grade transformation of follicular lymphoma: phenotypic tumor progression associated with diverse genetic lesions. Semin Cancer Biol 2003;13:191–202

876. Lossos IS, et al. Transformation of follicular lymphoma to diffuse large-cell lymphoma: alternative patterns with increased or decreased expression of c-myc and its regulated genes. Proc Natl Acad Sci USA 2002;99:8886–91

877. Matolcsy A, et al. Morphologic transformation of follicular lymphoma is associated with somatic mutation of the translocated Bcl-2 gene. Blood 1996;88: 3937–44

878. Lossos IS, Warnke R, Levy R. BCL-6 mRNA expression in higher grade transformation of follicle center lymphoma: correlation with somatic mutations in the 5′ regulatory region of the BCL-6 gene. Leukemia 2002;16:1857–62

879. Knutsen T. Cytogenetic mechanisms in the pathogenesis and progression of follicular lymphoma. Cancer Surv 1997;30:163–92

880. Rohatiner A, Lister TA. Management of follicular lymphoma. Curr Opin Oncol 1994;6:473–9

881. Natkunam Y, et al. Immunophenotypic and genotypic characterization of progression in follicular lymphomas. Appl Immunohistochem Mol Morphol 2004;12:97–104

882. Mohamed AN, et al. Chromosomal analyses of 52 cases of follicular lymphoma with t(14;18), including blastic/blastoid variant. Cancer Genet Cytogenet 2001;126:45–51

883. Martinez-Climent JA, et al. Transformation of follicular lymphoma to diffuse large cell lymphoma is associated with a heterogeneous set of DNA copy number and gene expression alterations. Blood 2003;101:3109–17

884. Pittaluga S, et al. Mantle cell lymphoma: a clinico-pathological study of 55 cases. Histopathology 1995;26:17–24

885. Meusers P, et al. Multicentre randomized therapeutic trial for advanced centrocytic lymphoma: anthracycline does not improve the prognosis. Hematol Oncol 1989;7:365–80

886. Schraders M, et al. Novel chromosomal imbalances in mantle cell lymphoma detected by genome-wide array-based comparative genomic hybridization. Blood 2005;105:1686–93

887. Hiddemann W, Dreyling M. Mantle cell lymphoma: therapeutic strategies are different from CLL. Curr Treat Options Oncol 2003;4:219–26

888. Lenz G, Dreyling M, Hiddemann W. Mantle cell lymphoma: established therapeutic options and future directions. Ann Hematol 2004;83:71–7

889. Berinstein NL, Mangel J. Integrating monoclonal antibodies into the management of mantle cell lymphoma. Semin Oncol 2004;31(Suppl 2):2–6

890. Brugger W. Clearing minimal residual disease with rituximab consolidation therapy. Semin Oncol 2004;31(Suppl 2):33–7

891. Martinez-Climent JA, et al. Loss of a novel tumor suppressor gene locus at chromosome 8p is associated with leukemic mantle cell lymphoma. Blood 2001;98:3479–82

892. Argatoff LH, et al. Mantle cell lymphoma: a clinicopathologic study of 80 cases. Blood 1997;89:2067–78

893. Norton AJ, et al. Mantle cell lymphoma: natural history defined in a serially biopsied population over a 20-year period. Ann Oncol 1995;6:249–56

894. Bernard M, et al. Blastic variant of mantle cell lymphoma: a rare but highly aggressive subtype. Leukemia 2001;15:1785–91

895. Bea S, et al. Increased number of chromosomal imbalances and high-level DNA amplifications in mantle cell lymphoma are associated with blastoid variants. Blood 1999;93:4365–74

896. Raty R, et al. Predictive factors for blastoid transformation in the common variant of mantle cell lymphoma. Eur J Cancer 2003;39:321–9

897. Pinyol M, et al. Deletions and loss of expression of p16INK4a and p21Waf1 genes are associated with aggressive variants of mantle cell lymphomas. Blood 1997;89:272–80

898. Pinyol M, et al. p16(INK4a) gene inactivation by deletions, mutations, and hypermethylation is associated with transformed and aggressive variants of non-Hodgkin's lymphomas. Blood 1998;91:2977–84

899. Andriko JA, et al. Is lymphoplasmacytic lymphoma/immunocytoma a distinct entity? A clinicopathologic study of 20 cases. Am J Surg Pathol 2001;25:742–51

900. Papamichael D, et al. Immunocytoma: a retrospective analysis from St Bartholomew's Hospital – 1972 to 1996. J Clin Oncol 1999;17:2847–53

901. Mansoor A, et al. Cytogenetic findings in lymphoplasmacytic lymphoma/Waldenström macroglobulinemia. Chromosomal abnormalities are associated with the polymorphous subtype and an aggressive clinical course. Am J Clin Pathol 2001;116:543–9

902. Schop RF, et al. Waldenström macroglobulinemia neoplastic cells lack immunoglobulin heavy chain locus translocations but have frequent 6q deletions. Blood 2002;100:2996–3001

903. Facon T, et al. Prognostic factors in Waldenstrom's macroglobulinemia: a report of 167 cases. J Clin Oncol 1993;11:1553–8

904. Morel P, et al. Prognostic factors in Waldenström macroglobulinemia: A report on 323 patients with the description of a new scoring system and its validation on 253 other patients. Blood 2000;96:852–8

905. Stalnikiewicz L, et al. Prognostic factors in Waldenström's macroglobulinemia: description of the complications during the evolution-preliminary results on 101 patients. Semin Oncol 2003;30:216–9

906. Leblond V, Tournilhac O, Morel P. Waldenström's macroglobulinemia: prognostic factors and recent therapeutic advances. Clin Exp Med 2004;3:187–98

907. Oscier D, Owen R, Johnson S. Splenic marginal zone lymphoma. Blood Rev 2005;19:39–51

908. Troussard X, et al. Splenic lymphoma with villous lymphocytes: clinical presentation, biology and prognostic factors in a series of 100 patients. Groupe Francais d'Hematologie Cellulaire (GFHC). Br J Haematol 1996;93:731–6

909. Chacon JI, et al. Splenic marginal zone lymphoma: clinical characteristics and prognostic factors in a series of 60 patients. Blood 2002;100:1648–54

910. Parry-Jones N, et al. Prognostic features of splenic lymphoma with villous lymphocytes: a report on 129 patients. Br J Haematol 2003;120:759–64

911. Thieblemont C, Felman P, et al. Treatment of splenic marginal zone B-cell lymphoma: an analysis of 81 patients. Clin Lymphoma 2002;3:41–7

912. Camacho FI, et al. Progression to large B-cell lymphoma in splenic marginal zone lymphoma: a description of a series of 12 cases. Am J Surg Pathol 2001;25:1268–76

913. Martinez-Climent JA, et al. Genomic abnormalities acquired in the blastic transformation of splenic marginal zone B-cell lymphoma. Leuk Lymphoma 2003;44:459–64

914. Lloret E, et al. Splenic marginal zone lymphoma with increased number of blasts: an aggressive variant? Hum Pathol 1999;30:1153–60

915. Ott MM, et al. Marginal zone B-cell lymphomas (MZBL) arising at different sites represent different biological entities. Genes Chromosomes Cancer 2000;28:380–6

916. Thieblemont C, et al. Splenic marginal-zone lymphoma: a distinct clinical and pathological entity. Lancet Oncol 2003;4:95–103

917. Bertoni F, et al. Genetic alterations underlying the pathogenesis of MALT lymphoma. Hematol J 2002;3:10–3

918. Bertoni F, Cotter FE, Zucca E. Molecular genetics of extranodal marginal zone (MALT-type) B-cell lymphoma. Leuk Lymphoma 1999;35:57–68

919. Zucca E, et al. Molecular analysis of the progression from Helicobacter pylori-associated chronic gastritis to mucosa-associated lymphoid-tissue lymphoma of the stomach. N Engl J Med 1998;338:804–10

920. Wotherspoon AC, Finn TM, Isaacson PG. Trisomy 3 in low-grade B-cell lymphomas of mucosa-associated lymphoid tissue. Blood 1995;85:2000–4

921. Ott G, et al. The t(11;18)(q21;q21) chromosome translocation is a frequent and specific aberration in low-grade but not high-grade malignant non-Hodgkin's lymphomas of the mucosa-associated lymphoid tissue (MALT-) type. Cancer Res 1997;57:3944–8

922. Auer IA, et al. t(11;18)(q21;q21) is the most common translocation in MALT lymphomas. Ann Oncol 1997;8:979–85

923. Liu H, et al. Resistance of t(11;18) positive gastric mucosa-associated lymphoid tissue lymphoma to

Helicobacter pylori eradication therapy. Lancet 2001; 357:39–40

924. Inagaki H, et al. Gastric MALT lymphomas are divided into three groups based on responsiveness to _Helicobacter pylori_ eradication and detection of API2–MALT1 fusion. Am J Surg Pathol 2004;28: 1560–7

925. Preudhomme C, Fenaux P. The clinical significance of mutations of the P53 tumour suppressor gene in haematological malignancies. Br J Haematol 1997; 98:502–11

926. de Jong D, Boot H, Taal B. Histological grading with clinical relevance in gastric mucosa-associated lymphoid tissue (MALT) lymphoma. Recent Results Cancer Res 2000;156:27–32

927. de Jong D, et al. Histological grading in gastric lymphoma: pretreatment criteria and clinical relevance. Gastroenterology 1997;112:1466–74

928. Cavalli F, et al. MALT lymphomas. Hematology (Am Soc Hematol Educ Program) 2001:241–58

929. Thieblemont C, et al. Mucosa-associated lymphoid tissue lymphoma is a disseminated disease in one third of 158 patients analyzed. Blood 2000;95:802–6

930. Chan JK, Ng CS, Isaacson PG. Relationship between high-grade lymphoma and low-grade B-cell mucosa-associated lymphoid tissue lymphoma (MALToma) of the stomach. Am J Pathol 1990;136:1153–64

931. Peng H, et al. Genetic evidence for a clonal link between low and high-grade components in gastric MALT B-cell lymphoma. Histopathology 1997;30: 425–9

932. Catovsky D, Matutes E. Splenic lymphoma with circulating villous lymphocytes/splenic marginal-zone lymphoma. Semin Hematol 1999;36:148–54

933. Nathwani BN, et al. Nodal monocytoid B-cell lymphoma (nodal marginal-zone B-cell lymphoma). Semin Hematol 1999;36:128–38

934. Nathwani BN, et al. Marginal zone B-cell lymphoma: A clinical comparison of nodal and mucosa-associated lymphoid tissue types. Non-Hodgkin's Lymphoma Classification Project. J Clin Oncol 1999; 17:2486–92

935. Matolcsy A, et al. Distinct clonal origin of low-grade MALT-type and high-grade lesions of a multifocal gastric lymphoma. Histopathology 1999;34:6–8

936. Zucca E, et al. The gastric marginal zone B-cell lymphoma of MALT type. Blood 2000;96:410–9

937. Isaacson PG. Gastric MALT lymphoma: from concept to cure. Ann Oncol 1999;10:637–45

938. Zinzani PL, et al. Nongastrointestinal low-grade mucosa-associated lymphoid tissue lymphoma: analysis of 75 patients. J Clin Oncol 1999;17:1254

939. Rosenwald A, et al. Exclusive detection of the t(11;18)(q21;q21) in extranodal marginal zone B cell lymphomas (MZBL) of MALT type in contrast to other MZBL and extranodal large B cell lymphomas. Am J Pathol 1999;155:1817–21

940. Dierlamm J, et al. Detection of t(11;18)(q21;q21) by interphase fluorescence in situ hybridization using API2 and MLT specific probes. Blood 2000;96:2215–8

941. Remstein ED, et al. Mucosa-associated lymphoid tissue lymphomas with t(11;18)(q21;q21) and mucosa-associated lymphoid tissue lymphomas with aneuploidy develop along different pathogenetic pathways. Am J Pathol 2002;161:63–71

942. Asatiani E, et al. Monoclonal gammopathy in extranodal marginal zone lymphoma (ENMZL) correlates with advanced disease and bone marrow involvement. Am J Hematol 2004;77:144

943. Mollejo M, et al. Monocytoid B cells. A comparative clinical pathological study of their distribution in different types of low-grade lymphomas. Am J Surg Pathol 1994;18:1131–9

944. Coiffier B. Diffuse large cell lymphoma. Curr Opin Oncol 2001;13:325–34

945. Coiffier B. Treatment of diffuse large B-cell lymphoma. Curr Hematol Rep 2005;4:7–14

946. Nakamine H, et al. Prognostic significance of clinical and pathologic features in diffuse large B-cell lymphoma. Cancer 1993;71:3130–7

947. Conconi A, et al. Prognostic models for diffuse large B-cell lymphoma. Hematol Oncol 2000;18:61–73

948. Suki S, et al. Risk classification for large cell lymphoma using lactate dehydrogenase, beta-2 microglobulin, and thymidine kinase. Leuk Lymphoma 1995;18:87–92

949. Aviles A, et al. Beta 2 microglobulin level as an indicator of prognosis in diffuse large cell lymphoma. Leuk Lymphoma 1992;7:135–8

950. Pavlidis AN, et al. Serum tumor markers in non-Hodgkin's lymphomas and chronic lymphocytic leukemia. Int J Biol Markers 1993;8:14–20

951. Vitolo U, et al. MACOP-B treatment in diffuse large-cell lymphoma: identification of prognostic groups in an Italian multicenter study. J Clin Oncol 1992;10:219–27

952. Yan Y, et al. Clinical and prognostic significance of bone marrow involvement in patients with diffuse aggressive B-cell lymphoma. J Clin Oncol 1995;13:1336–42

953. Mitterbauer-Hohendanner G, et al. Prognostic significance of molecular staging by PCR-amplification of immunoglobulin gene rearrangements in diffuse large B-cell lymphoma (DLBCL). Leukemia 2004;18:1102–7

954. Baars JW, et al. Diffuse large B-cell non-Hodgkin lymphomas: the clinical relevance of histological subclassification. Br J Cancer 1999;79:1770–6

955. Aki H, et al. T-cell-rich B-cell lymphoma: a clinicopathologic study of 21 cases and comparison with 43 cases of diffuse large B-cell lymphoma. Leuk Res 2004;28:229–36

956. Bouabdallah R, et al. T-cell/histiocyte-rich large B-cell lymphomas and classical diffuse large B-cell lymphomas have similar outcome after chemotherapy: a matched-control analysis. J Clin Oncol 2003;21:1271–7

957. Zinzani PL, et al. Identification of outcome predictors in diffuse large B-cell lymphoma. Immunohistochemical profiling of homogeneously treated de novo tumors with nodal presentation on tissue micro-arrays. Haematologica 2005;90:341–7

958. de Leval L, Harris NL. Variability in immunophenotype in diffuse large B-cell lymphoma and its clinical relevance. Histopathology 2003;43:509–28

959. Fang JM, et al. CD10 antigen expression correlates with the t(14;18)(q32;q21) major breakpoint region in diffuse large B-cell lymphoma. Mod Pathol 1999;12:295–300

960. Chang CC, et al. Immunohistochemical expression patterns of germinal center and activation B-cell markers correlate with prognosis in diffuse large B-cell lymphoma. Am J Surg Pathol 2004;28:464–70

961. de Leval L, et al. Diffuse large B-cell lymphoma of bone: an analysis of differentiation-associated

antigens with clinical correlation. Am J Surg Pathol 2003;27:1269–77

962. de Jong D, et al. Very late relapse in diffuse large B-cell lymphoma represents clonally related disease and is marked by germinal center cell features. Blood 2003;102:324–7

963. Slymen DJ, et al. Immunobiologic factors predictive of clinical outcome in diffuse large-cell lymphoma. J Clin Oncol 1990;8:986–93

964. Tominaga K, et al. Proliferation in non-Hodgkin's lymphomas as determined by immunohistochemical double staining for Ki-67. Hematol Oncol 1992;10: 163–9

965. Aref S, et al. The interplay between c-Myc oncogene expression and circulating vascular endothelial growth factor (sVEGF), its antagonist receptor, soluble Flt-1 in diffuse large B cell lymphoma (DLBCL): relationship to patient outcome. Leuk Lymphoma 2004;45:499–506

966. Tzankov A, et al. Prognostic significance of CD44 expression in diffuse large B cell lymphoma of activated and germinal centre B cell-like types: a tissue microarray analysis of 90 cases. J Clin Pathol 2003; 56:747–52

967. Inagaki H, et al. Prognostic significance of CD44v6 in diffuse large B-cell lymphoma. Mod Pathol 1999; 12:546–52

968. Donoghue S, et al. Immunohistochemical localization of caspase-3 correlates with clinical outcome in B-cell diffuse large-cell lymphoma. Cancer Res 1999; 59:5386–91

969. Muramatsu M, et al. Rearrangement of the BCL6 gene in B-cell lymphoid neoplasms: comparison with lymphomas associated with BCL2 rearrangement. Br J Haematol 1996;93:911–20

970. Aisenberg AC, Wilkes BM, Jacobson JO. The bcl-2 gene is rearranged in many diffuse B-cell lymphomas. Blood 1988;71:969–72

971. Leroy K, et al. p53 gene mutations are associated with poor survival in low and low-intermediate risk diffuse large B-cell lymphomas. Ann Oncol 2002;13: 1108–15

972. Wilson WH, et al. Relationship of p53, bcl-2, and tumor proliferation to clinical drug resistance in non-Hodgkin's lymphomas. Blood 1997;89:601–9

973. Zhang A, et al. Prognostic clinicopathologic factors, including immunologic expression in diffuse large B-cell lymphomas. Pathol Int 1999;49:1043–52

974. Moller MB, et al. Disrupted p53 function as predictor of treatment failure and poor prognosis in B- and T-cell non-Hodgkin's lymphoma. Clin Cancer Res 1999;5:1085–91

975. Gascoyne RD. Emerging prognostic factors in diffuse large B cell lymphoma. Curr Opin Oncol 2004;16: 436–41

976. Lossos IS, et al. Ongoing immunoglobulin somatic mutation in germinal center B cell-like but not in activated B cell-like diffuse large cell lymphomas. Proc Natl Acad Sci USA 2000;97:10209–13

977. Huang JZ, et al. The t(14;18) defines a unique subset of diffuse large B-cell lymphoma with a germinal center B-cell gene expression profile. Blood 2002;99:2285–90

978. Ramuz O, et al. Identification of TCL1A as an immunohistochemical marker of adverse outcome in diffuse large B-cell lymphomas. Int J Oncol 2005; 26:151–7

979. Moller MB, Pedersen NT, Christensen BE. Diffuse large B-cell lymphoma: clinical implications of extranodal versus nodal presentation – a population-based study of 1575 cases. Br J Haematol 2004;124:151–9

980. Dufau JP, et al. Intravascular large B-cell lymphoma with bone marrow involvement at presentation and haemophagocytic syndrome: two Western cases in favour of a specific variant. Histopathology 2000;37:509–12

981. Grange F, et al. Prognostic factors in primary cutaneous large B-cell lymphomas: a European multicenter study. J Clin Oncol 2001;19:3602–10

982. Sundram U, et al. Expression of the bcl-6 and MUM1/IRF4 proteins correlate with overall and disease-specific survival in patients with primary cutaneous large B-cell lymphoma: a tissue microarray study. J Cutan Pathol 2005;32:227–34

983. Goodlad JR, et al. Primary cutaneous diffuse large B-cell lymphoma: prognostic significance of clinicopathological subtypes. Am J Surg Pathol 2003;27: 1538–45

984. Touroutoglou N, et al. Testicular lymphoma: late relapses and poor outcome despite doxorubicin-based therapy. J Clin Oncol 1995;13:1361–7

985. Darby S, Hancock BW. Localised non-Hodgkin lymphoma of the testis: The Sheffield Lymphoma Group experience. Int J Oncol 2005;26:1093–9

986. Aviles A, et al. Testicular lymphoma: organ-specific treatment did not improve outcome. Oncology 2004; 67:211–14

987. Caroli E, Acqui M, Ferrante L. Primary cerebral lymphoma: a retrospective study in 22 immunocompetent patients. Tumori 2004;90:294–8

988. Braaten KM, et al. BCL-6 expression predicts improved survival in patients with primary central nervous system lymphoma. Clin Cancer Res 2003;9: 1063–9

989. Chang CC, et al. Expression of p53, c-Myc, or Bcl-6 suggests a poor prognosis in primary central nervous system diffuse large B-cell lymphoma among immunocompetent individuals. Arch Pathol Lab Med 2003; 127:208–12

990. Cazals-Hatem D, et al. Primary mediastinal large B-cell lymphoma. A clinicopathologic study of 141 cases compared with 916 nonmediastinal large B-cell lymphomas, a GELA ('Groupe d'Etude des Lymphomes de l'Adulte') study. Am J Surg Pathol 1996;20:877–88

991. Savage KJ, et al. The molecular signature of mediastinal large B-cell lymphoma differs from that of other diffuse large B-cell lymphomas and shares features with classical Hodgkin's lymphoma. Blood 2003

992. Rosenwald A, et al. Molecular diagnosis of primary mediastinal B cell lymphoma identifies a clinically favorable subgroup of diffuse large B cell lymphoma related to Hodgkin lymphoma. J Exp Med 2003;198: 851–62

993. Malpeli G, et al. Primary mediastinal B-cell lymphoma: hypermutation of the BCL6 gene targets motifs different from those in diffuse large B-cell and follicular lymphomas. Haematologica 2004;89:1091–9

994. Todeschini G, et al. Primary mediastinal large B-cell lymphoma (PMLBCL): long-term results from a retrospective multicentre Italian experience in 138 patients treated with CHOP or MACOP-B/VACOP-B. Br J Cancer 2004;90:372–6

995. Yamaguchi M, et al. De novo CD5-positive diffuse large B-cell lymphoma: clinical characteristics and therapeutic outcome. Br J Haematol 1999;105:1133–9

996. Yamaguchi M, et al. De novo CD5+ diffuse large B-cell lymphoma: a clinicopathologic study of 109 patients. Blood 2002;99:815–21

997. Harada S, et al. Molecular and immunological dissection of diffuse large B cell lymphoma: CD5+, and CD5– with CD10+ groups may constitute clinically relevant subtypes. Leukemia 1999;13:1441–7

998. Kroft SH, et al. De novo CD5+ diffuse large B-cell lymphomas. A heterogeneous group containing an unusual form of splenic lymphoma. Am J Clin Pathol 2000;114:523–33

999. Tagawa H, et al. Genome-wide array-based comparative genomic hybridization of diffuse large B-cell lymphoma: comparison between CD5-positive and CD5-negative cases. Cancer Res 2004;64:5948–55

1000. Yoshioka T, et al. Cytogenetic features of de novo CD5-positive diffuse large B-cell lymphoma: Chromosome aberrations affecting 8p21 and 11q13 constitute major subgroups with different overall survival. Genes Chromosomes Cancer 2005;42:149–57

1001. Colomo L, et al. Diffuse large B-cell lymphomas with plasmablastic differentiation represent a heterogeneous group of disease entities. Am J Surg Pathol 2004;28:736–47

1002. Delecluse HJ, et al. Plasmablastic lymphomas of the oral cavity: a new entity associated with the human immunodeficiency virus infection. Blood 1997;89: 1413–20

1003. Blum KA, Lozanski G, Byrd JC. Adult Burkitt leukemia and lymphoma. Blood 2004;104:3009–20

1004. Mead GM, et al. An international evaluation of CODOX-M and CODOX-M alternating with IVAC in adult Burkitt's lymphoma: results of United Kingdom Lymphoma Group LY06 study. Ann Oncol 2002;13:1264–74

1005. Thomas DA, et al. Hyper-CVAD program in Burkitt's-type adult acute lymphoblastic leukemia. J Clin Oncol 1999;17:2461–70

1006. Divine M, et al. Is the small non-cleaved-cell lymphoma histologic subtype a poor prognostic factor in adult patients? A case-controlled analysis. The Groupe d'Etude des Lymphomes de l'Adulte. J Clin Oncol 1996;14:240–8

1007. Lee EJ, et al. Brief-duration high-intensity chemotherapy for patients with small noncleaved-cell lymphoma or FAB L3 acute lymphocytic leukemia: results of cancer and leukemia group B study 9251. J Clin Oncol 2001;19:4014–22

1008. Magrath I, et al. Adults and children with small non-cleaved-cell lymphoma have a similar excellent outcome when treated with the same chemotherapy regimen. J Clin Oncol 1996;14:925–34

1009. Sweetenham JW, et al. Adult Burkitt's and Burkitt-like non-Hodgkin's lymphoma – outcome for patients treated with high-dose therapy and autologous stem-cell transplantation in first remission or at relapse: results from the European Group for Blood and Marrow Transplantation. J Clin Oncol 1996;14: 2465–72

1010. Yokohama A, et al. Durable remission induced by rituximab-containing chemotherapy in a patient with primary refractory Burkitt's lymphoma. Ann Hematol 2004;83:120–3

1011. Patte C, et al. High survival rate in advanced-stage B-cell lymphomas and leukemias without CNS involvement with a short intensive polychemotherapy: results from the French Pediatric Oncology Society of a randomized trial of 216 children. J Clin Oncol 1991;9:123–32

1012. Reiter A, et al. Improved treatment results in childhood B-cell neoplasms with tailored intensification of therapy: A report of the Berlin–Frankfurt–Münster Group Trial NHL-BFM 90. Blood 1999;94:3294–306

1013. Patte C, et al. The Societé Française d'Oncologie Pédiatrique LMB89 protocol: highly effective multi-agent chemotherapy tailored to the tumor burden and initial response in 561 unselected children with B-cell lymphomas and L3 leukemia. Blood 2001; 97:3370–9

1014. Patte C, et al. Improved survival rate in children with stage III and IV B cell non-Hodgkin's lymphoma and leukemia using multi-agent chemotherapy: results of a study of 114 children from the French Pediatric Oncology Society. J Clin Oncol 1986;4:1219–26

1015. Garcia JL, et al. Abnormalities on 1q and 7q are associated with poor outcome in sporadic Burkitt's lymphoma. A cytogenetic and comparative genomic hybridization study. Leukemia 2003;17:2016–24

1016. Barlogie B, et al. Plasma cell myeloma – new biological insights and advances in therapy. Blood 1989;73: 865–79

1017. Kyle RA. Why better prognostic factors for multiple myeloma are needed. Blood 1994;83:1713–16

1018. Kumar SK, et al. Clinical course of patients with relapsed multiple myeloma. Mayo Clin Proc 2004; 79:867–74

1019. Rajkumar SV, et al. Cytogenetic abnormalities correlate with the plasma cell labeling index and extent of bone marrow involvement in myeloma. Cancer Genet Cytogenet 1999;113:73–7

1020. Fonseca R, et al. Clinical and biologic implications of recurrent genomic aberrations in myeloma. Blood 2003;101:4569–75

1021. Fonseca R, et al. The recurrent IgH translocations are highly associated with nonhyperdiploid variant multiple myeloma. Blood 2003;102:2562–7

1022. Shaughnessy J, et al. Continuous absence of metaphase-defined cytogenetic abnormalities, especially of chromosome 13 and hypodiploidy, ensures long-term survival in multiple myeloma treated with Total Therapy I: interpretation in the context of global gene expression. Blood 2003;101:3849–56

1023. Alexanian R, et al. Treatment for multiple myeloma. Combination chemotherapy with different melphalan dose regimens. J Am Med Assoc 1969;208:1680–5

1024. Segeren CM, et al. Overall and event-free survival are not improved by the use of myeloablative therapy following intensified chemotherapy in previously untreated patients with multiple myeloma: a prospective randomized phase 3 study. Blood 2003;101: 2144–51

1025. Powles R, et al. Outcome assessment of a population-based group of 195 unselected myeloma patients under 70 years of age offered intensive treatment. Bone Marrow Transplant 1997;20:435–43

1026. Attal M, et al. A prospective, randomized trial of autologous bone marrow transplantation and chemotherapy in multiple myeloma. Intergroupe Français du Myelome. N Engl J Med 1996;335:91–7

1027. Yakoub-Agha I, et al. Thalidomide in patients with advanced multiple myeloma: a study of 83 patients – report of the Intergroupe Francophone du Myelome (IFM). Hematol J 2002;3:185–92

1028. Schaar CG, et al. Early response to therapy and survival in multiple myeloma. Br J Haematol 2004; 125:162–6

1029. Lincz LF, et al. Tumour kinetics in multiple myeloma before, during, and after treatment. Leuk Lymphoma 2001;40:373–84

1030. Sukpanichnant S, et al. Diagnostic criteria and histologic grading in multiple myeloma: histologic and immunohistologic analysis of 176 cases with clinical correlation. Hum Pathol 1994;25:308–18

1031. Harrison CJ, et al. Cytogenetics of multiple myeloma: interpretation of fluorescence in situ hybridization results. Br J Haematol 2003;120:944–52

1032. Kyle RA, Elveback LR. Management and prognosis of multiple myeloma. Mayo Clin Proc 1976;51:751–60

1033. Garcia-Sanz R, et al. Proliferative activity of plasma cells is the most relevant prognostic factor in elderly multiple myeloma patients. Int J Cancer 2004;112:884–9

1034. Perez-Simon JA, et al. Prognostic value of numerical chromosome aberrations in multiple myeloma: A FISH analysis of 15 different chromosomes. Blood 1998;91:3366–71

1035. Kroger N, et al. Deletion of chromosome band 13q14 as detected by fluorescence in situ hybridization is a prognostic factor in patients with multiple myeloma who are receiving allogeneic dose-reduced stem cell transplantation. Blood 2004;103:4056–61

1036. Avet-Loiseau H, et al. Monosomy 13 is associated with the transition of monoclonal gammopathy of undetermined significance to multiple myeloma. Intergroupe Francophone du Myelome. Blood 1999; 94:2583–9

1037. Avet-Loiseau H, et al. Oncogenesis of multiple myeloma: 14q32 and 13q chromosomal abnormalities are not randomly distributed, but correlate with natural history, immunological features, and clinical presentation. Blood 2002;99:2185–91

1038. Fonseca R, et al. Myeloma and the t(11;14) (q13;q32); evidence for a biologically defined unique subset of patients. Blood 2002;99:3735–41

1039. Facon T, et al. Chromosome 13 abnormalities identified by FISH analysis and serum beta2-microglobulin produce a powerful myeloma staging system for patients receiving high-dose therapy. Blood 2001;97:1566–71

1040. Moreau P, et al. Recurrent 14q32 translocations determine the prognosis of multiple myeloma, especially in patients receiving intensive chemotherapy. Blood 2002;100:1579–83

1041. Gutierrez NC, et al. Prognostic and biological significance of chromosomal imbalances assessed by comparative genomic hybridization in multiple myeloma. Blood 2004

1042. Gutierrez NC, et al. Differences in genetic changes between multiple myeloma and plasma cell leukemia demonstrated by comparative genomic hybridization. Leukemia 2001;15:840–5

1043. Liu P, et al. Activating mutations of N- and K-ras in multiple myeloma show different clinical associations: analysis of the Eastern Cooperative Oncology Group Phase III Trial. Blood 1996;88:2699–706

1044. Kyle RA, et al. Long-term follow-up of 241 patients with monoclonal gammopathy of undetermined significance: the original Mayo Clinic series 25 years later. Mayo Clin Proc 2004;79:859–66

1045. Kyle RA, et al. Long-term follow-up of IgM monoclonal gammopathy of undetermined significance. Blood 2003;102:3759–64

1046. Perez-Andres M, et al. Clonal plasma cells from monoclonal gammopathy of undetermined significance, multiple myeloma and plasma cell leukemia show different expression profiles of molecules involved in the interaction with the immunological bone marrow microenvironment. Leukemia 2005;19:449–55

1047. Dispenzieri A, et al. POEMS syndrome: definitions and long-term outcome. Blood 2003;101:2496–506

1048. Kluin PM, et al. Peripheral T/NK-cell lymphoma: a report of the IXth Workshop of the European Association for Haematopathology. Histopathology 2001;38:250–70

1049. Jaffe ES, Krenacs L, Raffeld M. Classification of cytotoxic T-cell and natural killer cell lymphomas. Semin Hematol 2003;40:175–84

1050. Jaffe ES, Krenacs L, Raffeld M. Classification of T-cell and NK-cell neoplasms based on the REAL classification. Ann Oncol 1997;8(Suppl 2):17–24

1051. Gorczyca W, et al. An approach to diagnosis of T-cell lymphoproliferative disorders by flow cytometry. Cytometry 2002;50:177–90

1052. Coiffier B, et al. T-cell lymphomas: immunologic, histologic, clinical, and therapeutic analysis of 63 cases. J Clin Oncol 1988;6:1584–9

1053. Armitage JO, et al. Clinical significance of immunophenotype in diffuse aggressive non-Hodgkin's lymphoma. J Clin Oncol 1989;7:1783–90

1054. Brown DC, et al. The prognostic significance of immunophenotype in high-grade non-Hodgkin's lymphoma. Histopathology 1989;14:621–7

1055. Cheng AL, et al. Direct comparisons of peripheral T-cell lymphoma with diffuse B-cell lymphoma of comparable histological grades – should peripheral T-cell lymphoma be considered separately? J Clin Oncol 1989;7:725–31

1056. Lippman SM, et al. The prognostic significance of the immunotype in diffuse large-cell lymphoma: a comparative study of the T-cell and B-cell phenotype. Blood 1988;72:436–41

1057. Bartlett NL, Longo DL. T-small lymphocyte disorders. Semin Hematol 1999;36:164–70

1058. Matutes E, et al. T-cell chronic lymphocytic leukaemia: the spectrum of mature T-cell disorders. Nouv Rev Fr Hematol 1988;30:347–51

1059. Matutes E. T-cell prolymphocytic leukemia. Cancer Control 1998;5:19–24

1060. Matutes E. Chronic T-cell lymphoproliferative disorders. Rev Clin Exp Hematol 2002;6:401–20; discussion 449–50

1061. Garand R, et al. Indolent course as a relatively frequent presentation in T-prolymphocytic leukaemia. Groupe Français d'Hématologie Cellulaire. Br J Haematol 1998;103:488–94

1062. Pawson R, et al. Treatment of T-cell prolymphocytic leukemia with human CD52 antibody. J Clin Oncol 1997;15:2667–72

1063. Dhodapkar MV, et al. Clinical spectrum of clonal proliferations of T-large granular lymphocytes: a T-cell clonopathy of undetermined significance? Blood 1994;84:1620–7

1064. Lamy T, Loughran TP Jr. Clinical features of large granular lymphocyte leukemia. Semin Hematol 2003;40:185–95

1065. Battiwalla M, et al. HLA-DR4 predicts haematological response to cyclosporine in T-large granular lymphocyte lymphoproliferative disorders. Br J Haematol 2003;123:449–53

1066. Kwong YL, Wong KF. Association of pure red cell aplasia with T large granular lymphocyte leukaemia. J Clin Pathol 1998;51:672–5

1067. Gentile TC, et al. CD3+, CD56+ aggressive variant of large granular lymphocyte leukemia. Blood 1994;84:2315–21

1068. Battiwalla M, Sauntharajah Y, et al. Treatment of T-LGL (large granular lymphocytic disease) with cyclosporine A. Long term follow-up. Blood 2002; 100(Suppl 1):669(abstr)

1069. Pandolfi F, Loughran TP, et al. Clinical course and prognosis of the lymphoproliferative disease of granular lymphocytes. A multicenter study. Cancer 1990;65:341–8

1070. Macon WR, et al. Natural killer-like T-cell lymphomas: aggressive lymphomas of T-large granular lymphocytes. Blood 1996;87:1474–83

1071. Poiesz BJ, et al. Detection and isolation of type C retrovirus particles from fresh and cultured lymphocytes of a patient with cutaneous T-cell lymphoma. Proc Natl Acad Sci USA 1980;77:7415–19

1072. Blattner WA, et al. The human type-C retrovirus, HTLV, in Blacks from the Caribbean region, and relationship to adult T-cell leukemia/lymphoma. Int J Cancer 1982;30:257–64

1073. Takatsuki K, et al. Clinical diversity in adult T-cell leukemia–lymphoma. Cancer Res 1985;45(9 Suppl): 4644s–4645s

1074. Kawano F, et al. Variation in the clinical courses of adult T-cell leukemia. Cancer 1985;55:851–6

1075. Shimoyama M. Diagnostic criteria and classification of clinical subtypes of adult T-cell leukaemia-lymphoma. A report from the Lymphoma Study Group (1984–87). Br J Haematol 1991;79:428–37

1076. Bazarbachi A, et al. New therapeutic approaches for adult T-cell leukaemia. Lancet Oncol 2004;5:664–72

1077. Yamaguchi K, Watanabe T. Human T lymphotropic virus type-I and adult T-cell leukemia in Japan. Int J Hematol 2002;76(Suppl 2):240–5

1078. Shimoyama M. Treatment of patients with adult T-cell leukemia–lymphoma: an overview. In Takatsuki K, Hinuma Y, Yoshida M, eds. Advances in Adult T-cell Leukemia and HTLV-1 Research. Tokyo: Japan Scientific Societies Press, 1992:43–6

1079. Shimoyama M. Chemotherapy of ATL. In Takatsuki K, ed. Adult T-cell Leukemia. Oxford: Oxford University Press, 1994:221–36

1080. Jaffe ES, et al. The pathologic spectrum of adult T-cell leukemia/lymphoma in the United States.

Human T-cell leukemia/lymphoma virus-associated lymphoid malignancies. Am J Surg Pathol 1984;8: 263–75

1081. Ohshima K, et al. Survival of patients with HTLV-I-associated lymph node lesions. J Pathol 1999;189: 539–45

1082. Yamaguchi T, et al. Clinicopathological features of cutaneous lesions of adult T-cell leukaemia/lymphoma. Br J Dermatol 2005;152:76–81

1083. Siegel RS, Gartenhaus RB, Kuzel TM. Human T-cell lymphotropic-I-associated leukemia/lymphoma. Curr Treat Options Oncol 2001;2:291–300

1084. Kim K, et al. Clinical features of peripheral T-cell lymphomas in 78 patients diagnosed according to the Revised European–American lymphoma (REAL) classification. Eur J Cancer 2002;38:75–81

1085. Lopez-Guillermo A, et al. Peripheral T-cell lymphomas: initial features, natural history, and prognostic factors in a series of 174 patients diagnosed according to the R.E.A.L. Classification. Ann Oncol 1998;9:849–55

1086. Mounier N, et al. Prognostic factors in patients with aggressive non-Hodgkin's lymphoma treated by front-line autotransplantation after complete remission: a cohort study by the Groupe d'Etude des Lymphomes de l'Adulte. J Clin Oncol 2004;22: 2826–34

1087. Steinberg AD, et al. NIH conference. Angioimmunoblastic lymphadenopathy with dysproteinemia. Ann Intern Med 1988;108:575–84

1088. Schetelig J, et al. Long-term disease-free survival in patients with angioimmunoblastic T-cell lymphoma after high-dose chemotherapy and autologous stem cell transplantation. Haematologica 2003;88:1272–8

1089. Massone C, et al. Subcutaneous, blastic natural killer (NK), NK/T-cell, and other cytotoxic lymphomas of the skin: a morphologic, immunophenotypic, and molecular study of 50 patients. Am J Surg Pathol 2004;28:719–35

1090. Takahara M, et al. P53, N- and K-Ras, and beta-catenin gene mutations and prognostic factors in nasal NK/T-cell lymphoma from Hokkaido, Japan. Hum Pathol 2004;35:86–95

1091. Tancrede-Bohin E, et al. Prognostic value of blood eosinophilia in primary cutaneous T-cell lymphomas. Arch Dermatol 2004;140:1057–61

1092. Grange F, et al. Prognostic factors in primary cutaneous lymphomas other than mycosis fungoides and the Sezary syndrome. The French Study Group on Cutaneous Lymphomas. Blood 1999;93:3637–42

1093. Jones D, et al. CD4⁻CD8⁻'Double-negative' cutaneous T-cell lymphomas share common histologic features and an aggressive clinical course. Am J Surg Pathol 2002;26:225–31

1094. Toro JR, et al. Gamma-delta T-cell phenotype is associated with significantly decreased survival in cutaneous T-cell lymphoma. Blood 2003;101:3407–12

1095. Foss F. Overview of cutaneous T-cell lymphoma: prognostic factors and novel therapeutic approaches. Leuk Lymphoma 2003;44(Suppl 3):S55–61

1096. Salhany KE, et al. Transformation of cutaneous T cell lymphoma to large cell lymphoma. A clinicopathologic and immunologic study. Am J Pathol 1988; 132:265–77

1097. Cerroni L, et al. Clinicopathologic and immunologic features associated with transformation of mycosis fungoides to large-cell lymphoma. Am J Surg Pathol 1992;16:543–52

1098. Diamandidou E, et al. Transformation of mycosis fungoides/Sezary syndrome: clinical characteristics and prognosis. Blood 1998;92:1150–9

1099. Vergier B, et al. Transformation of mycosis fungoides: clinicopathological and prognostic features of 45 cases. French Study Group of Cutaneious Lymphomas. Blood 2000;95:2212–18

1100. Vega F, et al. Clonal heterogeneity in mycosis fungoides and its relationship to clinical course. Blood 2002;100:3369–73

1101. Foulc P, N'Guyen JM, Dreno B. Prognostic factors in Sezary syndrome: a study of 28 patients. Br J Dermatol 2003;149:1152–8

1102. Mao X, et al. Molecular cytogenetic characterization of Sezary syndrome. Genes Chromosomes Cancer 2003;36:250–60

1103. Kadin ME. The spectrum of Ki-1+ cutaneous lymphomas. Curr Probl Dermatol 1990;19:132–43

1104. Kadin ME, Carpenter C. Systemic and primary cutaneous anaplastic large cell lymphomas. Semin Hematol 2003;40:244–56

1105. Bekkenk MW, et al. Primary and secondary cutaneous CD30(+) lymphoproliferative disorders: a report from the Dutch Cutaneous Lymphoma Group on the long-term follow-up data of 219 patients and guidelines for diagnosis and treatment. Blood 2000; 95:3653–61

1106. Paulli M, et al. CD30/Ki-1-positive lymphoproliferative disorders of the skin – clinicopathologic correlation and statistical analysis of 86 cases: a multicentric study from the European Organization for Research and Treatment of Cancer Cutaneous Lymphoma Project Group. J Clin Oncol 1995;13:1343–54

1107. Beljaards RC, et al. Prognostic significance of CD30 (Ki-1/Ber-H2) expression in primary cutaneous large-cell lymphomas of T-cell origin. A clinicopathologic and immunohistochemical study in 20 patients. Am J Pathol 1989;135:1169–78

1108. Bekkenk MW, et al. Peripheral T-cell lymphomas unspecified presenting in the skin: analysis of prognostic factors in a group of 82 patients. Blood 2003; 102:2213–9

1109. Macaulay WL. Lymphomatoid papulosis. A continuing self-healing eruption, clinically benign – histologically malignant. Arch Dermatol 1968;97:23–30

1110. Wang HH, Lach L, Kadin ME. Epidemiology of lymphomatoid papulosis. Cancer 1992;70:2951–7

1111. Beljaards RC, Willemze R. The prognosis of patients with lymphomatoid papulosis associated with malignant lymphomas. Br J Dermatol 1992;126:596–602

1112. Silva MM, et al. Lymphomatoid papulosis followed by Hodgkin's disease. Int J Dermatol 1998;37:541–3

1113. Zackheim HS, et al. Lymphomatoid papulosis associated with mycosis fungoides: a study of 21 patients including analyses for clonality. J Am Acad Dermatol 2003;49:620–3

1114. Gonzalez CL, et al. T-cell lymphoma involving subcutaneous tissue. A clinicopathologic entity commonly associated with hemophagocytic syndrome. Am J Surg Pathol 1991;15:17–27

1115. Kumar S, et al. Subcutaneous panniculitic T-cell lymphoma is a tumor of cytotoxic T lymphocytes. Hum Pathol 1998;29:397–403

1116. Go RS, Wester SM. Immunophenotypic and molecular features, clinical outcomes, treatments, and prognostic factors associated with subcutaneous panniculitis-like T-cell lymphoma: a systematic analysis of 156 patients reported in the literature. Cancer 2004;101:1404–13

1117. Natkunam Y, et al. Aggressive cutaneous NK and NK-like T-cell lymphomas: clinicopathologic, immunohistochemical, and molecular analyses of 12 cases. Am J Surg Pathol 1999;23:571–81

1118. Stein H, et al. CD30(+) anaplastic large cell lymphoma: a review of its histopathologic, genetic, and clinical features. Blood 2000;96:3681–95

1119. Ma Z, et al. Inv(2)(p23q35) in anaplastic large-cell lymphoma induces constitutive anaplastic lymphoma kinase (ALK) tyrosine kinase activation by fusion to ATIC, an enzyme involved in purine nucleotide biosynthesis. Blood 2000;95:2144–9

1120. Lamant L, et al. A new fusion gene TPM3-ALK in anaplastic large cell lymphoma created by a (1;2)(q25;p23) translocation. Blood 1999;93:3088–95

1121. Hernandez L, et al. TRK-fused gene (TFG) is a new partner of ALK in anaplastic large cell lymphoma producing two structurally different TFG–ALK translocations. Blood 1999;94:3265–8

1122. Falini B. Anaplastic large cell lymphoma: pathological, molecular and clinical features. Br J Haematol 2001;114:741–60

1123. Lamant L, et al. High incidence of the t(2;5)(p23;q35) translocation in anaplastic large cell lymphoma and its lack of detection in Hodgkin's disease. Comparison of cytogenetic analysis, reverse transcriptase-polymerase chain reaction, and P-80 immunostaining. Blood 1996;87:284–91

1124. Shiota M, Mori S. Anaplastic large cell lymphomas expressing the novel chimeric protein p80NPM/ALK: a distinct clinicopathologic entity. Leukemia 1997; 11(Suppl 3):538–40

1125. Benharroch D, et al. ALK-positive lymphoma: a single disease with a broad spectrum of morphology. Blood 1998;91:2076–84

1126. Falini B, et al. ALK expression defines a distinct group of T/null lymphomas ('ALK lymphomas') with a wide morphological spectrum. Am J Pathol 1998; 153:875–86

1127. ten Berge RL, et al. ALK-negative anaplastic large-cell lymphoma demonstrates similar poor prognosis to peripheral T-cell lymphoma, unspecified. Histopathology 2003;43:462–9

1128. Zinzani PL, et al. Anaplastic large-cell lymphoma: clinical and prognostic evaluation of 90 adult patients. J Clin Oncol 1996;14:955–62

1129. Vecchi V, et al. Anaplastic large cell lymphoma (Ki-1+/CD30+) in childhood. Med Pediatr Oncol 1993;21:402–10

1130. Reiter A, et al. Successful treatment strategy for Ki-1 anaplastic large-cell lymphoma of childhood: a prospective analysis of 62 patients enrolled in three consecutive Berlin-Frankfurt-Munster group studies. J Clin Oncol 1994;12:899–908

1131. Tilly H, et al. Primary anaplastic large-cell lymphoma in adults: clinical presentation, immunophenotype, and outcome. Blood 1997;90:3727–34

1132. Falini B, et al. Lymphomas expressing ALK fusion protein(s) other than NPM–ALK. Blood 1999;94:3509–15

1133. Onciu M, et al. ALK-positive anaplastic large cell lymphoma with leukemic peripheral blood involvement is a clinicopathologic entity with an unfavorable prognosis. Report of three cases and review of the literature. Am J Clin Pathol 2003;120:617–25

1134. Rassidakis GZ, et al. Differential expression of BCL-2 family proteins in ALK-positive and ALK-negative anaplastic large cell lymphoma of T/null-cell lineage. Am J Pathol 2001;159:527–35

1135. van Leeuwen FE, et al. Long-term risk of second malignancy in survivors of Hodgkin's disease treated during adolescence or young adulthood. J Clin Oncol 2000;18:487–97

1136. Specht L, Nissen NI. Prognostic factors in Hodgkin's disease stage IV. Eur J Haematol 1988;41:359–67

1137. Specht L, Nissen NI. Prognostic factors in Hodgkin's disease stage III with special reference to tumour burden. Eur J Haematol 1988;41:80–7

1138. Lister TA, et al. Report of a committee convened to discuss the evaluation and staging of patients with Hodgkin's disease: Cotswolds meeting. J Clin Oncol 1989;7:1630–6

1139. Lister TA, Crowther D. Staging for Hodgkin's disease. Semin Oncol 1990;17:696–703

1140. Sureda A, et al. Prognostic factors affecting long-term outcome after stem cell transplantation in Hodgkin's lymphoma autografted after a first relapse. Ann Oncol 2005

1141. MacLennan KA, et al. Relationship of histopathologic features to survival and relapse in nodular sclerosing Hodgkin's disease. A study of 1659 patients. Cancer 1989;64:1686–93

1142. d'Amore ES, et al. Lack of prognostic value of histopathologic parameters in Hodgkin's disease, nodular sclerosis type. A study of 123 patients with limited stage disease who had undergone laparotomy and were treated with radiation therapy. Arch Pathol Lab Med 1992;116:856–61

1143. van Spronsen DJ, et al. Disappearance of prognostic significance of histopathological grading of nodular sclerosing Hodgkin's disease for unselected patients, 1972–92. Br J Haematol 1997;96:322–7

1144. Hess JL, et al. Histopathologic grading of nodular sclerosis Hodgkin's disease. Lack of prognostic significance in 254 surgically staged patients. Cancer 1994;74:708–14

1145. Ferry JA, et al. Hodgkin disease, nodular sclerosis type. Implications of histologic subclassification. Cancer 1993;71:457–63

1146. von Wasielewski S, et al. Nodular sclerosing Hodgkin disease: new grading predicts prognosis in intermediate and advanced stages. Blood 2003;101:4063–9

1147. Petrella T, et al. CD 15 antigen in Hodgkin's disease. Pathol Res Pract 1989;185:886–90

1148. von Wasielewski R, et al. Classical Hodgkin's disease. Clinical impact of the immunophenotype. Am J Pathol 1997;151:1123–30

1149. Molin D, et al. Mast cell infiltration correlates with poor prognosis in Hodgkin's lymphoma. Br J Haematol 2002;119:122–4

1150. von Wasielewski R, et al. Tissue eosinophilia correlates strongly with poor prognosis in nodular sclerosing Hodgkin's disease, allowing for known prognostic factors. Blood 2000;95:1207–13

1151. Colby TV, Hoppe RT, Warnke RA. Hodgkin's disease: a clinicopathologic study of 659 cases. Cancer 1982;49:1848–58

1152. Feugier P, et al. Comparison of initial characteristics and long-term outcome of patients with lymphocyte-predominant Hodgkin lymphoma and classical Hodgkin lymphoma at clinical stages IA and IIA prospectively treated by brief anthracycline-based chemotherapies plus extended high-dose irradiation. Blood 2004;104:2675–81

1153. Khoury JD, et al. Bone marrow involvement in patients with nodular lymphocyte predominant Hodgkin lymphoma. Am J Surg Pathol 2004;28:489–95

1154. Delabie J, et al. Histiocyte-rich B-cell lymphoma. A distinct clinicopathologic entity possibly related to lymphocyte predominant Hodgkin's disease, paragranuloma subtype. Am J Surg Pathol 1992;16:37–48

1155. Bennett MH, et al. Non-Hodgkin's lymphoma arising in patients treated for Hodgkin's disease in the BNLI: a 20-year experience. British National Lymphoma Investigation. Ann Oncol 1991;2(Suppl 2):83–92

1156. de Jong D, et al. T-cell rich b-cell non-hodgkin's lymphoma: a progressed form of follicle centre cell lymphoma and lymphocyte predominance hodgkin's disease. Histopathology 1996;28:15–24

1157. Greaves MF, et al. Immunologically defined subclasses of acute lymphoblastic leukaemia in children: their relationship to presentation features and prognosis. Br J Haematol 1981;48:179–97

1158. Baccarani M, et al. Adolescent and adult acute lymphoblastic leukemia: prognostic features and outcome of therapy. A study of 293 patients. Blood 1982;60:677–84

1159. Amadori S, et al. Long-term survival in adolescent and adult acute lymphoblastic leukemia. Cancer 1983;52:30–4

1160. Pui CH, Campana D, Evans WE. Childhood acute lymphoblastic leukaemia – current status and future perspectives. Lancet Oncol 2001;2:597–607

1161. Gustafsson G, Kreuger A. Sex and other prognostic factors in acute lymphoblastic leukemia in childhood. Am J Pediatr Hematol Oncol 1983;5:243–50

1162. Miller DR, et al. Prognostic factors and therapy in acute lymphoblastic leukemia of childhood: CCG-141. A report from Children's Cancer Study Group. Cancer 1983;51:1041–9

1163. Pui CH, Evans WE. Acute lymphoblastic leukemia. N Engl J Med 1998;339:605–15

1164. Pieters R, et al. Relation of cellular drug resistance to long-term clinical outcome in childhood acute lymphoblastic leukaemia. Lancet 1991;338:399–403

1165. Kaspers GJ, et al. In vitro cellular drug resistance and prognosis in newly diagnosed childhood acute lymphoblastic leukemia. Blood 1997;90:2723–9

1166. Den Boer ML, et al. Patient stratification based on prednisolone–vincristine–asparaginase resistance profiles in children with acute lymphoblastic leukemia. J Clin Oncol 2003;21:3262–8

1167. Chessells JM, et al. Gender and treatment outcome in childhood lymphoblastic leukaemia: report from the MRC UKALL trials. Br J Haematol 1995;89:364–72

1168. Sather H, et al. Differences in prognosis for boys and girls with acute lymphoblastic leukaemia. Lancet 1981;1:739–43

1169. George SL, et al. A reappraisal of the results of stopping therapy in childhood leukemia. N Engl J Med 1979;300:269–73

1170. Pui CH, et al. Sex differences in prognosis for children with acute lymphoblastic leukemia. J Clin Oncol 1999;17:818–24

1171. Szklo M, et al. The changing survivorship of white and black children with leukemia. Cancer 1978;42:59–66

1172. Bhatia S. Influence of race and socioeconomic status on outcome of children treated for childhood acute lymphoblastic leukemia. Curr Opin Pediatr 2004;16:9–14

1173. Pollock BH, et al. Racial differences in the survival of childhood B-precursor acute lymphoblastic leukemia: a Pediatric Oncology Group Study. J Clin Oncol 2000;18:813–23

1174. Pui CH, et al. Risk of adverse events in children completing treatment for acute lymphoblastic leukemia: St. Jude Total Therapy studies VIII, IX, and X. J Clin Oncol 1991;9:1341–7

1175. Pui CH, et al. Outcome of treatment for childhood cancer in black as compared with white children. The St Jude Children's Research Hospital experience, 1962 through 1992. J Am Med Assoc 1995;273:633–7

1176. Bhatia S, et al. Racial and ethnic differences in survival of children with acute lymphoblastic leukemia. Blood 2002;100:1957–64

1177. Chilcote RR, et al. Mediastinal mass in acute lymphoblastic leukemia. Med Pediatr Oncol 1984;12:9–16

1178. Hammond D, et al. Analysis of prognostic factors in acute lymphoblastic leukemia. Med Pediatr Oncol 1986;14:124–34

1179. Miller DR, et al. Prognostic importance of morphology (FAB classification) in childhood acute lymphoblastic leukaemia (ALL). Br J Haematol 1981;48:199–206

1180. Palmer MK, et al. A score at diagnosis for predicting length of remission in childhood acute lymphoblastic leukaemia. Br J Cancer 1980;42:841–9

1181. Viana MB, Maurer HS, Ferenc C. Subclassification of acute lymphoblastic leukaemia in children: analysis of the reproducibility of morphological criteria and prognostic implications. Br J Haematol 1980; 44:383–8

1182. van Eys J, et al. The French–American–British (FAB) classification of leukemia. The Pediatric Oncology Group experience with lymphocytic leukemia. Cancer 1986;57:1046–51

1183. Pui CH. Childhood leukemias. N Engl J Med 1995; 332:1618–30

1184. Lilleyman JS, et al. Cytomorphology of childhood lymphoblastic leukaemia: a prospective study of 2000 patients. United Kingdom Medical Research Council's Working Party on Childhood Leukaemia. Br J Haematol 1992;81:52–7

1185. Kanerva J, et al. Reemphasis on lymphoblast L2 morphology as a poor prognostic factor in childhood acute lymphoblastic leukemia. Med Pediatr Oncol 1999;33:388–94

1186. Pullen DJ, et al. Pediatric oncology group utilization of immunologic markers in the designation of acute lymphocytic leukemia subgroups: influence on treatment response. Ann NY Acad Sci 1984;428:26–48

1187. Pui CH, et al. Clinical significance of CD10 expression in childhood acute lymphoblastic leukemia. Leukemia 1993;7:35–40

1188. Crist W, et al. Prognostic importance of the pre-B-cell immunophenotype and other presenting features in B-lineage childhood acute lymphoblastic leukemia: a Pediatric Oncology Group study. Blood 1989;74:1252–9

1189. Borowitz MJ, et al. Prognostic significance of fluorescence intensity of surface marker expression in childhood B-precursor acute lymphoblastic leukemia. A Pediatric Oncology Group Study. Blood 1997;89: 3960–6

1190. Jackson JF, et al. Favorable prognosis associated with hyperdiploidy in children with acute lymphocytic leukemia correlates with extra chromosome 6. A Pediatric Oncology Group study. Cancer 1990; 66:1183–9

1191. Harris MB, et al. Trisomy of leukemic cell chromosomes 4 and 10 identifies children with B-progenitor cell acute lymphoblastic leukemia with a very low risk of treatment failure: a Pediatric Oncology Group study. Blood 1992;79:3316–24

1192. Heerema NA, et al. Prognostic impact of trisomies of chromosomes 10, 17, and 5 among children with acute lymphoblastic leukemia and high hyperdiploidy (> 50 chromosomes). J Clin Oncol 2000;18: 876–87

1193. Forestier E, et al. Prognostic impact of karyotypic findings in childhood acute lymphoblastic leukaemia: a Nordic series comparing two treatment periods. For the Nordic Society of Paediatric Haematology and Oncology (NOPHO) Leukaemia Cytogenetic Study Group. Br J Haematol 2000;110:147–53

1194. Pui CH, et al. Clinical presentation, karyotypic characterization, and treatment outcome of childhood acute lymphoblastic leukemia with a near-haploid or hypodiploid less than 45 line. Blood 1990;75:1170–7

1195. Walters R, et al. The importance of cytogenetic studies in adult acute lymphocytic leukemia. Am J Med 1990;89:579–87

1196. Crist W, et al. Philadelphia chromosome positive childhood acute lymphoblastic leukemia: clinical and cytogenetic characteristics and treatment outcome. A Pediatric Oncology Group study. Blood 1990;76: 489–94

1197. Ribeiro RC, et al. Clinical and biologic hallmarks of the Philadelphia chromosome in childhood acute lymphoblastic leukemia. Blood 1987;70:948–53

1198. Arico M, et al. Outcome of treatment in children with Philadelphia chromosome-positive acute lymphoblastic leukemia. N Engl J Med 2000;342: 998–1006

1199. Fletcher JA, et al. Translocation (9;22) is associated with extremely poor prognosis in intensively treated children with acute lymphoblastic leukemia. Blood 1991;77:435–9

1200. Carroll AJ, et al. Pre-B cell leukemia associated with chromosome translocation 1;19. Blood 1984; 63:721–4

1201. Arthur DC, et al. Translocation 4;11 in acute lymphoblastic leukemia: clinical characteristics and prognostic significance. Blood 1982;59:96–9

1250. Head DR. Revised classification of acute myeloid leukemia. Leukemia 1996;10:1826–31

1251. de Greef GE, et al. Criteria for defining a complete remission in acute myeloid leukaemia revisited. An analysis of patients treated in HOVON-SAKK co-operative group studies. Br J Haematol 2005;128:184–91

1252. Thiele J, Kvasnicka HM, Schmitt-Graeff A. Acute panmyelosis with myelofibrosis. Leuk Lymphoma 2004;45:681–7

1253. Thiele J, et al. Acute panmyelosis with myelofibrosis: a clinicopathological study on 46 patients including histochemistry of bone marrow biopsies and follow-up. Ann Hematol 2004;83:513–21

1254. Tucker J, et al. Immunophenotype of blast cells in acute myeloid leukemia may be a useful predictive factor for outcome. Hematol Oncol 1990;8:47–58

1255. Killick S, et al. Outcome of biphenotypic acute leukemia. Haematologica 1999;84:699–706

1256. Legrand O, et al. Adult biphenotypic acute leukaemia: an entity with poor prognosis which is related to unfavourable cytogenetics and P-glycoprotein overexpression. Br J Haematol 1998;100:147–55

1257. Grimwade D. The clinical significance of cytogenetic abnormalities in acute myeloid leukaemia. Best Pract Res Clin Haematol 2001;14:497–529

1258. Mrozek K, Heerema NA, Bloomfield CD. Cytogenetics in acute leukemia. Blood Rev 2004;18:115–36

1259. Mrozek K, et al. Clinical significance of cytogenetics in acute myeloid leukemia. Semin Oncol 1997;24:17–31

1260. Slovak ML, et al. Karyotypic analysis predicts outcome of preremission and postremission therapy in adult acute myeloid leukemia: a Southwest Oncology Group/Eastern Cooperative Oncology Group Study. Blood 2000;96:4075–83

1261. Tallman MS. Acute promyelocytic leukemia as a paradigm for targeted therapy. Semin Hematol 2004;41(Suppl 4):27–32

1262. Fenaux P, Chevret S, de Botton S. Treatment of older adults with acute promyelocytic leukaemia. Best Pract Res Clin Haematol 2003;16:495–501

1263. Fenaux P, Chomienne C, Degos L. Acute promyelocytic leukemia: biology and treatment. Semin Oncol 1997;24:92–102

1264. Fenaux P, Degos L. Differentiation therapy for acute promyelocytic leukemia. N Engl J Med 1997;337:1076–7

1265. Fenaux P, et al. Cytogenetics and their prognostic value in de novo acute myeloid leukaemia: a report on 283 cases. Br J Haematol 1989;73:61–7

1266. Mrozek K, et al. Adult patients with de novo acute myeloid leukemia and t(9;11)(p22;q23) have a superior outcome to patients with other translocations involving band 11q23: a cancer and leukemia group B study. Blood 1997;90:4532–8

1267. Buchner T, et al. Double induction strategy for acute myeloid leukemia: the effect of high-dose cytarabine with mitoxantrone instead of standard-dose cytarabine with daunorubicin and 6-thioguanine: a randomized trial by the German AML Cooperative Group. Blood 1999;93:4116–24

1268. Kottaridis PD, et al. The presence of a FLT3 internal tandem duplication in patients with acute myeloid leukemia (AML) adds important prognostic information to cytogenetic risk group and response to the first cycle of chemotherapy: analysis of 854 patients from the United Kingdom Medical Research Council AML 10 and 12 trials. Blood 2001;98:1752–9

1269. Kottaridis PD, Gale RE, Linch DC. Prognostic implications of the presence of FLT3 mutations in patients with acute myeloid leukemia. Leuk Lymphoma 2003;44:905–13

1270. Beaupre DM, Kurzrock R. RAS and leukemia: from basic mechanisms to gene-directed therapy. J Clin Oncol 1999;17:1071–9

1271. Dohner K, et al. Prognostic significance of partial tandem duplications of the MLL gene in adult patients 16 to 60 years old with acute myeloid leukemia and normal cytogenetics: a study of the Acute Myeloid Leukemia Study Group Ulm. J Clin Oncol 2002;20:3254–61

1272. Nakano Y, et al. Prognostic value of p53 gene mutations and the product expression in de novo acute myeloid leukemia. Eur J Haematol 2000;65:23–31

1273. Karakas T, et al. The coexpression of the apoptosis-related genes bcl-2 and wt1 in predicting survival in adult acute myeloid leukemia. Leukemia 2002;16:846–54

1274. List AF. Role of multidrug resistance and its pharmacological modulation in acute myeloid leukemia. Leukemia 1996;10:937–42

1275. Murren JR. Modulating multidrug resistance: can we target this therapy? Clin Cancer Res 2002;8:633–5

1276. Ostergaard M, et al. WT1 gene expression: an excellent tool for monitoring minimal residual disease in 70% of acute myeloid leukaemia patients – results from a single-centre study. Br J Haematol 2004;125: 590–600

1277. Avvisati G, ten Cate JW, Mandelli F. Acute promyelocytic leukaemia. Br J Haematol 1992;81:315–20

1278. Avvisati G, et al. AIDA (all-*trans* retinoic acid + idarubicin) in newly diagnosed acute promyelocytic leukemia: a Gruppo Italiano Malattie Ematologiche Maligne dell'Adulto (GIMEMA) pilot study. Blood 1996;88:1390–8

1279. Degos L. Differentiation therapy in acute promyelocytic leukemia: European experience. J Cell Physiol 1997;173:285–7

1280. de Botton S, et al. Outcome of childhood acute promyelocytic leukemia with all-*trans*-retinoic acid and chemotherapy. J Clin Oncol 2004;22:1404–12

1281. Pulsoni A, et al. Clinicobiological features and outcome of acute promyelocytic leukemia occurring as a second tumor: the GIMEMA experience. Blood 2002;100:1972–6

1282. Avvisati G, Tallman MS. All-trans retinoic acid in acute promyelocytic leukaemia. Best Pract Res Clin Haematol 2003;16:419–32

1283. Larson RA, et al. Evidence for a 15;17 translocation in every patient with acute promyelocytic leukemia. Am J Med 1984;76:827–41

1284. Brunel V, et al. Variant and masked translocations in acute promyelocytic leukemia. Leuk Lymphoma 1996;22:221–8

1285. Corey SJ, et al. A non-classical translocation involving 17q12 (retinoic acid receptor alpha) in acute promyelocytic leukemia (APML) with atypical features. Leukemia 1994;8:1350–3

1286. Bloomfield CD, et al. Long-term survival of patients with acute myeloid leukemia: a third follow-up of the Fourth International Workshop on Chromosomes in Leukemia. Cancer 1997;80(11 Suppl):2191–8

1287. Sainty D, et al. A new morphologic classification system for acute promyelocytic leukemia distinguishes cases with underlying PLZF/RARA gene rearrangements. Groupe Français de Cytogénétique Hématologique, UK Cancer Cytogenetics Group and BIOMED 1 European Coomunity-Concerted Action Molecular Cytogenetic Diagnosis in Haematological Malignancies. Blood 2000;96:1287–96

1288. Parmar S, Tallman MS. Acute promyelocytic leukaemia: a review. Expert Opin Pharmacother 2003; 4:1379–92

1289. Onida F, et al. Prognostic factors and scoring systems in chronic myelomonocytic leukemia: a retrospective analysis of 213 patients. Blood 2002;99:840–9

1290. Solal-Celigny P, et al. Chronic myelomonocytic leukemia according to FAB classification: analysis of 35 cases. Blood 1984;63:634–8

1291. Fenaux P, et al. Prognostic factors in adult chronic myelomonocytic leukemia: an analysis of 107 cases. J Clin Oncol 1988;6:1417–24

1292. Fenaux P, et al. Chronic and subacute myelomonocytic leukaemia in the adult: a report of 60 cases with special reference to prognostic factors. Br J Haematol 1987;65:101–6

1293. Storniolo AM, et al. Chronic myelomonocytic leukemia. Leukemia 1990;4:766–70

1294. Tefferi A, et al. Chronic myelomonocytic leukemia: natural history and prognostic determinants. Mayo Clin Proc 1989;64:1246–54

1295. Germing U, Kundgen A, Gattermann N. Risk assessment in chronic myelomonocytic leukemia (CMML). Leuk Lymphoma 2004;45:1311–18

1296. Germing U, et al. Problems in the classification of CMML – dysplastic versus proliferative type. Leuk Res 1998;22:871–8

1297. Onida F, Beran M. Chronic myelomonocytic leukemia: myeloproliferative variant. Curr Hematol Rep 2004;3:218–26

1298. Anonymous. Chronic myelomonocytic leukemia: single entity or heterogeneous disorder? A prospective multicenter study of 100 patients. Groupe Français de Cytogénétique Hématologique. Cancer Genet Cytogenet 1991;55:57–65

1299. Worsley A, et al. Prognostic features of chronic myelomonocytic leukaemia: a modified Bournemouth score gives the best prediction of survival. Br J Haematol 1988;68:17–21

1300. Bennett JM, et al. Proposals for the classification of the myelodysplastic syndromes. Br J Haematol 1982;51:189–99

1352. Huntly BJ, et al. Imatinib improves but may not fully reverse the poor prognosis of patients with CML with derivative chromosome 9 deletions. Blood 2003;102:2205–12

1353. Quintas-Cardama A, et al. Imatinib mesylate therapy may overcome the poor prognostic significance of deletions of derivative chromosome 9 in patients with chronic myelogenous leukemia. Blood 2005;105:2281–6

1354. Thiele J, et al. Prognostic features at diagnosis of chronic myeloid leukaemia with special emphasis on histological parameters. Med Oncol Tumor Pharmacother 1988;5:49–60

1355. Thiele J, et al. Bone marrow features and clinical findings in chronic myeloid leukemia – a comparative, multicenter, immunohistological and morphometric study on 614 patients. Leuk Lymphoma 2000;36:295–308

1356. Buesche G, et al. Marrow fibrosis, indicator of therapy failure in chronic myeloid leukemia – prospective long-term results from a randomized-controlled trial. Leukemia 2003;17:2444–53

1357. Cervantes F, Rozman C, Feliu E. Prognostic evaluation of initial bone marrow histopathological features in chronic granulocytic leukemia. Acta Haematol 1989;82:12–5

1358. Buesche G, et al. Treatment intensity significantly influencing fibrosis in bone marrow independently of the cytogenetic response: meta-analysis of the long-term results from two prospective controlled trials on chronic myeloid leukemia. Leukemia 2004;18:1460–7

1359. Bueso-Ramos CE, et al. Imatinib mesylate therapy reduces bone marrow fibrosis in patients with chronic myelogenous leukemia. Cancer 2004;101:332–6

1360. Thiele J, et al. Changing patterns of histological subgroups during therapy of Ph1+ chronic myelogenous leukaemia. Histopathology 2000;37:355–62

1361. Bernstein R. Cytogenetics of chronic myelogenous leukemia. Semin Hematol 1988;25:20–34

1362. Kardinal CG, Bateman JR, Weiner J. Chronic granulocytic leukemia. Review of 536 cases. Arch Intern Med 1976;136:305–13

1363. Sokal JE. Prognosis in chronic myeloid leukaemia: biology of the disease vs. treatment. Baillières Clin Haematol 1987;1:907–29

1364. Faderl S, et al. Chronic myelogenous leukemia: biology and therapy. Ann Intern Med 1999;131:207–19

1365. Faderl S, et al. The biology of chronic myeloid leukemia. N Engl J Med 1999;341:164–72

1366. Kantarjian HM, et al. Treatment of chronic myelogenous leukemia in accelerated and blastic phases with daunorubicin, high-dose cytarabine, and granulocyte-macrophage colony-stimulating factor. J Clin Oncol 1992;10:398–405

1367. Beard MD, et al. Blast crisis of chronic myeloid leukaemia (CML). I. Presentation simulating acute lymphoid leukaemia (ALL). Br J Haematol 1976;34:167–78

1368. Cervantes F, et al. 'Lymphoid' blast crisis of chronic myeloid leukaemia is associated with distinct clinico-haematological features. Br J Haematol 1998;100:123–8

1369. Druker BJ, et al. Efficacy and safety of a specific inhibitor of the BCR–ABL tyrosine kinase in chronic myeloid leukemia. N Engl J Med 2001;344:1031–7

1370. O'Brien SG, et al. Imatinib compared with interferon and low-dose cytarabine for newly diagnosed chronic-phase chronic myeloid leukemia. N Engl J Med 2003;348:994–1004

1371. Sawyers CL, et al. Imatinib induces hematologic and cytogenetic responses in patients with chronic myelogenous leukemia in myeloid blast crisis: results of a phase II study. Blood 2002;99:3530–9

1372. Shah NP, et al. Multiple BCR-ABL kinase domain mutations confer polyclonal resistance to the tyrosine kinase inhibitor imatinib (STI571) in chronic phase and blast crisis chronic myeloid leukemia. Cancer Cell 2002;2:117–25

1373. Marin D, et al. Survival of patients with chronic-phase chronic myeloid leukaemia on imatinib after failure on interferon alfa. Lancet 2003;362:617–9

1374. Cortes JE, et al. Prognostic significance of cytogenetic clonal evolution in patients with chronic myelogenous leukemia on imatinib mesylate therapy. Blood 2003;101:3794–800

1375. Marktel S, et al. Chronic myeloid leukemia in chronic phase responding to imatinib: the occurrence of additional cytogenetic abnormalities predicts disease progression. Haematologica 2003;88:260–7

1376. Lange T, et al. BCR–ABL transcripts are early predictors for hematological relapse in chronic myeloid leukemia after hematopoietic cell transplantation with reduced intensity conditioning. Leukemia 2004; 18:1468–75

1377. Passweg JR, et al. Validation and extension of the EBMT Risk Score for patients with chronic myeloid leukaemia (CML) receiving allogeneic haematopoietic stem cell transplants. Br J Haematol 2004;125: 613–20

1378. Olavarria E, et al. Response to imatinib in patients who relapse after allogeneic stem cell transplantation for chronic myeloid leukemia. Leukemia 2003;17: 1707–12

1379. Na IK, et al. Quantitative RT-PCR of Wilms tumor gene transcripts (WT1) for the molecular monitoring of patients with accelerated phase bcr/abl + CML. Leuk Res 2005;29:343–5

1380. Najean Y, Rain JD. The very long-term evolution of polycythemia vera: an analysis of 318 patients initially treated by phlebotomy or 32P between 1969 and 1981. Semin Hematol 1997;34:6–16

1381. Chievitz E, Thiede T. Complications and causes of death in polycythaemia vera. Acta Med Scand 1962; 172:513–23

1382. Bilgrami S, Greenberg BR. Polycythemia rubra vera. Semin Oncol 1995;22:307–26

1383. Murphy S. Diagnostic criteria and prognosis in polycythemia vera and essential thrombocythemia. Semin Hematol 1999;36(Suppl 2):9–13

1384. Kiladjian JJ, et al. Long-term outcomes of polycythemia vera patients treated with pipobroman as initial therapy. Hematol J 2003;4:198–207

1385. Wasserman LR, et al. Influence of therapy on causes of death in polycythemia vera. Trans Assoc Am Physicians 1981;94:30–8

1386. Gruppo-Italiano-Studio-Policitemia. Polycythemia vera: the natural history of 1213 patients followed for 20 years. Gruppo Italiano Studio Policitemia. Ann Intern Med 1995;123:656–64

1387. Tefferi A. A contemporary approach to the diagnosis and management of polycythemia vera. Curr Hematol Rep 2003;2:237–41

1388. Polycythemia GIS. Polycythemia vera: the natural history of 1213 patients followed for 20 years. Gruppo

Italiano Studio Policitemia. Ann Intern Med 1995; 123:656–64

1389. Kurosawa M, Iwasaki H. Megakaryoblastic transformation of polycythemia vera with hypercalcemia. Ann Hematol 2002;81:668–71

1390. West WO. Hydroxyurea in the treatment of polycythemia vera: a prospective study of 100 patients over a 20-year period. South Med J 1987;80:323–7

1391. Nand S, et al. Leukemogenic risk of hydroxyurea therapy in polycythemia vera, essential thrombocythemia, and myeloid metaplasia with myelofibrosis. Am J Hematol 1996;52:42–6

1392. Georgii A, Buesche G, Kreft A. The histopathology of chronic myeloproliferative diseases. Baillières Clin Haematol 1998;11:721–49

1393. Murphy S, et al. Experience of the Polycythemia Vera Study Group with essential thrombocythemia: a final report on diagnostic criteria, survival, and leukemic transition by treatment. Semin Hematol 1997;34: 29–39

1394. Shibata K, et al. Essential thrombocythemia terminating in acute leukemia with minimal myeloid differentiation – a brief review of recent literature. Acta Haematol 1994;91:84–8

1395. Tefferi A. Myelofibrosis with myeloid metaplasia. N Engl J Med 2000;342:1255–65

1396. Cervantes F, et al. Myelofibrosis with myeloid metaplasia in young individuals: disease characteristics, prognostic factors and identification of risk groups. Br J Haematol 1998;102:684–90

1397. Rozman C, et al. Life expectancy of patients with chronic nonleukemic myeloproliferative disorders. Cancer 1991;67:2658–63

1398. Dupriez B, et al. Prognostic classification of myelofibrosis with myeloid metaplasia. Br J Haematol 1989; 73:136–7

1399. Cervantes F, et al. Identification of 'short-lived' and 'long-lived' patients at presentation of idiopathic myelofibrosis. Br J Haematol 1997;97:635–40

1400. Silverstein MN, Brown AL Jr, Linman JW. Idiopathic myeloid metaplasia. Its evolution into acute leukemia. Arch Intern Med 1973;132:709–12

1401. Bouroncle BA, Doan CA. Myelofibrosis. Clinical, hematologic and pathologic study of 110 patients. Am J Med Sci 1962;243:697–715